Complete Canadian
Diabetes
Cookbook

Complete Canadian
Diabetes
Cookbook

Edited by
Katherine E. Younker
MBA, RD, Certified Diabetes Educator

Published in cooperation with

 CANADIAN DIABETES ASSOCIATION | ASSOCIATION CANADIENNE DU DIABÈTE

Robert ROSE

For a list of contributing authors, see page 364.
For complete cataloguing information, see page 365.

Disclaimer
The recipes in this book have been carefully tested by our kitchen and
our tasters. To the best of our knowledge, they are safe and nutritious
for ordinary use and users. For those people with food or other allergies,
or who have special food requirements or health issues, please read the
suggested contents of each recipe carefully and determine whether or
not they may create a problem for you. All recipes are used at the risk
of the consumer.

We cannot be responsible for any hazards, loss or damage that may
occur as a result of any recipe use.

For those with special needs, allergies, requirements or health
problems, in the event of any doubt, please contact your medical adviser
prior to the use of any recipe.

Design & Production: PageWave Graphics Inc.
Photography: Mark T. Shapiro

Cover image: Old-Fashioned Beef Stew (see recipe, page 80)

We acknowledge the financial support of the Government of Canada
through the Book Publishing Industry Development Program (BPIDP)
for our publishing activities.

Published by Robert Rose Inc.
120 Eglinton Avenue East, Suite 800, Toronto, Ontario, Canada M4P 1E2
Tel: (416) 322-6552 Fax: (416) 322-6936

Printed in Canada

3 4 5 6 7 8 9 10 CPL 16 15 14 13 12 11 10

Contents

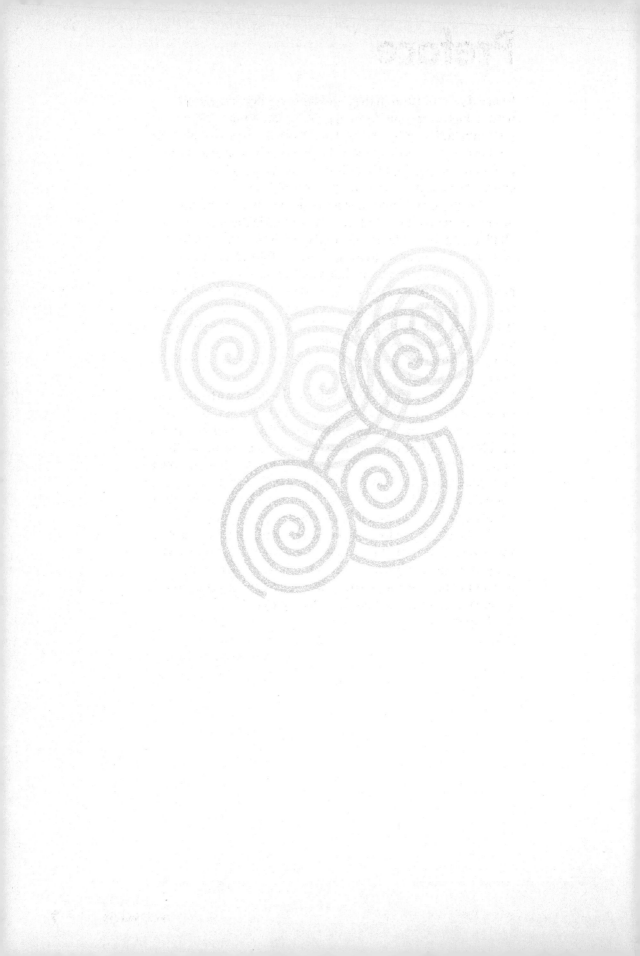

Children born to mothers who have had gestational diabetes during that pregnancy are also at increased risk of developing type 2 diabetes later in life.

4. Am I overweight? Overweight and obesity are common health problems worldwide. Studies have shown that 80% of people with type 2 diabetes are overweight. Extra body weight makes it harder for your pancreas to function, and the body may become more resistant to insulin. The risk is greater when the extra weight is located around the middle. Reducing body weight by as little as 5% to 7% can prevent or delay the development of diabetes when added to regular physical activity.

Other risk factors include:
- a history of impaired fasting glucose or impaired glucose tolerance;
- being a member of a high-risk population (e.g., people of Aboriginal, Hispanic, South Asian, Asian or African descent);
- the presence of high blood pressure;
- the presence of elevated blood fat levels (high cholesterol or triglycerides);
- the presence of any disease of the blood vessels (vascular disease);
- in women, the presence of polycystic ovarian disease;
- the presence of acanthosis nigricans (darkening of the skin);
- a family history of schizophrenia; and
- the presence of any complication related to diabetes (such as heart disease).

PREVENTING DIABETES

Eating a well-balanced low-fat diet, including high-fiber carbohydrate choices and moderate portion sizes, can help to promote a healthy weight, and together with regular physical activity can help reduce the risk of diabetes for the population at large.

We also know that there are many people who already have elevated blood glucose levels, defined as either **impaired fasting glucose** or **impaired glucose tolerance** (now often referred to as **pre-diabetes**). Impaired fasting glucose is defined as blood glucose (sugar) between 6.1 and 6.9 mmol/L after an overnight fast. Impaired glucose tolerance is defined as blood glucose between 6.1 and 6.9 mmol/L after an overnight fast or values of between 7.8–11.0 two hours after being given a glucose drink containing 75 g of carbohydrate. [1] Studies of people with

[1] Canadian Diabetes Association 2003, "Clinical Practice Guidelines for the Prevention and Management of Diabetes in Canada," www.diabetes.ca/cpg2003 (2003).

either of these conditions have found that improved eating habits and regular exercise have prevented or delayed the development of diabetes in these individuals.

How much activity is enough?
Health Canada reports that "a brisk walk for 30 minutes, or similar activity, five times a week, can lower the risk of developing type 2 diabetes" (www.healthcanada.ca/diabetes). Active living is integral to the lives of people of *all* ages. Adults over the age of 60, who have the highest prevalence of type 2 diabetes, have been found to benefit positively from increasing their daily physical activity.

MANAGEMENT OF DIABETES
Current recommendations for blood glucose targets are lower than ever and are closer to the recommendations for those without diabetes. Studies have shown that risk for developing all types of diabetes complications increases proportionately to the elevation in blood glucose levels. For those with diabetes, blood glucose targets are 4 to 7 mmol/L before meals and 5 to 10 mmol/L two hours after eating. For those without diabetes, normal ranges are 4 to 6 mmol/L before meals and 5 to 8 mmol/L two hours after eating. People with diabetes may have symptoms such as increased thirst and urination, numbness or tingling in the hands and feet, fatigue, dry mouth and tongue, and weight loss, or they may exhibit no symptoms at all.

There are three types of diabetes. Type 1 diabetes, found in about 10% of cases, usually occurs in children and young adults and requires insulin for management, as the pancreatic cells that produced the insulin are no longer able to produce it. Dietary management and regular activity are additional key treatments.

Type 2 diabetes accounts for almost 90% of people diagnosed with diabetes and is usually seen in adults, although with growing obesity rates it is now being diagnosed in children. The pancreas does not produce enough insulin for the individual, or the insulin is not used effectively. Type 2 diabetes is managed with a personalized meal plan, physical activity and the addition of oral diabetes medications and/or insulin.

Gestational diabetes occurs in 2% to 4% of all pregnancies. It is usually managed by meal planning, exercise and sometimes insulin. Gestational diabetes increases the risk for type 2 diabetes in both the mother and children later in life.

Once diagnosed, managing diabetes requires daily attention. Food intake, activity, blood glucose monitoring and healthy lifestyle choices are all part of the package.

Nutrition Principles for Canadians with Diabetes

Canada's Guidelines for Healthy Eating apply to all Canadians, including those with diabetes. These guidelines are:

1. Eat a variety of foods.
2. Emphasize cereals, breads, other grain products, vegetables and fruit.
3. Choose lower-fat dairy products, leaner meats and food prepared with little or no fat.
4. Achieve and maintain a healthy body weight by enjoying regular physical activity and healthy eating.
5. Limit salt, alcohol and caffeine.

More detailed recommendations for people with diabetes come from "The Guidelines for the Nutritional Management of Diabetes Mellitus in the New Millennium: A Position Statement by the Canadian Diabetes Association." These guidelines state: "A major goal for diabetes care is to improve glycemic control by balancing food intake with endogenous and/or exogenous insulin levels. For people with type 1 diabetes, insulin doses need to be adjusted to balance with nutritionally adequate food intake and physical activity. For individuals with type 2 diabetes, impaired glucose tolerance or impaired fasting glucose, attention to food portions, and weight management combined with physical activity may help improve glycemic control."[2] The guidelines provide advice on a variety of nutrients of concern to those with diabetes.

CARBOHYDRATE

Recommendations regarding carbohydrate indicate that 50% to 60% of energy (calories) should be obtained from carbohydrate. Carbohydrate sources, including grains & starches, fruits, milk & alternatives, other choices, vegetables and even added sugars should be part of your meal plan. Added sugars (sucrose, fructose, glucose, etc.), as opposed to those found naturally in vegetables, fruit and milk products, may comprise up to 10% of the total daily energy intake.

FIBER

A fiber intake of at least 25 to 35 g per day is recommended for adults. High-fiber food choices are preferred, particularly those with a low glycemic index (see page 30). Fiber should

[2] "The Guidelines for the Nutritional Management of Diabetes Mellitus in the New Millennium: A Position Statement by the Canadian Diabetes Association," *Canadian Journal of Diabetes Care* 23: 3 (1999), 56–69.

be chosen from a variety of sources, and it is suggested that choosing at least 5 to 10 g from soluble fiber sources (such as oatmeal or apples) can help to reduce serum (blood) cholesterol.

PROTEIN

Recommendations regarding protein suggest a moderate intake, with some emphasis on vegetable protein sources such as beans, lentils and soybeans. An intake of 0.86 g per kg is suggested each day. For an 80 kg (176 lb) person this would translate into 70 g of protein per day, from all sources. A moderate protein intake is helpful in the management of nephropathy (kidney disease) for people with diabetes.

FAT

In keeping with recommendations for all Canadians, an intake of less than 30% of energy from fat, and less than 10% from the combination of saturated and trans fat, is recommended. A high fat intake can increase the risk of cardiovascular disease by helping to raise blood lipids (cholesterol), promote weight gain and impair glucose tolerance. Intake of processed foods containing saturated and trans fats should be limited. Monounsaturated fats (from canola, olive and peanut oil) are recommended where possible, and polyunsaturated fat should be limited to less than 10% of fat (see page 21). As well, intake of fatty fish containing omega-3 fatty acids (such as salmon and mackerel) at least once a week has been found to be helpful in lowering triglyceride levels.

ALCOHOL

An alcohol intake of less than 5% of energy or fewer than 2 drinks per day (fewer than 14 regular drinks per week for men and fewer than 9 per week for women) is suggested. Use of alcohol should be discussed with the diabetes health care team, as it can further aggravate conditions such as hypertension (high blood pressure) and dyslipidemia (high blood fat levels) and can disrupt liver function. Consumption of alcohol can cause either hyperglycemia (high blood glucose) or hypoglycemia (low blood sugar). Due to the risk of hypoglycemia, it is recommended that people with diabetes consume a source of carbohydrate with alcohol. They should also inform family and friends regarding the risk and wear identification such as a Medic Alert® bracelet.

SWEETENERS

Both "nutritive" sweeteners (sugar, fructose, aspartame and sugar alcohols) and "non-nutritive" sweeteners (acesulfame potassium, sucralose, saccharin and cyclamate) can play roles in the diet of the person with diabetes. Sugar alcohols such as sorbitol, xylitol, mannitol, maltitol, lactitol and isomalt may be used in moderation with little effect on blood glucose (sugar) levels. In large amounts, they may cause flatulence (gas) and diarrhea. Health Canada has provided an acceptable daily intake for aspartame and the "non-nutritive" sweeteners acesulfame potassium, sucralose, saccharin and cyclamate. These amounts are based on body weight, and for most individuals with diabetes moderate use of these sweeteners is acceptable. Discuss sweetener use with the dietitian on your diabetes health care team. For more information on sweeteners see the Canadian Diabetes Association website: www.diabetes.ca.

VITAMINS AND MINERALS

The recommended intake of vitamins and minerals for people with diabetes is the same as for all Canadians. Most individuals can obtain adequate amounts of these nutrients by consuming a well-balanced diet. Some nutrients, such as vitamins C and E and beta-carotene (which can be converted to vitamin A), may be protective against the development of complications of diabetes. When vitamins and minerals are obtained from plant sources, other components in the plant called phytochemicals are consumed as well. These phytochemicals are also thought to protect against disease.

Sodium restriction to 2 to 4 g (2000 to 4000 mg) may help to control hypertension (high blood pressure) in those people who are salt sensitive.

To determine individual requirements, the Canadian Diabetes Association recommends that all persons with diabetes receive nutrition counseling from a Registered Dietitian. Work with your diabetes health care team to review your dietary intake and a meal plan that will best suit your lifestyle.

Healthy Eating and Balanced Blood Glucose (Sugars)

Healthy eating together with regular activity and, if needed, the use of diabetes medication (oral diabetes pills and/or insulin) are the keys to keeping blood glucose (sugars) in the target range. The Canadian Diabetes Association (CDA) recommends several guidelines for meal planning, which are important for good health and good glycemic (blood glucose) control:

Did you ...
* choose foods from a variety of food groups at each meal?
  * Grains & Starches
  * Vegetables & Fruits
  * Milk & Alternatives
  * Meat & Alternatives
* have 3 meals today, including breakfast?
* have portion sizes that will help you reach or maintain a healthy body weight?
* space your meals 4 to 6 hours apart from each other?

These guidelines can help to start you on the way to healthy eating and balanced blood glucose (sugar) levels.

Breakfast is the most important meal of the day. This is also true for people with diabetes. "Breaking the fast" is essential to provide energy and carbohydrate to begin the day. We need to put some fuel in the tank so the body can perform during the waking hours. For those with diabetes, not eating breakfast makes it difficult to perform, especially because the only fuel for the brain is glucose. If you have diabetes, which is managed by following a meal plan, skipping breakfast can sometimes make the blood glucose higher. Why? When the body is not supplied with a source of glucose, the brain will signal the body to produce it. The liver must then find sources of glucose, which may include breaking down protein and fat tissue. If your diabetes is managed by oral diabetes medication and/or insulin, skipping breakfast after taking your medication may put you at risk for hypoglycemia or low blood glucose (sugar).

Managing portion sizes is another key to diabetes meal planning. Control or reduction of portion sizes can promote weight loss and glycemic control. Most people with type 2 diabetes are overweight. Recent research has shown that weight control can help to delay the onset of type 2 diabetes, which may be an important consideration if other family members do not already have diabetes. Once diabetes is present, loss of body weight in the range of 5% to 7% has been shown to improve blood glucose (sugar) control and decrease risk factors associated with the complications of diabetes. Reduction and management of fat intake to less than 30% of food intake is a successful strategy for long-term weight management.

Managing portion sizes of carbohydrate from meal to meal also contributes directly to the maintenance of euglycemia (normal blood glucose).

Spacing your meals 4 to 6 hours apart works to help maintain blood glucose (sugar) levels and manage appetite. When meals are too close together (less than 4 hours) it may be difficult for most people to achieve a healthy blood glucose before the next meal, as the blood glucose may not have returned to the ideal range (4 to 7 mmol/L). When meals are spaced too far apart (more than 6 hours), people with diabetes may be at risk for hypoglycemia (low blood glucose or sugar) or may have difficulty controlling their appetite and thus "forget" to manage portion sizes.

What about snacks? The need for snacks should be reviewed on an individual basis in consultation with the dietitian on your diabetes health care team. For many individuals with diabetes who have a habit of consuming three substantial meals per day, there may not be a need for snacks. Others who work in a physically demanding environment or who are very active, are pregnant or are young with a limited stomach capacity may require between-meal and/or evening snacks to help maintain good blood glucose (sugar) control. The best method of determining this is through home blood glucose (sugar) monitoring and consultation with your dietitian.

Reducing Sodium

Many people with diabetes also have hypertension (elevated blood pressure). Reducing sodium intake is one way to lower blood pressure. Salt (or sodium chloride) contains about 2400 mg of sodium per tsp. Reducing sodium intake to 2000 to 4000 mg can help reduce blood pressure levels in those individuals who are salt sensitive. There are several ways to reduce the sodium in your diet:

- Avoid using the salt shaker on the table.
- Modify your recipes: avoid adding salt, and where appropriate substitute herbs, spices or flavored vinegar.
- Read the nutrition labels on packages and choose products that are lower in sodium.
- Use reduced-sodium or no-salt-added products, such as reduced-sodium soya sauce, teriyaki sauce, MSG and other condiments.
- Choose low-sodium soup mixes, or make your own.
- Choose whole, fresh, unprocessed foods and avoid canned and convenience ones when possible. If you choose canned products such as vegetables, drain and rinse the liquid from the food before using.
- Avoid processed meats (such as wieners and ham) or choose sodium-reduced types.
- Limit foods packed in brines, such as pickles, sauerkraut, olives, etc.
- Choose crackers and snack foods that are reduced in sodium.
- Reduce your use of condiments such as mustard, horseradish, ketchup and Worcestershire sauce.

The Canadian Diabetes Association recommends that all people with diabetes receive nutrition counseling from a Registered Dietitian. Work with your diabetes health care team to review your dietary intake and develop a meal plan that will best suit your lifestyle. Ask your physician for a referral or call your local diabetes center to make an appointment.

Vitamins, Minerals, Fiber and Phytochemicals

Vitamins, minerals and fiber are all part of the nutrients we need every day. Are you getting the right amount? The new Nutrition Facts table on labels in Canada appears in a standard format, making it easier to see how much of certain key nutrients a product provides. Wonderful information about the new labeling system and how to use it in meal planning can be found at www.healthyeatingisinstore.ca.

When we talk about nutrients such as **vitamins** and **minerals**, what do "good source" and "excellent source" mean? According the to Canadian Food Inspection Agency, each vitamin and mineral has a Recommended Daily Intake (RDI) for both children under two and adults. On food labels, this is presented as a percent of the Daily Value (% DV). A food must contain at least 5% of the DV of a nutrient for it to appear on the label, unless it is a mandatory nutrient. When a food or recipe indicates that it is a "good source" of a particular nutrient, it must contain at least 15% of the RDI for that nutrient (30% for vitamin C). An "excellent source" contains greater than 25% of the RDI for that nutrient (50% for vitamin C).

Remember that vitamins C and E and beta carotene (vitamin A) are thought to be antioxidant vitamins and may be protective against a number of diseases and potentially some of the complications of diabetes. Choosing foods high in these nutrients is a part of a healthy lifestyle.

Fiber, the indigestible portion of plant foods, can be either soluble or insoluble. It is an important nutrient for a variety of reasons. Soluble fiber is found in fruits and vegetables, barley, legumes, oats, rye and seeds. When soluble fiber is consumed, it slows the digestion of food and may help to control blood glucose (rise) after meals. Regular consumption of soluble fiber may help to lower cholesterol levels. Insoluble fiber, found in cereals, whole grains, beans and lentils, seeds, fruits and vegetables helps to promote regular elimination and may be helpful in reducing cancer risk. Choose high-fiber foods at every meal whenever possible. On food labels, "high fiber" foods are identified as those that contain 4 g of or more of dietary fiber per serving. "Very high fiber" foods contain 6 g or more of dietary fiber per serving. If you need more fiber, be sure to choose one of the many high-fiber recipes in this book.

Phytochemicals are substances found in plants that appear to help increase resistance against disease. They are found in a variety of different plants and have many types of action in the human body. A few examples are carotenoids (such as beta carotene in carrots and lycopene in tomatoes), flavonoids (found in berries, celery, onions, grapes, soybeans and whole wheat products), lignans (part of the fiber found in flaxseed), phenolic acids (found in coffee beans, apples, blueberries, oranges, potatoes and soybeans) and phytoesterols (found in soybeans and lentils).

When choosing to consume food sources of vitamins and minerals, you also obtain the benefit of fiber and phytochemicals. Thus, choosing to "eat" your vitamins and minerals offers benefits that no supplement can match.

Choosing to Sweeten

On average, "added sugars" contain 5 g of carbohydrate per tsp (5 mL), 0 g of protein and 0 g of fat and have an energy value of about 20 calories. (You will find the specific information listed on the nutrition panel on the label of these products.) The Canadian Diabetes Association suggests that added sugars can compose up to 10% of energy intake for a person with diabetes. What does that mean? In practical terms, if you are someone with an energy intake of about 1500 calories per day, about 150 could come from added sugars. This would equal about 7½ tsp (37 mL/38 g) of added sugar per day. If your energy intake is about 2000 calories, then 200 calories or about 10 tsp (50 mL/50 g) could come from added sugars.

When choosing to include added sugars, keep in mind that many packaged products contain added sugar, and this should be taken into consideration when choosing how much additional added sugar to include. For example, ketchup, salad dressings, creamed corn, coating mixes, cereals and many other items may contain sugar in a variety of forms. Use of products such as these can quickly "use up" those added sugars.

Remember that added sugars are a part of many recipes (including some in this book) in a variety of forms, including granulated white or brown sugar, corn syrup, honey, maple syrup and molasses. When these items are added to a recipe, the carbohydrate content is increased. For example, the recipe Quinoa Wraps with Hoisin Vegetables on page 291 contains 2 tbsp (25 mL) of honey, which contributes about 5 g of carbohydrate per serving or about 1 tsp (5 mL) of added sugar per serving. By replacing the honey in this recipe with a granulated sugar substitute, you can reduce the carbohydrate content by about 5 g per serving. This may alter the taste slightly, but if you are trying to limit your carbohydrate intake at a meal, it is an easy way to keep within your target.

WHAT SHOULD YOU CHOOSE?
This decision depends on several factors:

1. **Your carbohydrate target for the meal.** If you are trying to balance your intake by consuming a certain amount of carbohydrate or food choices from a meal plan, it may be beneficial to use a sugar substitute. If, however, you can adjust your insulin or other food choices to account for the extra carbohydrate, you may choose to leave in the added sugar.

2. Personal taste preference. You may wish to choose those products with added sugars over those containing sugar substitutes. If you prefer added sugars, you may have to be more particular with your portion sizes to maintain your carbohydrate goals.

3. Change of recipe texture or results. In many cases, using a sugar substitute in products such as baked goods can alter the recipe texture, color and appearance. When using sugar substitutes, be sure to follow the manufacturer's directions exactly for best results. Most companies have toll-free information lines you can call for help.

Reducing Fat

Reducing fat in the diet helps decrease the risk of diabetes in those not yet diagnosed, improves metabolic syndrome and lowers daily energy (calorie) intake to promote weight loss. Many Canadians consume more fat than recommended. On average, 1 tsp (5 mL) of fat contains 0 g of carbohydrate, 0 g of protein and 5 g of fat and has an energy value of about 45 calories. (You will find the specific information listed on the nutrition panel on the labels of these products.) It is recommended that fat contribute no more than 30% of energy intake for a person with diabetes, with less than 10% of energy intake from saturated and trans fat.

In practical terms, if you are someone with an energy intake of about 1500 calories per day, about 450 could come from fat. This would equal about 10 tsp (50 mL/50 g) of fat per day from all sources and, of that, 3 tsp (15 mL/less than 15 g) from saturated fat. If your energy intake is about 2000 calories, then 600 calories or about 13 tsp (65 mL/65 g) of fat would supply about 30%. Saturated fat should supply less than 4 tsp (20 mL/20 g) in a 2000-calorie diet.

Fat of various types is found in many foods — protein-containing foods, milk products, dressings and sauces — and is added to many baked and prepared products. Check the product label to see how much fat is found in the product and choose the lower-fat ones.

Most protein-containing foods and milk products contain fat in the form of saturated fat. To limit your intake of saturated fat from these sources,

- Choose lean cuts of meat and trim fat before cooking. Remove poultry skin and avoid food preparation methods such as deep frying, pan frying and those where fat is added.
- Avoid prepared packaged meats such as deli meats and wieners unless they are fat-reduced.
- Choose lower-fat dairy products, such as cheese with a milk fat (M.F.) of 20% or less on the label.
- Choose lower-fat milk such as skim, 1% or 2%.

Baked goods, prepared items and fast foods with hydrogenated vegetable oils or shortening contain trans fatty acids, which are similar to saturated fat and have the same effect on blood lipid (cholesterol) levels. To avoid products containing hydrogenated vegetable oils and shortening,

- Choose baked goods prepared with soft margarine or vegetable oils such as canola, olive or peanut oil.

- Look at the labels for products that contain less than 1 tsp (5 mL/5 g) of fat per serving.
- Prepare your own baked goods at home.

When using fat, keep the following in mind:

- Choose oils such as canola, olive or peanut oil.
- Choose a non-hydrogenated unsaturated margarine in a soft tub on which the polyunsaturated and monounsaturated fats listed on the label are at least 75% of the total fat. Look for "non-hydrogenated" or "no trans fat" on the label.
- Low-fat margarine or butter is not suitable for baking or frying due to its high water content.
- If you have added fat during cooking, limit the amount of fat you include at the table.
- Nuts and seeds contain unsaturated fat, but are very high in energy. Enjoy them sparingly if you are trying to manage your weight.
- Remember that all fats supply an equal amount of energy, so even if the fat is unsaturated it is wise to limit its use. This is particularly important if you are trying to lose or maintain weight.

Beyond the Basics: Meal Planning for Healthy Eating, Diabetes Prevention and Management

Beyond the Basics: Meal Planning for Healthy Eating, Diabetes Prevention and Management is a new guide that replaces the Good Health Eating Guide, which had been part of the meal planning system for diabetes in Canada since early 1982. The Beyond the Basics guide is compatible with Canada's Good Guide to Healthy Eating and Canada's Guidelines for Healthy Eating. The Beyond the Basics guide provides information on a variety of foods by classifying those containing similar macronutrients (carbohydrate, protein, fat and energy [calories]) into one of eight groups, as shown below.

GRAINS & STARCHES

These foods all contribute to a rise in blood glucose and are a key part of a diabetes meal plan. Some choices contain dietary fiber, either soluble or insoluble (or in combination), both of which play important roles in good health and diabetes meal planning.

One Grains & Starches choice contains 15 g carbohydrate, 2 g protein and 0 g fat. Examples of one choice are:

- 1 slice bread
- ½ bagel (3-inch/7.5 cm diameter), ¼ large bagel
- ½ cup (125 mL) cold cereal flakes
- ¾ cup (175 mL) cooked cereal
- ½ cup (125 mL) pasta, couscous or bulgur
- ½ medium potato, boiled or baked
- ⅓ cup (75 mL) sweet potato
- 1 cup (250 mL) soup

FRUITS

All fruits and fruit juices contain carbohydrate as naturally occurring sugar. They are an important source of vitamins and minerals in the diet, and all raise blood glucose levels. The CDA recommends choosing fruit over juice for the benefit of about 2 g fiber per serving and because liquids containing sugar raise blood glucose quickly.

One Fruits choice contains 15 g carbohydrate, 0 g protein and 0 g fat. Examples of one choice are:

- 1 medium apple
- 1 small banana
- 1 large peach or nectarine
- 1 small grapefruit, all colors
- 2 medium kiwis
- ¾ cup (175 mL) or 2 slices fresh pineapple
- 15 grapes
- ¼ cup (50 mL) dates or figs
- ¼ cup (50 mL) dried fruit (raisins)
- ½ cup (125 mL) unsweetened juice (apple, orange)

MILK & ALTERNATIVES

This group contains milk and yogurt choices. All forms of milk contain carbohydrate in the form of lactose, the naturally occurring sugar in milk. Milk is an important source of calcium in the diet of many Canadians and also provides other vitamins and minerals, such as vitamin D, phosphorus and riboflavin.

One Milk & Alternatives choice contains 15 g carbohydrate, 8 g protein and variable fat. Examples of one choice are:

- 1 cup (250 mL) skim, 1% or 2% milk
- 1 cup (250 mL) buttermilk
- ½ cup (125 mL) canned or evaporated milk
- 1 cup (250 mL) fluid soy milk
- ¾ cup (175 mL) yogurt (flavored, nonfat, artificial sweetener)

OTHER CHOICES (SWEET FOODS AND SNACKS)

This group contains foods with added sugar from a variety of sources, which are also a part of meal planning for diabetes. As with all other foods containing carbohydrate, they contribute to a rise in blood glucose. Nutrition guidelines suggest that added sugars can comprise up to 10% of the carbohydrate in the diet of people with diabetes. Added sugars contribute little in the way of nutrients to meal planning, but when substituted for other carbohydrates they increase meal plan flexibility and choice.

One Other Choices serving contains 15 g carbohydrate and variable protein and fat. Examples of one serving are:

- 1 tbsp (15 mL) sugar or brown sugar
- 1 tbsp (15 mL) honey, molasses or maple, corn or chocolate syrup

- 1 tbsp (15 mL) jam, jelly or marmalade
- 5 hard candies
- 3 cups (750 mL) air-popped lower-fat popcorn
- 7 large lower-fat pretzels or 30 lower-fat pretzel sticks
- ½ cup (125 mL) regular soft drink

VEGETABLES

Vegetables are a good source of vitamins, minerals, fiber and phytochemicals. Most are low in carbohydrate and can be eaten freely. Most Canadians do not consume the recommended number of vegetable servings per day.

Below are examples of one serving of vegetables. Try to have five servings a day.

- 4 spears asparagus
- 1 cup (250 mL) yellow or green beans
- 1 cup (250 mL) broccoli
- 1 cup (250 mL) cabbage
- 1 cup (250 mL) carrots
- 1 cup (250 mL) celery
- 1 cup (250 mL) cucumber
- 1 cup (250 mL) leeks
- 1 cup (250 mL) mushrooms
- 1 cup (250 mL) peppers
- 1 cup (250 mL) spinach
- 1 cup (250 mL) zucchini
- 1 cup (250 mL) beets
- ½ cup (125 mL) parsnips
- ½ cup (125 mL) peas
- ½ cup (125 mL) rutabaga (turnips)
- ½ cup (125 mL) squash

MEAT & ALTERNATIVES

This group is made up of choices such as fish, lean meat, poultry, cheese and some foods from plant sources, such as peanut butter, soybeans, tofu and lentils. Most of these foods contain no carbohydrate and do not directly affect blood glucose levels. In addition to providing protein, many of the animal forms contain minerals such as iron and fats such as omega-3 fatty acids, while the vegetable forms may contain plant sterols and phytochemicals.

One Meat & Alternatives choice contains 0 g carbohydrate, 7 g protein and 3 to 5 g fat. Examples of one choice are:

- 1 oz (30 g) fresh fish or shellfish
- 1 oz (30 g) canned fish
- 1 oz (30 g) lean meat or skinless poultry
- 1 oz (30 g) lean ground meat or poultry
- 1 oz (30 g) lean non-processed deli meat
- 1 oz (30 g) cheese (less than 7% M.F.)
- 1 large egg
- ½ cup (125 mL) hummus
- 2 tbsp (25 mL) peanut butter

FATS

Fats add energy to the diet, and some provide a source of essential fatty acids. Although fats contribute energy, it is very important for people with diabetes to watch both the amount and the type of fat they choose. Monounsaturated fats, found in some plant oils (canola, olive and peanut), are the preferred choice. Choose foods with saturated and trans fats less often. They should be limited to about 10% of the energy intake, or the equivalent of about 4 to 5 Fats choices (or tsp) per day.

One Fats choice contains 0 g carbohydrate, 0 g protein and 5 g fat. Examples of one choice are:

- 1 tsp (5 mL) oil
- 1 tsp (5 mL) butter
- 1 tsp (5 mL) soft regular margarine
- 1 tbsp (15 mL) cheese spread
- 1 slice bacon
- 1 tbsp (15 mL) nuts or seeds
- 2 tbsp (25 mL) lower-fat salad dressing
- 2 tbsp (25 mL) reduced-fat sour cream
- ½ tbsp (7 mL) tahini

EXTRAS

This group adds variety to diabetes meal planning. The foods in this group include items that are low in both calories and carbohydrate.

One Extras choice contains less than 5 g carbohydrate and 20 calories. Examples of one choice are:

- 2 anchovy fillets
- Garlic
- Pimentos or hot peppers
- Gelatin or sugar-free jelly powder
- Herbs and spices

- Sugar substitute
- 1 tsp (5 mL) ketchup
- 1 tsp (15 mL) barbecue sauce
- 1 tbsp (15 mL) carob powder
- Black coffee
- Clear or herbal tea
- Club soda
- Sugar-free soft drinks
- Sugar-free crystal drinks

The new Beyond the Basics guide will be available in April 2005. A resource manual containing a more detailed list of foods and other material will be available in 2006. These will be available from your health care team at your local diabetes center, a dietitian at your local hospital or community center or the provincial branch or national office of the Canadian Diabetes Association.

Carbohydrate Counting

Carbohydrate counting is a method of meal management used by people with diabetes as an alternative to following a meal plan. People choosing to count carbohydrate are often those who use a rapid-acting insulin, which they can adjust depending on their carbohydrate consumption. Those with type 2 diabetes managed by meal planning (with or without oral diabetes medication) may use this method to aim for carbohydrate targets at meals. This method increases flexibility in meal planning for many people.

One advantage of the newer rapid-acting insulins is that they can be taken after meals, permitting people to judge how much insulin to take based on how much they have eaten.

WHAT ARE THE PRINCIPLES OF CARBOHYDRATE COUNTING?

Carbohydrate found in foods is known to be the primary source of glucose in the blood. Although both of the other macronutrients, protein and fat, can be broken down into carbohydrate, this will not usually occur except when there is inadequate carbohydrate available to the body for energy.

There are several forms of carbohydrate, some of which contribute to blood glucose and some of which do not. These are sugars, starch, dietary fiber and "sugar alcohols." The latter are usually seen in products developed for people with diabetes, such as "no sugar added" candies; small amounts sometimes occur naturally in foods.

Dietary fiber, primarily undigested by the body, is one of the components of carbohydrate that does not raise the blood glucose. Therefore, when counting carbohydrate, it is important to remove the dietary fiber from the total carbohydrate to determine the "available carbohydrate." **Available carbohydrate is the carbohydrate that will contribute to a rise in blood glucose.**

ARE THERE CONCERNS WITH CARBOHYDRATE COUNTING?

People who choose to count carbohydrate should always keep good nutrition in mind. With increased meal flexibility, some food choices may provide less nutrition. For example, high-fat, high-carbohydrate desserts may take the place of more nutritious choices such as fresh fruit with meals. As a consequence, those using insulin may require larger amounts of rapid-acting insulin to achieve blood glucose targets, and over time this may lead to weight gain. Making these choices can also have an impact on weight and blood lipid (cholesterol) levels. Finally, substituting low-nutrient foods for healthier selections may deprive the body of a number of essential nutrients, such as calcium, vitamins A and C, fiber and a whole host of others.

WORKING WITH A DIETITIAN

Work with the dietitian from your diabetes health care team if you are thinking about using carbohydrate counting as a method of meal planning. Together you can review the essentials of carbohydrate counting, look at your regular intake to determine an appropriate carbohydrate/insulin ratio and work through any difficulties that result when you begin.

Those choosing to count carbohydrate learn to adjust their meal intake to meet their individual targets, or if using insulin may adjust their dose to cover their carbohydrate intake. If you plan your meals and snacks by counting carbohydrate, there are two ways to do this.

Method 1

Use the Beyond the Basics meal planning guide. Using this guide, one serving of carbohydrate equals 15 g of carbohydrate or 1 Carbohydrate choice (the combined value of the Grains & Starches, Fruits, Milk & Alternatives, Other Choices and Vegetables choices). The available carbohydrate has been considered when determining the Carbohydrate choices found in each recipe.

For example, the recipe for Tex-Mex Pork Chops with Black Bean–Corn Salsa on page 216 contains 2 Carbohydrate choices. Therefore, it provides about 30 g of carbohydrate per serving. (Carbohydrate choices are rounded to the nearest ½ choice.)

You can use this information to make sure you are meeting your carbohydrate targets. If you are taking insulin, your carbohydrate-to-insulin ratio may be based on the number of Carbohydrate choices you choose.

Method 2

Look at the nutrient information listed on recipes or product labels. Simply take the amount of carbohydrate listed and subtract the fiber. This provides you with the amount of available carbohydrate per recipe. For example, on page 216, the nutrition information for the Tex-Mex Pork Chops with Black Bean–Corn Salsa recipe indicates:

Calories	400
Carbohydrate	45 g
Fiber	12 g
Protein	35 g

Fat, total	10 g
Fat, saturated	2 g
Sodium	218 mg
Cholesterol	51 mg

Carbohydrate 45 g – Fiber 12 g =
Available carbohydrate 33 g = 2 carbohydrate choices

Using this information together with the carbohydrate from the other foods in your meal, you can estimate the total amount of available carbohydrate to see if you are meeting your carbohydrate targets or to determine how much insulin to take based on your carbohydrate-to-insulin ratio. It is important to work with the dietitian on your diabetes health care team to determine your individual carbohydrate-to-insulin ratio and to become comfortable with this method of meal planning. Keep healthy eating and good nutrition in mind.

The Glycemic Index

The glycemic index is a scale that ranks carbohydrate-rich foods by how much they raise blood glucose levels compared to a standard food. After we eat foods containing carbohydrate, blood glucose levels rise; the extent of that rise is called the glycemic response. The glycemic index of different foods has been compared to a standard glucose response, and the effect of these foods on blood glucose has been given a value (see table below).

Many factors contribute to a food's glycemic effect: the soluble fiber contained in the food; how resistant the carbohydrate-containing food is to digestion; how the food has been cooked or prepared; and whether the food is eaten alone or as part of a mixed meal.

By choosing foods that have a low glycemic index more often, people with diabetes may experience less of a rise in blood glucose after meals or snacks. In some instances, people who have regularly chosen foods low on the glycemic index have required less insulin. Low-glycemic-index foods are often higher in vitamins, minerals and fiber and provide increased satiety. Some research also indicates that people at risk for diabetes may reduce their risk by regularly choosing foods that have a low glycemic index.

More information on the glycemic index can be found on the Canadian Diabetes Association website: www.diabetes.ca.

GLYCEMIC INDEX EXCHANGES
Low Glycemic Index (choose more often) to High Glycemic Index (choose less often)

Pearl barley	25	Couscous	65
Legumes	25–48	Shredded Wheat®	69
Spaghetti	41	Whole wheat bread	69
Parboiled rice	47	White wheat bread	70
Bran Buds with Psyllium®	47	Cornmeal	70
Bulgur (cracked wheat)	48	Mashed potato	70–83
Red River Cereal®	49	Corn chips	73
Rye kernel-pumpernickel bread	50	Puffed Wheat®	74
Yams	51	French fries	75
Oat bran	55	Jelly beans	80
Polished rice	56	Cornflakes®	84
Pita bread	57	Puffed Rice®	86
White/whole/canned potatoes	61	Rice cakes	88
		Glucose	100

References: Wolever, T.M.S., Glycemic Index Workshop, 2000.

Recipe Analysis

The recipes were analyzed using the Nutriwatch Nutrient Analysis Program (Canadian Nutrient file 2000), Version 6.120E, Delphi 1, copyright 2000, Elizabeth Warwick. Where necessary, additional data was supplemented using the online USDA database found at www.nal.usda.gov/fnic/foodcomp/.

In the analyses,

- Imperial measures and weights were used, except where metric measurements were listed.
- The larger number of servings were used when there was a range.
- The first ingredient and amount were used where alternatives were specified.
- Optional ingredients were not included.
- Calculations including meat and poultry used lean portions without skin.
- Soft margarine and canola oil were used where the type of fat was not specified.
- The milk and cheese listed for the specific recipe has been used; however, in most instances you should be able to successfully use lower-fat milk and cheese to further reduce the fat content.
- Nutrient values were rounded to the nearest whole number for presentation in the text. In determining the Beyond the Basics choices, the values shown in the table below were used in calculation, prior to rounding.

Food Group	Carbohydrate (g)	Protein (g)	Fat (g)
Grains & Starches	15	2	0
Fruits	15	1	0
Milk & Alternatives	15	8	variable
Other Choices	15	variable	variable
Vegetables	most are free	0	0
Meat & Alternatives	0	7	5
Fats	0	0	5
Extras	<5	0	0

Editor's note: No-sugar-added yogurt is suggested in sidebars to complete a number of meals. Your personal carbohydrate targets for a meal may permit you to use a regular yogurt instead.

Appetizers, Dips and Spreads

Appetizers are a delicious way to begin a meal or entertain guests. Many can be prepared ahead and "cooked" just when guests arrive, allowing the host or hostess to enjoy company rather than "fuss" with food.

A collection of appetizers together with low-fat crackers or whole grain bread can actually be used in combination to make a meal.

When preparing to entertain, keep in mind, some friends with diabetes may need to watch the timing of meals and snacks.

It is always prudent for hosts to provide both alcoholic and non-alcoholic drinks to provide choice for those who need to drive or who may have to limit alcohol for medical reasons. Sugar-free soft drinks combined with Crystal-Light® or light (reduced carbohydrate) cranberry cocktail are delicious alcohol-free alternatives.

Tips

Buy snow peas that are firm and crisp, and have no blemishes.

Medium-sized scallops would also be delicious for this very sophisticated hors d'oeuvre.

Make Ahead

If serving cold, prepare and refrigerate early in day.

Shrimp and Snow Pea Tidbits

16	snow peas	16
2 tsp	vegetable oil	10 mL
1 tsp	crushed garlic	5 mL
1 tbsp	chopped fresh parsley	15 mL
16	medium shrimp, peeled, deveined, tail left on	16

1. Steam or microwave snow peas until barely tendercrisp. Rinse with cold water. Drain and set aside.

2. In nonstick skillet, heat oil; sauté garlic, parsley and shrimp just until shrimp turn pink, 3 to 5 minutes.

3. Wrap each snow pea around shrimp; fasten with toothpick. Serve warm or cold.

Choices Per Serving

½   Meat & Alternative

Nutritional Analysis Per Serving			
Calories	39	Fat, total	2 g
Carbohydrate	1 g	Fat, saturated	0 g
Fiber	0 g	Sodium	27 mg
Protein	4 g	Cholesterol	28 mg

SERVES 4 TO 6 OR
MAKES 18 HORS
D'OEUVRES

Preheat broiler

Baking sheet sprayed with nonstick vegetable spray

Tip

Tender beef is delicious with this sweet Asian sauce.

Make Ahead

Refrigerate chicken in marinade early in day. Wrap chicken around mushroom caps and broil just before serving.

Oriental Chicken–Wrapped Mushrooms

1 tbsp	rice wine vinegar	15 mL
1 tbsp	vegetable oil	15 mL
2 tbsp	soya sauce	25 mL
1 tsp	crushed garlic	5 mL
2 tbsp	finely chopped onion	25 mL
1 tsp	sesame oil	5 mL
2 tbsp	water	25 mL
2 tbsp	brown sugar	25 mL
½ tsp	sesame seeds (optional)	2 mL
¾ lb	boneless skinless chicken breast	375 g
18	medium mushroom caps (without stems)	18

1. In bowl, combine vinegar, oil, soya sauce, garlic, onion, sesame oil, water, sugar, and sesame seeds (if using); mix well.

2. Cut chicken into strips about 3 inches (8 cm) long and 1 inch (2.5 cm) wide to make 18 strips. Add to bowl and marinate for 20 minutes, stirring occasionally.

3. Wrap each chicken strip around mushroom; secure with toothpick. Place on baking sheet. Broil for approximately 5 minutes or until chicken is no longer pink inside. Serve immediately.

Choices Per Serving

½ Carbohydrate

2 Meat & Alternatives

Nutritional Analysis Per Serving

Calories	130	Fat, total	5 g
Carbohydrate	7 g	Fat, saturated	1 g
Fiber	0 g	Sodium	329 mg
Protein	15 g	Cholesterol	36 mg

● ● ● ● ● ● ● ● ● ● ● ● ● ● ●

Preheat oven to
400°F (200°C)

● ● ● ● ● ● ● ● ● ● ● ● ● ● ●

Tips

This filling can be
used to stuff medium
mushrooms. Just remove
the mushroom stems.

You can reduce the
fat content of this recipe
by choosing low-fat
cheeses. One-eighth of
the recipe (or 4 cherry
tomatoes) is a good
source of vitamin C.

● ● ● ● ● ● ● ● ● ● ● ● ● ● ●

Make Ahead

Make early in day and
refrigerate. Bake just
before serving.

Warm Cherry Tomatoes Stuffed with Garlic and Cheese

24	cherry tomatoes	24
½ cup	dry bread crumbs	125 mL
2 tbsp	chopped green onion	25 mL
½ tsp	chopped garlic	2 mL
2 tbsp	chopped fresh parsley	25 mL
1 tbsp	margarine, melted	15 mL
⅓ cup	shredded mozzarella cheese	75 mL
1 tbsp	grated Parmesan cheese	15 mL

1. Cut slice from top of each tomato; carefully scoop out seeds and most of the pulp.

2. In bowl, combine bread crumbs, onion, garlic, parsley, margarine and mozzarella until well mixed.

3. Spoon into tomatoes; sprinkle with Parmesan. Place on baking sheet and bake for approximately 10 minutes or until stuffing is golden.

Choices Per Serving

½ Carbohydrate
½ Meat & Alternative
½ Fat

Nutritional Analysis Per Serving			
Calories	87	Fat, total	5 g
Carbohydrate	8 g	Fat, saturated	2 g
Fiber	1 g	Sodium	134 mg
Protein	4 g	Cholesterol	10 mg

Tips

Goat cheese, also known as chèvre, comes in a variety of shapes ranging from logs to pyramids and discs. Some are sprinkled with herbs and spices throughout. Use any variety.

Serve also as a dip or serve on celery sticks or in hollow cherry tomatoes.

Make Ahead

Prepare and refrigerate mixture up to a day before. Place on cucumber slices just before serving.

Smoked Salmon and Goat Cheese Cucumber Slices

3 oz	smoked salmon, diced	75 g
3 oz	goat cheese	75 g
2 tbsp	2% yogurt	25 mL
½ tsp	lemon juice	2 mL
4 tsp	chopped fresh dill (or ½ tsp/2 mL dried dillweed)	20 mL
25	slices (¼-inch/5 mm thick) cucumber	25

1. Reserve about 25 bits of salmon for garnish.

2. In bowl or using food processor, combine goat cheese, yogurt, remaining salmon, lemon juice and dill; mix with fork or using on/off motion just until combined but not puréed.

3. Place spoonful of filling on each cucumber slice. Garnish with bit of reserved salmon.

Choices Per Serving

1   Meat & Alternative

Nutritional Analysis Per Serving			
Calories	92	Fat, total	6 g
Carbohydrate	2 g	Fat, saturated	4 g
Fiber	0 g	Sodium	156 mg
Protein	8 g	Cholesterol	19 mg

Preheat oven to
425°F (220°C)

Baking sheet sprayed
with vegetable spray

Tip

If using fresh spinach,
use half the package
(5 oz/125 g), wash and
cook with water clinging
to leaves until wilted and
cooked (approximately
3 minutes). Drain, rinse
with cold water, squeeze
out excess moisture and
chop. Goat cheese can
replace the feta cheese.

Make Ahead

Prepare early in the
day, cover and keep
refrigerated until ready
to bake.

Greek Egg Rolls with Spinach and Feta

2 tsp	vegetable oil	10 mL
2 tsp	minced garlic	10 mL
¾ cup	diced onions	175 mL
1⅔ cup	diced mushrooms	400 mL
1 tsp	dried oregano	5 mL
Half	package (10 oz/300 g) frozen chopped spinach, thawed and drained	Half
2 oz	feta cheese, crumbled	50 g
10	egg roll wrappers	10

1. In nonstick skillet, heat oil over medium-high heat. Add garlic, onions, mushrooms and oregano; cook for 5 minutes or until softened. Add spinach and feta; cook, stirring, for 2 minutes or until well mixed and cheese melts.

2. Keeping rest of egg roll wrappers covered with a cloth to prevent drying out, put one wrapper on work surface with a corner pointing towards you. Put 2 tbsp (25 mL) of the filling in the center. Fold the lower corner up over the filling, fold the two side corners in over the filling and roll the bundle away from you. Place on prepared pan and repeat until all wrappers are filled. Bake for 12 to 14 minutes until browned, turning the egg rolls at the halfway point.

Choices Per Serving

1½ Carbohydrates

½ Fat

Nutritional Analysis Per Serving			
Calories	132	Fat, total	3 g
Carbohydrate	22 g	Fat, saturated	1 g
Fiber	1 g	Sodium	251 mg
Protein	5 g	Cholesterol	8 mg

Tips

If suggested seafood is not used, try a firm white fish such as swordfish, haddock, or monkfish.

A combination of seafood together with these vegetables make this appetizer packed with nutrients. It is an excellent source of vitamins C and B_{12} and a good source of vitamin A, magnesium, phosphorus, iron and niacin.

Make Ahead

Prepare early in the day and keep refrigerated. Mix before serving.

Seafood Garlic Antipasto

1 lb	scallops, squid or shrimp, or a combination, cut into pieces	500 g
3/4 cup	chopped snow peas	175 mL
3/4 cup	chopped red peppers	175 mL
1/2 cup	diced tomatoes	125 mL
1/3 cup	chopped red onions	75 mL
1/3 cup	minced coriander or dill	75 mL
1/4 cup	sliced black olives	50 mL
3 tbsp	lemon juice	45 mL
2 tbsp	olive oil	25 mL
1 1/2 tsp	minced garlic	7 mL
	Pepper to taste	

1. In a nonstick skillet sprayed with vegetable spray, cook the seafood over medium-high heat for 3 minutes, or until just done. Drain excess liquid, if any, and place seafood in serving bowl. Let cool slightly.

2. Add snow peas, red peppers, tomatoes, red onions, coriander and olives; mix well. Whisk together lemon juice, olive oil, garlic; pour over seafood mixture. Add pepper to taste. Chill for 1 hour before serving.

Choices Per Serving

1/2	Carbohydrate
2	Meat & Alternatives

Nutritional Analysis Per Serving

Calories	150	Fat, total	6 g
Carbohydrate	7 g	Fat, saturated	1 g
Fiber	1 g	Sodium	137 mg
Protein	17 g	Cholesterol	115 mg

Preheat broiler

Tips

Tuna packed in water
is a great substitute
for salmon.

You can also use the
mixture as a dip if you
purée it until smooth.

Serve 2 whole halves
as a light lunch.

Make Ahead

Make and refrigerate
salmon mixture up to
a day before. Stir before
spreading on muffins.

Salmon Swiss Cheese English Muffins

1	can (7½ oz/220 g) salmon, drained	1
¼ cup	light mayonnaise	50 mL
2 tbsp	chopped green onion	25 mL
2 tbsp	chopped red onion	25 mL
2 tbsp	diced celery	25 mL
2 tbsp	chopped fresh dill (or 1 tsp/5 mL) dried dillweed)	25 mL
2 tsp	lemon juice	10 mL
4	English muffins, split in half and toasted	4
⅓ cup	shredded Swiss cheese	75 mL

1. In food processor, combine salmon, mayonnaise, green and red onions, celery, dill and lemon juice. Using on/off motion, process just until chunky but not puréed.

2. Divide salmon mixture over muffins and spread evenly. Sprinkle with cheese. Broil just until cheese melts, approximately 2 minutes. To serve, slice each muffin into quarters.

Choices Per Serving	
1	Carbohydrate
1	Meat & Alternative
½	Fat

Nutritional Analysis Per Serving			
Calories	149	Fat, total	7 g
Carbohydrate	15 g	Fat, saturated	2 g
Fiber	0 g	Sodium	213 mg
Protein	8 g	Cholesterol	14 mg

Tips

To toast pine nuts, bake in 350°F (180°C) oven 8 to 10 minutes or until golden and fragrant. Or, in a nonstick skillet over high heat, toast until browned, about 2 to 3 minutes.

Avoid sun-dried tomatoes packed in oil; these have a lot of extra calories and fat.

Sun-dried tomatoes make this recipe a good source of lycopene.

Great as a topping with crackers, baguettes or as a dip for vegetables or baked tortilla chips.

● ● ● ● ● ● ● ● ● ● ● ● ● ● ● ●

Make Ahead

Prepare up to 3 days in advance.

Creamy Sun-Dried Tomato Dip

4 oz	dry-packed sun-dried tomatoes	125 g
¾ cup	5% ricotta cheese	175 mL
½ cup	chopped fresh parsley	125 mL
⅓ cup	basic vegetable stock (see recipe, page 55) or water	75 mL
3 tbsp	chopped black olives	45 mL
2 tbsp	olive oil	25 mL
2 tbsp	toasted pine nuts	25 mL
2 tbsp	grated Parmesan cheese	25 mL
1 tsp	minced garlic	5 mL

1. In a small bowl, pour boiling water to cover over sun-dried tomatoes. Let stand 15 minutes. Drain and chop.

2. In a food processor combine sun-dried tomatoes, ricotta, parsley, stock, olives, olive oil, pine nuts, Parmesan and garlic; process until well combined but still chunky. Makes 1¾ cups (425 mL).

Choices Per Serving	
½	Carbohydrate
½	Meat & Alternative
1	Fat

Nutritional Analysis Per Serving			
Calories	111	Fat, total	6 g
Carbohydrate	10 g	Fat, saturated	2 g
Fiber	0 g	Sodium	356 mg
Protein	6 g	Cholesterol	8 mg

Preheat oven to
450°F (230°C)

Tips

It works wonderfully as a
smoky-oniony dip for raw
vegetables and also as a
spread on sandwiches.

This dip can be served
immediately or it can
wait, covered and
unrefrigerated, for up
to 2 hours. If refrigerated,
let it come back to room
temperature and give
it a couple of stirs
before serving.

Melizzano Despina (Eggplant Dip)

1	medium eggplant (about 1 lb/500 g)	1
1 tsp	vegetable oil	5 mL
1	onion	1
2 tbsp	lemon juice	25 mL
¼ cup	olive oil	50 mL
	Few sprigs fresh parsley, chopped	
	Salt and pepper to taste	

1. Brush eggplant lightly with vegetable oil. Using a fork, pierce the skin lightly at 1-inch (2.5-cm) intervals. Place on a baking sheet and bake for 1 hour, or until eggplant is very soft and the skin is dark brown and caved in.

2. Transfer eggplant to a working surface. Cut off 1 inch (2 cm) at the stem end and discard (this part never quite cooks through). Peel the eggplant by picking at an edge from the cut end, then pulling upward. The skin should come off easily in strips.

3. Cut the eggplant lengthwise and place each half with the interior facing you. With a spoon scoop out the tongues of seed-pods, leaving as much of the flesh as possible. To remove the additional seed-pods hiding inside, cut each piece of eggplant in half and repeat the deseeding procedure. Once deseeded, let cleaned eggplant flesh sit to shed some of its excess water.

Choices Per Serving	
½	Carbohydrate
3	Fats

Nutritional Analysis Per Serving

Calories	166	Fat, total	15 g
Carbohydrate	9 g	Fat, saturated	2 g
Fiber	0 g	Sodium	4 mg
Protein	1 g	Cholesterol	0 mg

4. Transfer drained eggplant flesh to a bowl. Using a wooden spoon, mash and then whip the pulp until smooth and very soft. Coarsely grate onion directly into the eggplant (the onion juice that results is very important to this dip). Add lemon juice and whip with a wooden spoon until perfectly integrated. Keep beating and add olive oil in a very thin stream; the result should be a frothy, light colored emulsion. Season to taste with salt and pepper. Transfer to a serving bowl and garnish with chopped parsley.

Tips

To toast pine nuts, put in nonstick skillet over medium-high heat for 3 minutes, stirring occasionally. Or put them on a baking sheet and toast in a 400°F (200°C) oven for 5 minutes. Whichever method you choose, watch carefully — nuts burn quickly.

If basil is not available, use parsley or spinach leaves.

When choosing Grains & Starches choices to accompany this dip, look for crisps or crackers with less than 2 g of fat/serving.

Make Ahead

Prepare early in the day and keep covered and refrigerated.

Creamy Pesto Dip

1 cup	well-packed basil leaves	250 mL
2 tbsp	toasted pine nuts	25 mL
2 tbsp	grated Parmesan cheese	25 mL
2 tbsp	olive oil	25 mL
2 tsp	lemon juice	10 mL
1 tsp	minced garlic	5 mL
½ cup	5% ricotta cheese	125 mL
¼ cup	light sour cream	50 mL

1. Put basil, pine nuts, Parmesan, olive oil, lemon juice and garlic in food processor; process until finely chopped, scraping sides of bowl down once. Add ricotta and sour cream and process until smooth. Serve with pita or tortilla crisps, or fresh vegetables.

Choices Per Serving

½	Meat & Alternative
1	Fat

Nutritional Analysis Per Serving

Calories	72	Fat, total	6 g
Carbohydrate	2 g	Fat, saturated	2 g
Fiber	0 g	Sodium	53 mg
Protein	3 g	Cholesterol	9 mg

. . . .

Tips

This delicious, versatile and explosive sauce requires no cooking, and can live in the fridge nicely for 2 to 3 days, though it is best about an hour after it's freshly made. The hotness of the sauce can be regulated by modifying the amount of jalapeno pepper seeds used.

When working with hot peppers, be sure to wear gloves; otherwise, wash hands thoroughly.

Pico de Gallo (Mexican Hot Sauce)

1	medium tomato, cut into ¼-inch (0.5-cm) cubes	1
¼ cup	finely diced red onions	50 mL
2	jalapeno peppers, finely diced (with or without seeds, depending on desired hotness)	2
½ tsp	salt	2 mL
1 tbsp	lime juice	15 mL
1 tbsp	vegetable oil	15 mL
	Few sprigs fresh coriander, chopped	

1. In bowl combine tomato, onions, jalapeno, salt and lime juice. Stir to mix well. Add oil and stir again.

2. Transfer to a serving bowl and scatter chopped coriander on top. Let rest for about 1 hour, covered and unrefrigerated, for best flavor. Serve alongside main courses and appetizers.

Choices Per Serving

½   Fat

Nutritional Analysis Per Serving

Calories	44	Fat, total	4 g
Carbohydrate	3 g	Fat, saturated	0 g
Fiber	1 g	Sodium	365 mg
Protein	1 g	Cholesterol	0 mg

9- by 5-inch (2 L) loaf
pan lined with plastic
wrap

Tips

If using wild mushrooms,
try shiitake or cremini.
This can be served in
a serving bowl instead
of a loaf pan.

Most supermarkets
regularly carry a variety
of wild mushrooms. You
can vary the flavor of this
pâté by changing the
mushroom. A wonderful
alternative to traditional
meat pâté.

Make Ahead

Prepare up to 2 days
in advance.

Leek Mushroom Cheese Pâté

2 tsp	vegetable oil	10 mL
1½ tsp	minced garlic	7 mL
1½ cups	chopped leeks	375 mL
½ cup	finely chopped carrots	125 mL
12 oz	oyster or regular mushrooms, thinly sliced	375 g
2 tbsp	sherry or white wine	25 mL
2 tbsp	chopped fresh dill (or 2 tsp/10 mL dried)	25 mL
1½ tsp	dried oregano	7 mL
¼ tsp	coarsely ground black pepper	1 mL
2 oz	feta cheese, crumbled	50 g
2 oz	light cream cheese	50 g
½ cup	5% ricotta cheese	125 mL
2 tsp	freshly squeezed lemon juice	10 mL
2 tbsp	chopped fresh dill	25 mL

1. In a large nonstick frying pan sprayed with vegetable spray, heat oil over medium-high heat. Add garlic, leeks and carrots; cook 3 minutes, stirring occasionally. Stir in mushrooms, sherry, dill, oregano and pepper; cook, stirring occasionally, 8 to 10 minutes or until carrots are tender and liquid is absorbed. Remove from heat.

2. Transfer vegetable mixture to a food processor. Add feta, cream cheese, ricotta and lemon juice; purée until smooth. Spoon into prepared loaf pan. Cover and chill until firm.

3. Invert onto serving platter; sprinkle with chopped dill. Serve with crackers, bread or vegetables.

Choices Per Serving

½ Carbohydrate

½ Meat & Alternative

½ Fat

Nutritional Analysis Per Serving			
Calories	80	Fat, total	5 g
Carbohydrate	6 g	Fat, saturated	2 g
Fiber	1 g	Sodium	124 mg
Protein	4 g	Cholesterol	13 mg

● ● ● ● ● ● ● ● ● ● ● ● ● ● ●

Tips

Adjust the chili powder
to your taste.

Serve with pita bread,
vegetables or crackers.

● ● ● ● ● ● ● ● ● ● ● ● ● ● ●

Make Ahead

Make early in day and
squeeze more lemon
juice over top to
prevent discoloration.
Refrigerate. Stir just
before serving.

Avocado, Tomato and Chili Guacamole

Half	avocado, peeled	Half
¾ tsp	crushed garlic	4 mL
2 tbsp	chopped green onions	25 mL
1 tbsp	lemon juice	15 mL
¼ cup	finely diced sweet red pepper	50 mL
½ cup	chopped tomato	125 mL
Pinch	chili powder	Pinch

1. In bowl, combine avocado, garlic, onions, lemon juice, red pepper, tomato and chili powder; mash with fork, mixing well.

Choices
Per Serving

½   Fat

Nutritional Analysis Per Serving

Calories	35	Fat, total	3 g
Carbohydrate	3 g	Fat, saturated	0 g
Fiber	1 g	Sodium	5 mg
Protein	1 g	Cholesterol	0 mg

Preheat oven to
350°F (180°C)

Small casserole dish

Tips

The three cheeses in
this recipe make it a
good source of calcium.
Served with French
bread, this recipe can
make a delicious lunch.

Serve over French bread
or with vegetables.

Make Ahead

Prepare up to 1 day
in advance. Bake just
before serving.

Hot Three-Cheese Dill Artichoke Bake

1	can (14 oz/398 mL) artichoke hearts, drained and halved	1
½ cup	shredded part-skim mozzarella cheese (about 2 oz/50 g)	125 mL
⅓ cup	shredded Swiss cheese (about 1½ oz/35 g)	75 mL
⅓ cup	minced fresh dill (or 1 tsp/5 mL dried)	75 mL
¼ cup	light sour cream	50 mL
3 tbsp	light mayonnaise	45 mL
1 tbsp	freshly squeezed lemon juice	15 mL
1 tsp	minced garlic	5 mL
Pinch	cayenne pepper	Pinch
1 tbsp	grated Parmesan cheese	15 mL

1. In a food processor, combine artichoke hearts, mozzarella and Swiss cheeses, dill, sour cream, mayonnaise, lemon juice, garlic and cayenne. Process on and off just until combined but still chunky. Place in a small casserole dish. Sprinkle with Parmesan cheese.

2. Bake uncovered 10 minutes. Broil 3 to 5 minutes just until top is slightly browned. Serve warm with crackers.

Choices Per Serving

1	Meat & Alternative
½	Fat

Nutritional Analysis Per Serving			
Calories	116	Fat, total	8 g
Carbohydrate	3 g	Fat, saturated	4 g
Fiber	0 g	Sodium	218 mg
Protein	8 g	Cholesterol	21 mg

Tips

White navy pea beans can also be used. If you cook your own dry beans, ½ cup (125 mL) dry yields approximately 1½ cups (375 mL) of cooked beans.

The red pepper in this recipe makes it a good source of vitamin C.

Make Ahead

Prepare up to a day ahead; keep covered and refrigerated. Stir before using.

Tuna and White Bean Spread

1 cup	canned, cooked white kidney beans, drained	250 mL
1	can (6.5 oz/184 g) tuna in water, drained	1
1½ tsp	minced garlic	7 mL
2 tbsp	lemon juice	25 mL
2 tbsp	light mayonnaise	25 mL
¼ cup	5% ricotta cheese	50 mL
3 tbsp	minced red onions	45 mL
¼ cup	minced fresh dill (or 1 tsp/5 mL dried)	50 mL
1 tbsp	grated Parmesan cheese	15 mL
¼ cup	diced red pepper	50 mL

1. Place beans, tuna, garlic, lemon juice, mayonnaise and ricotta in food processor; pulse on and off until combined but still chunky. Place in serving bowl.

2. Stir onions, dill, Parmesan and red pepper into bean mixture.

Choices Per Serving

½ Carbohydrate

1 Meat & Alternative

Nutritional Analysis Per Serving

Calories	88	Fat, total	3 g
Carbohydrate	9 g	Fat, saturated	1 g
Fiber	0 g	Sodium	52 mg
Protein	7 g	Cholesterol	10 mg

Rosy Shrimp Spread

4 oz	light cream cheese, softened	125 g
¼ cup	light sour cream or plain yogurt	50 mL
2 tbsp	prepared chili sauce	25 mL
1 tsp	prepared horseradish	5 mL
	Hot pepper sauce, to taste	
1	can (4 oz/113 g) small shrimp, rinsed and drained	1
1 tbsp	minced green onion tops or chives	15 mL

Tips

Microwave cold cream cheese at Medium for 1 minute to soften.

This spread is equally good with crackers or vegetable dippers.

Instead of shrimp, try using 1 can (6 oz/170 g) crab.

Make Ahead

Spread can be prepared up to 2 days ahead, covered and refrigerated.

1. In a bowl, beat cream cheese until smooth. Stir in sour cream, chili sauce, horseradish and hot pepper sauce.

2. Fold in shrimp and green onions. Transfer to serving dish; cover and refrigerate until serving time.

Choices Per Serving

½ Meat & Alternative

Nutritional Analysis Per Serving

Calories	48	Fat, total	3 g
Carbohydrate	2 g	Fat, saturated	1 g
Fiber	0 g	Sodium	127 mg
Protein	4 g	Cholesterol	27 mg

Soups, Chowders and Stews

Soups come in a wonderful variety, can be served hot or cold, eaten as a starter or served as a complete meal. Most are chock full of vitamins and minerals and depending on the ingredients can also be a source of fiber.

Those containing vegetables are also are a good source of phytochemicals, the ingredients in plant foods which are thought to protect against disease. Science may not understand all the reasons yet, but what a tasty way to help your health.

Regular chicken and beef broth have been used in the majority of these recipes. If you are concerned about salt or sodium content, choose a reduced sodium broth or make one from scratch when the recipe calls for chicken or beef broth. 35%-less-salt bouillion envelopes contain about 649 mg of sodium per 1 cup (250 mL) serving as compared with about 900 mg in their regular counterparts.

continued on next page

**MAKES 6 CUPS
(1.5 L)
(1 cup/250 mL
per serving)**

Tip

Here's the perfect
stock for vegetarians.
It keeps for up to
6 months if frozen in
airtight containers.

Vegetable Stock

6 cups	water	1.5 L
1	large sweet potato, diced	1
2	large celery stalks, chopped	2
2	large leeks, cleaned and sliced	2
1	large onion, chopped	1
½ cup	chopped parsley	125 mL
2	large cloves garlic	2
2	bay leaves	2
¼ tsp	freshly ground black pepper	1 mL
⅛ tsp	salt	0.5 mL

1. In a saucepan over medium-high heat, combine water, potato, celery, leeks, onion, parsley, garlic, bay leaves, pepper and salt; bring to a boil. Reduce heat to low; simmer, covered, for 1½ hours.

2. Pour mixture through a strainer; discard solids. Refrigerate stock until cold. Stock can be kept, refrigerated, for up to 3 days or frozen in an airtight container.

**Choices
Per Serving**

1   Extra

Nutritional Analysis Per Serving			
Calories	8	Fat, total	0 g
Carbohydrate	2 g	Fat, saturated	0 g
Fiber	0 g	Sodium	47 mg
Protein	0 g	Cholesterol	0 mg

● ● ● ● ● ● ● ● ● ● ● ● ● ● ● ●

Tip

For fish or seafood stock,
use whatever pieces
you can find — including
fish heads and bones,
shrimp shells, or unused
pieces of flesh.

Fish Stock

6 cups	water	1.5 L
1½ lbs	fish or seafood pieces	750 g
1	large carrot, peeled and chopped	1
1	medium onion, quartered	1
1	large celery stalk, chopped	1
3	large cloves garlic	3
¼ tsp	freshly ground black pepper	1 mL
⅛ tsp	salt	0.5 mL
½ cup	chopped parsley	125 mL
2	bay leaves	2

1. In a saucepan over medium-high heat, combine water, fish/seafood pieces, carrot, onion, celery, garlic, pepper, salt, parsley, and bay leaves. Bring to a boil, skimming any foam that rises to the top. cover, reduce heat to low; simmer for 1½ hours.

2. Pour mixture through a strainer; discard solids. Refrigerate stock until cold; skim fat off surface. Stock can be refrigerated for up to 3 days or frozen in an airtight container.

**Choices
Per Serving**

Free Food

Nutritional Analysis Per Serving			
Calories	13	Fat, total	0 g
Carbohydrate	1 g	Fat, saturated	0 g
Fiber	0 g	Sodium	54 mg
Protein	2 g	Cholesterol	6 mg

Artichoke Leek Potato Soup

2 tsp	vegetable oil	10 mL
2 tsp	minced garlic	10 mL
1½ cups	chopped leeks	375 mL
3½ to 4 cups	basic vegetable stock (see recipe, below)	875 mL to 1 L
1½ cups	diced potatoes	375 mL
1 tsp	dried tarragon	5 mL
1	can (14 oz/398 mL) artichoke hearts, drained and halved	1

1. In a nonstick saucepan, heat oil over medium-low heat. Stir in garlic and leeks, cover and cook 5 minutes.

2. Stir in stock, potatoes, tarragon and artichoke hearts. Bring to a boil; reduce heat to medium-low, cover and cook 15 minutes, or until potato is tender.

3. In a food processor or blender, purée soup.

BASIC VEGETABLE STOCK

8 cups	fresh water or cooking water	2 L
2	stalks celery, chopped	2
2	large onions, chopped	2
2	large carrots, washed and chopped	2
4	cloves garlic, chopped	4
4	bay leaves	4
4	whole cloves (or pinch ground)	4
10	peppercorns, crushed	10
¼ cup	chopped fresh parsley (or ¼ tsp/1 mL dried)	50 mL
¼ tsp	salt (optional)	1 mL

1. Combine all ingredients in a large pot. Bring to simmer and cook, uncovered, for 45 minutes.

2. Remove from heat; let cool. Strain, discarding solids. Store in a container with tight-fitting lid. Stock will keep 1 week in refrigerator and several months if frozen.

Nutritional Analysis Per Serving			
Calories	156	Fat, total	3 g
Carbohydrate	31 g	Fat, saturated	0 g
Fiber	5 g	Sodium	112 mg
Protein	5 g	Cholesterol	0 mg

Choices Per Serving

1½	Carbohydrates
½	Fat

Tips

Choose the greenest asparagus with straight, firm stalks. The tips should be tightly closed and firm.

This soup can be served warm or cold.

Using low-sodium chicken stock in this recipe will reduce the sodium to 391 mg/serving.

Make Ahead

Make and refrigerate up to a day before and reheat gently before serving, adding more stock if too thick.

Asparagus and Leek Soup

¾ lb	asparagus	375 g
1½ tsp	vegetable oil	7 mL
1 tsp	crushed garlic	5 mL
1 cup	chopped onion	250 mL
2	leeks, sliced	2
3½ cups	chicken stock	875 mL
1 cup	diced peeled potato	250 mL
	Salt and pepper	
2 tbsp	grated Parmesan cheese	25 mL

1. Trim asparagus; cut stalks into pieces and set tips aside.

2. In large nonstick saucepan, heat oil; sauté garlic, onion, leeks and asparagus stalks just until softened, approximately 10 minutes.

3. Add stock and potato; reduce heat, cover and simmer for 20 to 25 minutes or until vegetables are tender. Purée in food processor until smooth. Taste and adjust seasoning with salt and pepper. Return to saucepan.

4. Steam or microwave reserved asparagus tips just until tender; add to soup. Serve sprinkled with Parmesan cheese.

Choices Per Serving

1	Carbohydrate
½	Fat

Nutritional Analysis Per Serving

Calories	118	Fat, total	3 g
Carbohydrate	20 g	Fat, saturated	1 g
Fiber	3 g	Sodium	918 mg
Protein	5 g	Cholesterol	2 mg

Tips

Increase curry to $1\frac{1}{2}$ tsp (7 mL) for more intense flavor.

This soup is high in fiber and is an excellent source of Vitamins A and C.

If you use a granulated sugar substitute to replace the honey in this soup, the carbohydrate content will be reduced by almost 7 g/serving.

Using low-sodium chicken stock in this recipe will reduce the sodium to 369 mg/serving.

● ● ● ● ● ● ● ● ● ● ● ● ● ●

Make Ahead

Prepare and refrigerate up to a day ahead and reheat gently before serving, adding more stock if too thick.

Curried Broccoli Sweet Potato Soup

2 tsp	vegetable oil	10 mL
$1\frac{1}{2}$ tsp	minced garlic	7 mL
$1\frac{1}{2}$ cups	chopped onions	375 mL
1 tsp	curry powder	5 mL
4 cups	chicken stock	1 L
4 cups	broccoli florets	1 L
3 cups	peeled, diced sweet potato	750 mL
2 tbsp	honey	25 mL

1. Heat oil in nonstick saucepan over medium heat. Add garlic, onions and curry; cook for 4 minutes or until softened. Add stock, broccoli and sweet potatoes; bring to a boil. Cover, reduce heat to low and simmer for 30 minutes or until vegetables are tender.

2. Transfer soup to food processor or blender; add honey and purée.

Choices Per Serving	
$2\frac{1}{2}$	Carbohydrates
$\frac{1}{2}$	Fat

Nutritional Analysis Per Serving			
Calories	216	Fat, total	3 g
Carbohydrate	45 g	Fat, saturated	0 g
Fiber	6 g	Sodium	971 mg
Protein	5 g	Cholesterol	0 mg

Broccoli and Lentil Soup

1½ tsp	vegetable oil	7 mL
2 tsp	crushed garlic	10 mL
1	medium onion, chopped	1
1	celery stalk, chopped	1
1	large carrot, chopped	1
4 cups	chicken stock	1 L
2½ cups	chopped broccoli	625 mL
¾ cup	dried green lentils	175 mL
2 tbsp	grated Parmesan cheese	25 mL

1. In large nonstick saucepan, heat oil; sauté garlic, onion, celery and carrot until softened, approximately 5 minutes.

2. Add stock, broccoli and lentils; cover and simmer for 30 minutes, stirring occasionally, or until lentils are tender.

3. Purée in food processor until creamy and smooth. Serve sprinkled with Parmesan.

Choices Per Serving

1 Carbohydrate
1 Meat & Alternative

Nutritional Analysis Per Serving

Calories	139	Fat, total	3 g
Carbohydrate	20 g	Fat, saturated	1 g
Fiber	4 g	Sodium	999 mg
Protein	10 g	Cholesterol	2 mg

Tips

This soup can be served hot or cold.

A dollop of yogurt on each bowlful enhances both the appearance and flavor.

Carrots make this soup an excellent source of vitamin A.

Using low-sodium chicken stock in this recipe will reduce the sodium to 329 mg/serving.

Make Ahead

Make and refrigerate up to a day before. If serving warm, reheat gently.

Dill Carrot Soup

1 lb	carrots, sliced (6 to 8 medium)	500 g
2 tsp	vegetable oil	10 mL
2 tsp	crushed garlic	10 mL
1 cup	chopped onion	250 mL
3½ cups	chicken stock	875 mL
¾ cup	2% milk	175 mL
2 tbsp	chopped fresh dill (or 1 tsp/5 mL dried dillweed)	25 mL
2 tbsp	chopped fresh chives or green onions	25 mL

1. In large saucepan of boiling water, cook carrots just until tender. Drain and return to saucepan; set aside.

2. In nonstick skillet, heat oil; sauté garlic and onion until softened, approximately 5 minutes. Add to carrots along with stock; cover and simmer for 25 minutes.

3. Purée in food processor until smooth, in batches if necessary. Return to saucepan; stir in milk, dill and chives.

Choices Per Serving

½ Carbohydrate

½ Fat

Nutritional Analysis Per Serving

Calories	89	Fat, total	3 g
Carbohydrate	13 g	Fat, saturated	1 g
Fiber	2 g	Sodium	863 mg
Protein	3 g	Cholesterol	2 mg

Slow cooker

Make Ahead

This soup can be assembled the night before it is cooked. Follow preparation directions in Steps 1 and 2. Cover and refrigerate overnight. The next day, continue cooking as directed in Steps 3 and 4.

Santa Fe Sweet Potato Soup

2	dried New Mexico chili peppers	2
2 cups	boiling water	500 mL
1 tbsp	vegetable oil	15 mL
2	onions, finely chopped	2
4	cloves garlic, minced	4
1	finely chopped jalapeno pepper, optional	1
1 tsp	salt, optional	5 mL
1 tsp	dried oregano leaves	5 mL
4 cups	peeled, cubed sweet potatoes, about ½ inch (1 cm)	1 L
6 cups	vegetable or chicken broth	1.5 L
2 cups	corn kernels, thawed if frozen	500 mL
1 tsp	grated lime zest	5 mL
2 tbsp	lime juice	25 mL
2	roasted red peppers, cut into thin strips	2
	Finely chopped cilantro	

1. In a heatproof bowl, soak chilies in boiling water for 30 minutes. Drain, discarding soaking liquid and stems. Pat dry, chop finely and set aside.

2. In a skillet, heat oil over medium heat. Add onions and cook, stirring, until softened. Add garlic, jalapeno pepper and salt, if using, oregano and reserved chilies and cook, stirring, for 1 minute. Transfer mixture to slow cooker stoneware. Add sweet potatoes and broth and stir to combine.

Choices Per Serving

| 2 | Carbohydrates |
| ½ | Fat |

Nutritional Analysis Per Serving

Calories	175	Fat, total	3 g
Carbohydrate	31 g	Fat, saturated	0 g
Fiber	4 g	Sodium	439 mg
Protein	7 g	Cholesterol	0 mg

3. Cover and cook on Low for 8 to 10 hours or on High for 4 to 6 hours, until sweet potatoes are tender. Strain vegetables, reserving broth. In a blender or food processor, purée vegetables with 1 cup (250 mL) reserved broth until smooth. Return mixture, along with reserved broth, to slow cooker stoneware. Or, using a hand-held blender, purée the soup in stoneware. Add corn, lime zest and juice. Cover and cook on High for 20 minutes, until corn is tender.

4. When ready to serve, ladle soup into individual bowls and garnish with red pepper strips and cilantro.

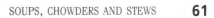

Tips

Sweet bell peppers and red onions make this a naturally sweet-tasting soup. Sugar may not be necessary.

Start with the lesser amount of stock, adding more to reach the consistency you prefer.

This soup is a very high source of fiber.

Make Ahead

Prepare up to 2 days in advance. Add more stock if too thick. Freeze up to 4 weeks.

Red Onion and Grilled Red Pepper Soup

3	large red bell peppers	3
2 tsp	vegetable oil	10 mL
2 tsp	minced garlic	10 mL
1 tbsp	packed brown sugar	15 mL
5 cups	thinly sliced red onions	1.25 L
3 to 3½ cups	basic vegetable stock (see recipe, page 46)	750 mL to 875 mL

GARNISH

⅓ cup	chopped fresh basil or parsley	75 mL
	Light sour cream (optional)	

1. Arrange oven rack 6 inches (15 cm) under broiler. Cook peppers on baking sheet, turning occasionally, 20 minutes or until charred. Cool. Discard stem, skin and seeds; cut peppers into thin strips. Set aside.

2. In a large nonstick saucepan, heat oil over medium-low heat. Add garlic, brown sugar and red onions; cook, stirring occasionally, 15 minutes or until onions are browned. Stir in stock and red pepper strips; cook 15 minutes longer.

3. In a blender or food processor, purée soup until smooth. Serve hot, garnished with chopped basil or parsley and a dollop of sour cream, if desired.

Choices Per Serving

2	Carbohydrates
½	Fat

Nutritional Analysis Per Serving			
Calories	187	Fat, total	3 g
Carbohydrate	39 g	Fat, saturated	0 g
Fiber	7 g	Sodium	64 mg
Protein	5 g	Cholesterol	0 mg

Tips

When tomatoes are in season make this delicious soup. Try using several different types to experiment with a variety of tastes.

This soup can be served hot or cold.

A dollop of light sour cream enhances each soup bowl.

● ● ● ● ● ● ● ● ● ● ● ● ● ● ● ●

Make Ahead

Prepare and refrigerate early in day, then serve cold or reheat gently.

Fresh Tomato Dill Soup

1 tbsp	olive oil	15 mL
1 tsp	crushed garlic	5 mL
1	medium carrot, chopped	1
1	celery stalk, chopped	1
1 cup	chopped onion	250 mL
2 cups	chicken stock	500 mL
5 cups	chopped ripe tomatoes	1.25 L
3 tbsp	tomato paste	45 mL
2 tsp	granulated sugar	10 mL
3 tbsp	chopped fresh dill	45 mL

1. In large nonstick saucepan, heat oil; sauté garlic, carrot, celery and onion until softened, approximately 5 minutes.

2. Add stock, tomatoes and tomato paste; reduce heat, cover and simmer for 20 minutes, stirring occasionally.

3. Purée in food processor until smooth. Add sugar and dill; mix well.

Choices Per Serving

1	Carbohydrate
½	Fat

Nutritional Analysis Per Serving

Calories	106	Fat, total	4 g
Carbohydrate	18 g	Fat, saturated	1 g
Fiber	4 g	Sodium	506 mg
Protein	3 g	Cholesterol	0 mg

● ● ● ● ● ● ● ● ● ● ● ● ● ● ● ●

Preheat broiler

Two baking sheets lined with aluminum foil and sprayed with vegetable spray

● ● ● ● ● ● ● ● ● ● ● ● ● ● ● ●

Tips

Regular fresh tomatoes can replace plum.

Dill or coriander can replace basil.

In the summer, grill tomatoes and 2 whole cobs of corn on barbecue.

● ● ● ● ● ● ● ● ● ● ● ● ● ● ● ●

Make Ahead

Prepare soup up to 2 days in advance, adding more stock, if necessary, when reheating. Freeze up to 4 weeks.

Roasted Tomato and Corn Soup

2½ lbs	plum tomatoes (about 10)	1.25 kg
1	can (12 oz/341 mL) corn, drained	1
2 tsp	vegetable oil	10 mL
2 tsp	minced garlic	10 mL
1 cup	chopped onions	250 mL
¾ cup	finely chopped carrots	175 mL
2½ cups	basic vegetable stock (see recipe, page 55)	625 mL
3 tbsp	tomato paste	45 mL
½ cup	chopped fresh basil (or 2 tsp/10 mL dried)	125 mL

1. Put tomatoes on one baking sheet. With rack 6 inches (15 cm) under broiler, broil tomatoes about 30 minutes, turning occasionally, or until charred on all sides. Meanwhile, spread corn on other baking sheet and broil, stirring occasionally, about 15 minutes or until slightly browned. (Some corn kernels will pop.) When cool enough to handle, chop tomatoes.

2. In a nonstick saucepan, heat oil over medium-high heat. Add garlic, onions and carrots; cook 5 minutes or until softened and beginning to brown. Add roasted tomatoes, stock, tomato paste and, if using, dried basil. (If using fresh basil, wait until Step 3.) Bring to a boil; reduce heat to medium-low, cover and cook 20 minutes or until vegetables tender.

3. In food processor or blender, purée soup. Return to saucepan; stir in corn and, if using, fresh basil.

Choices Per Serving

1½   Carbohydrates

½   Fat

Nutritional Analysis Per Serving

Calories	139	Fat, total	3 g
Carbohydrate	29 g	Fat, saturated	0 g
Fiber	5 g	Sodium	216 mg
Protein	4 g	Cholesterol	0 mg

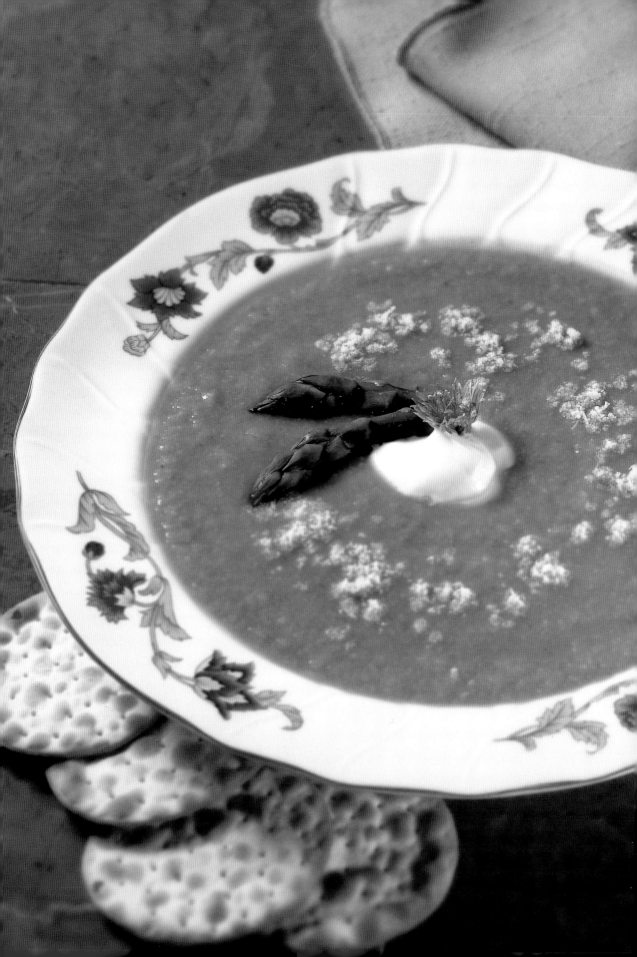

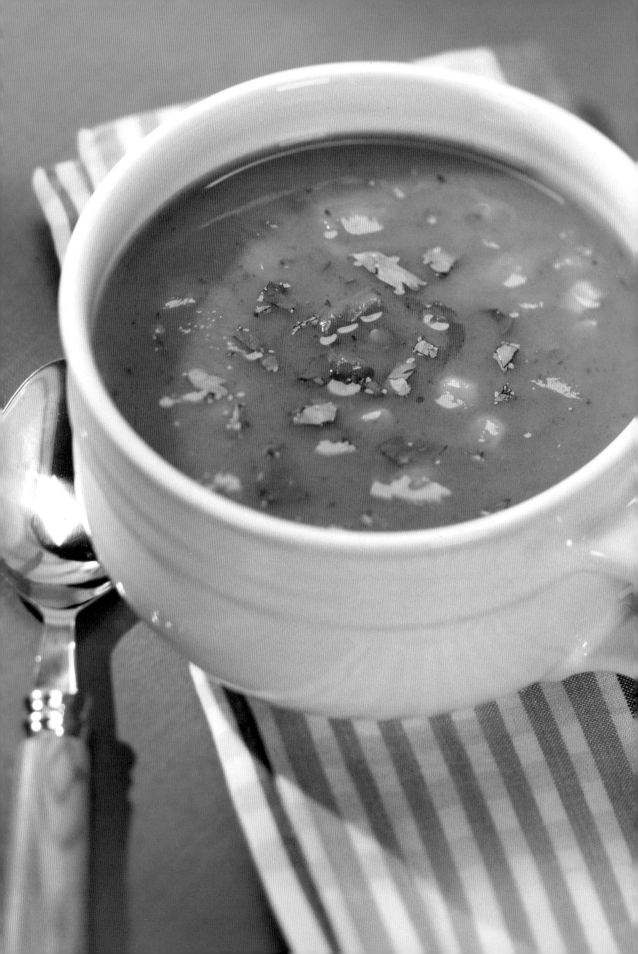

Vegetable Minestrone with Sun-Dried Tomato Pesto

Tips

Sun-Dried Tomato Pesto is optional, but it adds a wonderful jolt of flavor and dresses up the soup. You can also use whatever pesto you have on hand.

Refrigerate soup for up to five days or freeze in airtight containers for up to three months.

Rinse the canned Romano beans thoroughly to further reduce the sodium in this recipe.

If you don't have time to make the vegetable stock on page 53, using a low-sodium chicken stock will increase sodium to 827 mg. Regular stock increases sodium to 1971 mg/serving.

The vegetables in this soup make it an excellent source of vitamin A.

1 tbsp	olive oil	15 mL
2	large onions, chopped	2
3	cloves garlic, finely chopped	3
2	carrots, peeled and chopped	2
2	stalks celery, chopped	2
10 cups	vegetable stock (see recipe, page 53) or low-sodium chicken stock (approx.)	2.5 L
2 cups	shredded cabbage	500 mL
2 cups	small cauliflower florets	500 mL
1/3 cup	short fine noodles or other small-shaped pasta such as shells	75 mL
1 cup	frozen peas	250 mL
1	can (19 oz/540 mL) Romano or navy beans, drained and rinsed	1
3/4 cup	Sun-Dried Tomato Pesto (see recipe, page 119)	175 mL
	Freshly grated Parmesan cheese (optional)	

1. In a large stockpot or 32-cup (8 L) Dutch oven, heat oil over medium heat. Add onions, garlic, carrots and celery; cook, stirring occasionally, for 10 minutes or until softened.

2. Add stock and cabbage; bring to a boil over high heat. Reduce heat, cover and simmer for 20 minutes or just until vegetables are tender. Stir in cauliflower and pasta; simmer, covered, for 8 minutes or just until pasta is tender. Stir in peas and beans; cook for 2 minutes.

3. Ladle into bowls; swirl a generous tablespoon (15 mL) Sun-Dried Tomato Pesto into each. Sprinkle with Parmesan cheese, if desired. Soup thickens slightly as it cools; add more stock, if necessary.

Choices Per Serving

1	Carbohydrate
1/2	Meat & Alternative
1	Fat

Nutritional Analysis Per Serving

Calories	203	Fat, total	7 g
Carbohydrate	28 g	Fat, saturated	2 g
Fiber	6 g	Sodium	466 mg
Protein	9 g	Cholesterol	3 mg

Tips

Using a commercially prepared low-sodium chicken stock or vegetable stock reduces the sodium content of this recipe from 1051 mg to 727 mg.

If you have time to make the vegetable stock on page 53, you can reduce the sodium to 127 mg/serving — a savings of 600 mg!

Harvest Vegetable Barley Soup

2 tbsp	margarine or butter	25 mL
1	large onion, chopped	1
3	cloves garlic, finely chopped	3
1½ cups	diced peeled rutabaga	375 mL
½ tsp	dried thyme or marjoram leaves	2 mL
8 cups	low-sodium chicken stock or vegetable stock (see recipe, page 53) (approx.)	2 L
½ cup	pearl barley, rinsed	125 mL
1½ cups	diced peeled sweet potatoes	375 mL
1½ cups	diced zucchini	375 mL
	Salt and freshly ground black pepper	

1. In a large Dutch oven or stockpot, melt butter over medium heat. Add onion, garlic, rutabaga and thyme; cook, stirring often, for 5 minutes or until vegetables are lightly colored.

2. Stir in stock and barley; bring to a boil. Reduce heat, cover and simmer for 20 minutes. Add sweet potatoes and zucchini; simmer, covered, for 15 minutes or until barley is tender. Season with salt and pepper to taste.

Choices Per Serving

2 Carbohydrates

1 Meat & Alternative

Nutritional Analysis Per Serving

Calories	231	Fat, total	6 g
Carbohydrate	34 g	Fat, saturated	3 g
Fiber	5 g	Sodium	727 mg
Protein	11 g	Cholesterol	10 mg

Tip

If you have to watch your salt intake, keep in mind that store-bought canned bouillon, powder and cubed stocks are high in sodium. Making your own stock is a much healthier alternative. Take a look at the stock recipes on pages 53–55 and give them a try. For chicken and beef stocks, refrigerate overnight, remove any layers of fat and freeze in containers for later use.

Barley Minestrone with Pesto

1 cup	chopped onions	250 mL
1½ tsp	minced garlic	7 mL
1½ cups	diced unpeeled zucchini	375 mL
1 cup	diced unpeeled eggplant	250 mL
½ cup	diced carrots	125 mL
4¾ cups	vegetable stock (see recipe, page 53) or chicken stock	1.175 L
1	can (19 oz/540 mL) whole tomatoes, with juice	1
1½ cups	diced peeled potatoes	375 mL
1 cup	canned cooked white kidney beans, rinsed and drained	250 mL
⅓ cup	pearl barley	75 mL
2½ tsp	dried basil	12 mL
1	bay leaf	1
2 tbsp	pesto	25 mL
3 tbsp	grated low-fat Parmesan cheese	45 mL

1. In a large nonstick saucepan sprayed with vegetable spray, cook onions and garlic over medium-high heat for 2 minutes or until softened. Add zucchini, eggplant and carrots; cook for 5 minutes, stirring occasionally.

2. Add stock, tomatoes (with juice), potatoes, kidney beans, barley, basil and bay leaf. Bring to a boil, breaking tomatoes with back of a spoon. Reduce heat to medium-low; cook, covered, for 45 minutes or until barley is tender.

3. Ladle soup into bowls. Spoon a dollop of pesto in center of each serving; garnish with Parmesan cheese.

Nutritional Analysis Per Serving			
Calories	135	Fat, total	1 g
Carbohydrate	28 g	Fat, saturated	0 g
Fiber	5 g	Sodium	5 mg
Protein	5 g	Cholesterol	5 mg

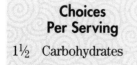

**Choices
Per Serving**

1½ Carbohydrates

Slow cooker

Make Ahead

This dish can be assembled the night before it is cooked. Follow preparation directions in Steps 1 and 2 and refrigerate overnight. The next day, transfer to slow cooker stoneware and continue cooking as directed in Step 3.

Sophisticated Mushroom Barley Soup

1	cup boiling water	250 mL
1	package (½ oz/14 g) dried wild mushrooms, such as porcini	1
2 tbsp	margarine or butter, divided	25 mL
3	onions, finely chopped	3
6	cloves garlic, minced	6
1 tsp	salt, optional	5 mL
1 tsp	cracked black peppercorns	5 mL
1½ lbs	button mushrooms, sliced	750 g
⅔ cup	pearl barley	150 mL
6 cups	low-sodium beef stock	1.5 L
1 cup	water	250 mL
1	bay leaf	1
¼ cup	low-sodium soya sauce	50 mL
	Finely chopped green onions or parsley (optional)	

1. In a heatproof bowl, combine boiling water and dried mushrooms. Let stand for 30 minutes, then strain through a fine sieve, reserving liquid. Chop mushrooms finely and set aside.

2. In a skillet, over medium heat, melt 1 tbsp (15 mL) butter. Add onions and cook until soft. Add garlic, optional salt and pepper and cook for 1 minute. Transfer mixture to slow cooker stoneware. In same pan, melt remaining butter and cook button mushrooms over medium-high heat until they begin to lose their liquid. Add dried mushrooms, toss to combine and cook for 1 minute. Transfer mixture to slow cooker stoneware. Add barley, reserved mushroom soaking liquid, stock, water, bay leaf and soya sauce.

3. Cover and cook on Low for 6 to 8 hours or on High for 3 to 4 hours. Discard bay leaf. Ladle into individual bowls and garnish with chopped green onions or parsley, if using.

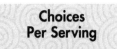

Choices Per Serving

1   Carbohydrate
½   Meat & Alternative

Nutritional Analysis Per Serving			
Calories	138	Fat, total	4 g
Carbohydrate	22 g	Fat, saturated	2 g
Fiber	3 g	Sodium	627 mg
Protein	6 g	Cholesterol	8 mg

Tips

Oyster or cremini mushrooms are the best to use here. If unavailable, substitute white common mushrooms.

Barley is available in "pearl" and "pot" varieties; whichever you use, cook until tender.

This soup is a good source of fiber.

Use some dried mushrooms to really highlight this dish.

Make Ahead

Prepare up to 2 days in advance. Add more stock when reheating if too thick. Freeze for up to 3 weeks.

Wild Mushroom and Barley Soup

2 tsp	vegetable oil	10 mL
2 tsp	minced garlic	10 mL
1 cup	chopped onions	250 mL
3½ cups	basic vegetable stock (see recipe, page 55)	875 mL
1	can (19 oz/540 mL) tomatoes, crushed	1
½ cup	barley	125 mL
½ tsp	dried thyme	2 mL
¼ tsp	freshly ground black pepper	1 mL
8 oz	wild mushrooms, sliced (see Tip, at left)	250 g

1. In a nonstick saucepan, heat oil over medium heat. Add garlic and onions; cook 4 minutes or until softened.

2. Stir in stock, tomatoes, barley, thyme and pepper. Bring to a boil; reduce heat to medium-low, cover and simmer 40 to 50 minutes, or until barley is tender.

3. Meanwhile, in a nonstick frying pan sprayed with vegetable spray, cook mushrooms over high heat, stirring, 8 minutes or until browned.

4. Stir mushrooms into soup and serve.

Choices Per Serving

1½	Carbohydrates
½	Fat

Nutritional Analysis Per Serving

Calories	135	Fat, total	2 g
Carbohydrate	28 g	Fat, saturated	0 g
Fiber	4 g	Sodium	289 mg
Protein	4 g	Cholesterol	0 mg

Tips

This soup is meant to be fairly thick; if too thick, add 1 to 2 cups (250 to 500 mL) water, stir and bring back to boil.

This recipe can be easily halved; but leftovers freeze well and can be reheated with minimal loss of flavor.

Like most beans, the kidney beans here make this soup rich in folic acid.

Fassolada (Greek Bean Soup)

2½ cups	dried white kidney beans	625 mL
1 tbsp	baking soda	15 mL
12 cups	water	3 L
1	onion, diced	1
1	large carrot, diced	1
½ cup	chopped fresh celery leaves, packed down (or 2 celery stalks, finely chopped)	125 mL
2 tbsp	tomato paste	25 mL
1 tsp	lemon juice	5 mL
1	medium tomato, blanched, skinned and chopped	1
1 tsp	dried rosemary, basil or oregano	5 mL
1 tsp	salt, optional	5 mL
½ tsp	black pepper	2 mL
¼ cup	chopped fresh parsley, packed down	50 mL
¼ cup	olive oil	50 mL
	Extra virgin olive oil, olive bits, diced red onion, and crumbled feta cheese as accompaniments	

1. In a large bowl cover beans with plenty of warm water. Add baking soda and mix well. (The water will foam and remove some of the gas from the beans.) Let soak for at least 3 hours, preferably overnight, unrefrigerated.

2. Drain beans and transfer to a soup pot. Add plenty of water and bring to a boil. Reduce heat to medium-low and simmer for 30 minutes, occasionally skimming froth that rises to the top.

Choices Per Serving

2	Carbohydrates
1	Meat & Alternative
½	Fat

Nutritional Analysis Per Serving

Calories	274	Fat, total	8 g
Carbohydrate	40 g	Fat, saturated	1 g
Fiber	10 g	Sodium	481 mg
Protein	14 g	Cholesterol	0 mg

3. Drain beans; rinse and drain again. Scrub pot, cleaning off foam stuck to the sides. Return the beans to the pot; add the 12 cups (3 L) water and place over high heat. Add onion, carrot, celery, tomato paste, lemon juice and tomato. Bring to boil, stirring; reduce heat to medium-low. Cook for $1\frac{1}{2}$ hours at a rolling bubble, stirring very occasionally until the beans and vegetables are very tender.

4. Add rosemary, optional salt, pepper, parsley and olive oil. Cook for another 5 minutes, stirring occasionally, and take off heat. Cover soup and let rest for 5 to 10 minutes. Season to taste with salt and pepper. Serve with any or all of suggested garnishes.

Tips

Canned, drained salmon can be used if fresh is unavailable.

Leftover cooked salmon can also be used.

Fresh basil can replace dill. If using dried herbs, use 1 tsp (5 mL) and add during cooking.

Using low-sodium chicken stock in this recipe will reduce the sodium to 380 mg/serving.

. . . .

Make Ahead

Prepare up to a day ahead, but do not add salmon until just ready to serve. Add more stock if soup is too thick.

Creamy Salmon Dill Bisque

6 oz	salmon fillet	150 g
2 tsp	margarine or butter	10 mL
1 tsp	minced garlic	5 mL
1 cup	chopped onions	250 mL
1 cup	chopped carrots	250 mL
½ cup	chopped celery	125 mL
1 tbsp	tomato paste	15 mL
2¼ cups	chicken stock	550 mL
1½ cups	peeled, chopped potatoes	375 mL
½ cup	2% milk	125 mL
¼ cup	chopped fresh dill	50 mL

1. In nonstick pan sprayed with vegetable spray, cook salmon over high heat for 3 minutes, then turn and cook 2 minutes longer, or until just barely done at center. Set aside.

2. Melt margarine in nonstick saucepan sprayed with vegetable spray over medium heat. Add garlic, onions, carrots, and celery; cook for 5 minutes or until onion is softened. Add tomato paste, stock and potatoes; bring to a boil. Cover, reduce heat to low and simmer for 20 minutes or until carrots and potatoes are tender.

3. Transfer soup to food processor or blender and purée. Return to saucepan and stir in milk and dill. Flake the cooked salmon. Add to soup and serve.

Choices Per Serving

1½ Carbohydrates

1½ Meat & Alternatives

Nutritional Analysis Per Serving			
Calories	220	Fat, total	6 g
Carbohydrate	31 g	Fat, saturated	1 g
Fiber	4 g	Sodium	895 mg
Protein	13 g	Cholesterol	23 mg

Tips

Stewing beef is often used in a soup like this. But I find that it takes a lot of cooking time before it becomes tender — and I'm always in a hurry. So I use more tender cuts of beef: either round or loin. Remember, too, that the smaller the cubes, the faster the meat tenderizes.

This hearty soup is an excellent source of vitamin A and folic acid.

Hearty Beef Soup with Lentils and Barley

6 oz	boneless round steak, cut into ½-inch (1 cm) cubes	175 g
2 tbsp	all-purpose flour	25 mL
½ cup	chopped onions	125 mL
1 tsp	minced garlic	5 mL
½ cup	chopped carrots	125 mL
½ cup	chopped green bell peppers	125 mL
½ cup	green lentils	125 mL
1	can (19 oz/540 mL) tomatoes, with juice	1
4½ cups	beef stock or chicken stock	1.125 L
⅓ cup	pearl barley	75 mL
2 tsp	packed brown sugar	10 mL
1½ tsp	dried basil	7 mL
2	bay leaves	2
¼ tsp	freshly ground black pepper	1 mL

1. In a bowl coat beef with flour; shake off excess. In a nonstick saucepan sprayed with vegetable spray, cook beef over medium-high heat for 5 minutes or until browned on all sides. Remove meat to a plate; respray pan. Add onions and garlic; cook for 2 minutes. Add carrots and green peppers; cook, stirring occasionally, for 4 minutes or until vegetables are softened.

2. Add browned beef, lentils, tomatoes, stock, barley, brown sugar, basil, bay leaves and pepper; bring to a boil, breaking up tomatoes with back of a spoon. Reduce heat to medium-low; cook, covered, for 45 minutes or until lentils and barley are tender. Ladle soup into bowls. Serve.

Choices Per Serving

3 Carbohydrates

2½ Meat & Alternatives

Nutritional Analysis Per Serving			
Calories	317	Fat, total	3 g
Carbohydrate	49 g	Fat, saturated	1 g
Fiber	7 g	Sodium	387 mg
Protein	26 g	Cholesterol	31 mg

Tips

Use either pot or pearl barley.

Common mushrooms should be firm and dry to the touch. They are very perishable and should be cooked within 48 hours.

Add a chunk of low-fat cheese, low-fat milk, ½ cup (125 mL) of unsweetened applesauce and cinnamon snap cookies for a delicious complete lunch.

Using low-sodium beef broth in this recipe will reduce the sodium to 473 mg/serving.

• • • • • • • • • • • • • • •

Make Ahead

Make and refrigerate up to a day before. Reheat gently just before serving, adding more stock if too thick.

Vegetable Beef Barley Soup

1 tbsp	vegetable oil	15 mL
2 tsp	crushed garlic	10 mL
1	medium onion, diced	1
2	celery stalks, diced	2
2	carrots, diced	2
2 cups	sliced mushrooms	500 mL
3½ cups	(approx) beef stock	875 mL
⅓ cup	barley	75 mL
2	small potatoes, peeled and diced	2
4 oz	stewing beef, diced	125 g
2 tbsp	chopped fresh parsley	25 mL

1. In large nonstick saucepan, heat oil; sauté garlic, onion, celery, carrots and mushrooms until tender, approximately 10 minutes.

2. Add stock, barley, potatoes and beef; cover, reduce heat and simmer approximately 50 minutes or until barley and potatoes are tender, stirring occasionally.

Choices Per Serving

2 Carbohydrates

1 Meat & Alternative

Nutritional Analysis Per Serving			
Calories	208	Fat, total	5 g
Carbohydrate	31 g	Fat, saturated	1 g
Fiber	4 g	Sodium	1009 mg
Protein	11 g	Cholesterol	13 mg

Cranberry Borscht

Slow cooker

Tip

For a vegetarian version, substitute concentrated vegetable stock for the beef broth. This soup is also good served hot.

Make Ahead

This dish can be assembled the night before it is cooked but without adding the cranberries, sugar, orange juice and zest and beet leaves. Follow preparation directions and refrigerate overnight in a large bowl. The next day, continue cooking as directed in Step 1. Or the soup can be cooked overnight in the slow cooker, finished the next morning and chilled during the day.

6	medium beets, peeled and cut into ½-inch (1 cm) cubes	6
	Leaves from the beets, washed, coarsely chopped and set aside in refrigerator	
4	cloves garlic, chopped	4
1	can (10 oz/284 mL) condensed beef broth (undiluted)	1
4 cups	water	1 L
1 tsp	salt, optional	5 mL
½ tsp	freshly ground black pepper	2 mL
1 cup	cranberries	250 mL
2 tbsp	granulated sugar	25 mL
	Zest and juice of 1 orange	
	Sour cream	
	Chopped dill (optional)	

1. In slow cooker stoneware, combine beets, garlic, beef stock, water, optional salt and pepper. Cover and cook on Low for 8 to 10 hours or on High for 4 to 5 hours, until vegetables are tender.

2. Add cranberries, sugar, orange zest and juice and beet leaves. Cover and cook on High for 30 minutes or until cranberries are popping from their skins.

3. In a blender or food processor, purée soup in batches. If serving cold, transfer to a large bowl and chill thoroughly, preferably overnight.

4. When ready to serve, spoon into individual bowls, top with sour cream and garnish with dill, if using.

Choices Per Serving

1 Carbohydrate

½ Fat

Nutritional Analysis Per Serving

Calories	77	Fat, total	2 g
Carbohydrate	14 g	Fat, saturated	1 g
Fiber	2 g	Sodium	548 mg
Protein	2 g	Cholesterol	5 mg

Tips

Try to ensure that mango is ripe. They can be stored in the refrigerator for up to 3 days. How can you tell if a mango is ripe? It should have a strong fragrance and feel slightly soft if you apply gentle pressure.

This soup can also be served at room temperature.

Make Ahead

Prepare up to 2 days in advance. Freeze up to 3 weeks.

Cold Mango Soup

2 tsp	vegetable oil	10 mL
1/2 cup	chopped onions	125 mL
2 tsp	minced garlic	10 mL
2 cups	basic vegetable stock (see recipe, page 55)	500 mL
2 1/2 cups	chopped ripe mango (about 2 large)	625 mL

GARNISH (OPTIONAL)

2% plain yogurt
Coriander leaves

1. In a nonstick saucepan, heat oil over medium heat. Add onions and garlic; cook, stirring, 4 minutes or until browned.

2. Add stock. Bring to a boil; reduce heat to medium-low and cook 5 minutes or until onions are soft.

3. Transfer mixture to a food processor. Add 2 cups (500 mL) of the mango. Purée until smooth. Stir in remaining chopped mango.

4. Chill 2 hours or until cold. Serve with a dollop of yogurt and garnish with coriander, if desired.

Choices Per Serving

1 1/2 Carbohydrates

1/2 Fat

Nutritional Analysis Per Serving			
Calories	110	Fat, total	3 g
Carbohydrate	23 g	Fat, saturated	0 g
Fiber	3 g	Sodium	38 mg
Protein	1 g	Cholesterol	0 mg

SERVES 4

Tips

Roasted red peppers taste wonderful, but they require some time to prepare. So when a recipe (like this one) calls for just a small amount, do what I do — use bottled roasted peppers. Look for those packaged in water (not oil) to avoid excess fat. Once opened, a jar of these peppers does not keep for very long, so freeze any unused peppers in small airtight containers.

Roasted peppers make this chowder an excellent source of vitamin C.

Corn Chowder with Wild Rice and Roasted Peppers

1 cup	chopped onions	250 mL
1½ tsp	minced garlic	7 mL
4 cups	vegetable stock (see recipe, page 53) or chicken stock	1 L
⅓ cup	wild rice	75 mL
1 cup	diced peeled potatoes	250 mL
⅛ tsp	salt	0.5 mL
⅛ tsp	freshly ground black pepper	0.5 mL
¾ cup	low-fat evaporated milk	175 mL
1 tbsp	all-purpose flour	15 mL
1	can (12 oz/341 mL) corn, drained or 2 cups/500 mL frozen corn, thawed	1
⅓ cup	chopped roasted red bell peppers	75 mL
⅓ cup	chopped fresh coriander, basil or dill	75 mL

1. In a nonstick saucepan sprayed with vegetable spray, cook onions and garlic over medium-high heat for 4 minutes or until softened. Add stock and wild rice; bring to a boil. Reduce heat to medium-low; cook, covered, for 15 minutes. Add potatoes, salt and pepper; cook, covered, for 20 minutes or until rice and potatoes are tender.

2. In a bowl whisk together evaporated milk and flour; add to soup. Add corn and roasted red peppers; cook for 3 minutes or until slightly thickened. Serve garnished with coriander.

Choices Per Serving

3 Carbohydrates
½ Meat & Alternative

Nutritional Analysis Per Serving			
Calories	233	Fat, total	2 g
Carbohydrate	48 g	Fat, saturated	1 g
Fiber	4 g	Sodium	376 mg
Protein	10 g	Cholesterol	4 mg

Tips

Frozen corn niblets would be fine to use. If time is available, make your own stock for a really delicious chowder.

Corn and potatoes are two vegetables that are considered Grains & Starches.

Make Ahead

Make and refrigerate early in day and reheat gently, adding more stock or milk if too thick.

Potato Corn Chowder

2 cups	corn niblets (canned or fresh)	500 mL
1½ tsp	margarine	7 mL
1 cup	chopped onions	250 mL
½ cup	chopped sweet red pepper	125 mL
1 tsp	crushed garlic	5 mL
1 cup	diced peeled potato	250 mL
1⅓ cups	chicken stock	325 mL
2 tbsp	all-purpose flour	25 mL
1½ cups	2% milk	375 mL
¼ tsp	Worcestershire sauce	1 mL
	Pepper	

1. In food processor, process 1 cup (250 mL) of the corn until puréed; add to remaining corn and set aside.

2. In large nonstick saucepan, melt margarine; sauté onions, red pepper and garlic for 5 minutes. Add potato and stock; simmer, covered, until potato is tender, approximately 15 minutes.

3. Add corn mixture to soup; cook for 5 minutes. Stir in flour and cook for 1 minute. Add milk, Worcestershire sauce, and pepper to taste; cook on medium heat for approximately 5 minutes or just until thickened.

Choices Per Serving

2   Carbohydrates

½   Meat & Alternative

Nutritional Analysis Per Serving			
Calories	176	Fat, total	4 g
Carbohydrate	32 g	Fat, saturated	1 g
Fiber	4 g	Sodium	441 mg
Protein	7 g	Cholesterol	6 mg

Clam and Pasta Chowder

2 tsp	vegetable oil	10 mL
1½ tsp	crushed garlic	7 mL
1 cup	chopped onions	250 mL
½ cup	finely chopped carrots	125 mL
⅔ cup	chopped sweet green peppers	150 mL
1½	cans (5 oz/140 mL) clams, reserving juice from 1 can	1½
1 cup	diced potatoes	250 mL
2½ cups	canned or fresh tomatoes, crushed	625 mL
2½ cups	seafood or chicken stock	625 mL
⅓ cup	tubetti or macaroni	75 mL

1. In large nonstick saucepan, heat oil; sauté garlic, onions, carrots and green peppers until tender, approximately 5 minutes.

2. Add juice of 1 can of clams, potatoes, tomatoes and stock. Cover and simmer for 20 minutes.

3. Add reserved clams and tubetti. Simmer for 10 minutes or until pasta is cooked.

Nutritional Analysis Per Serving

Calories	149	Fat, total	3 g
Carbohydrate	24 g	Fat, saturated	0 g
Fiber	3 g	Sodium	643 mg
Protein	8 g	Cholesterol	12 mg

Old-Fashioned Beef Stew

Tips

This comfort food is an excellent source of nutrients including vitamins A and C, B vitamins and iron, phosphorus, magnesium and zinc.

If you add the salt and use regular beef stock, sodium is 854 mg/serving.

¼ cup	all-purpose flour	50 mL
1 tsp	salt, optional	5 mL
½ tsp	pepper	2 mL
2 tbsp	vegetable oil (approx.)	25 mL
1½ lbs	stewing beef, cut into cubes 1½ inches (4 cm) square	750 g
2	medium onions, chopped	2
3	cloves garlic, finely chopped	3
1 tsp	dried thyme	5 mL
1 tsp	dried marjoram	5 mL
1	bay leaf	1
1 cup	red wine or additional beef stock	250 mL
3 tbsp	tomato paste	45 mL
3 cups	low-sodium beef stock (approx.)	750 mL
5	carrots	5
2	stalks celery	2
1½ lbs	potatoes (about 5)	750 g
12 oz	green beans	375 g
¼ cup	chopped fresh parsley	50 mL

1. Combine flour, optional salt and pepper in a heavy plastic bag. In batches, add beef to flour mixture and toss to coat. Transfer to a plate. Reserve remaining flour mixture.

2. In a Dutch oven, heat half the oil over medium-high heat; cook beef in batches, adding more oil as needed, until browned all over. Transfer to a plate.

3. Reduce heat to medium-low. Add onions, garlic, thyme, marjoram, bay leaf and remaining flour to pan; cook, stirring, for 4 minutes or until softened. Add wine and tomato paste; cook, stirring, to scrape up brown bits. Return beef and any accumulated juices to pan; pour in stock.

Choices Per Serving

2 Carbohydrates

4 Meat & Alternatives

Nutritional Analysis Per Serving			
Calories	419	Fat, total	13 g
Carbohydrate	38 g	Fat, saturated	4 g
Fiber	5 g	Sodium	359 mg
Protein	32 g	Cholesterol	55 mg

4. Bring to a boil, stirring, until slightly thickened. Reduce heat, cover and simmer over medium-low heat, stirring occasionally, for 1 hour.

5. Meanwhile, peel carrots and halve lengthwise. Cut carrots and celery into 1½-inch (4 cm) chunks. Peel potatoes and quarter. Add vegetables to pan. Cover and simmer for 30 minutes.

6. Trim ends of beans and cut into 2-inch (5 cm) lengths. Stir into stew mixture, adding more stock if necessary, until vegetables are just covered. Cover and simmer for 30 minutes more or until vegetables are tender. Remove bay leaf and stir in parsley. Adjust seasoning with salt and pepper to taste.

Tips

Here's a soothing dish to serve for casual get-togethers. This stew requires no more preparation time than a stir-fry or one-pot dish. Cutting the meat into smaller pieces also shortens the cooking time.

Sodium content totals 1097 mg/serving with optional salt.

This nutritious recipe is an excellent source of 8 vitamins and 3 minerals.

Variation

Lean stewing beef can be substituted for the pork. For a vegetarian dish, replace meat with cubes of firm tofu. Add along with kidney beans.

Make-Ahead Southwestern Pork Stew

4 tsp	olive oil, divided	20 mL
1 lb	lean stewing pork, cut into ¾-inch (2 cm) cubes	500 g
2	medium onions, chopped	2
3	cloves garlic, finely chopped	3
4 tsp	chili powder	20 mL
1½ tsp	dried oregano leaves	7 mL
1 tsp	ground cumin	5 mL
¾ tsp	salt, optional	4 mL
½ tsp	hot pepper flakes	2 mL
3 tbsp	all-purpose flour	45 mL
2 cups	low-sodium beef or chicken stock	500 mL
1	can (28 oz/796 mL) tomatoes, including juice, chopped	1
2	bell peppers (assorted colors), cubed	2
2 cups	frozen corn kernels	500 mL
1	can (19 oz/540 mL) kidney beans or black beans, drained and rinsed	1
	Chopped cilantro (optional)	

1. In a Dutch oven or large saucepan, heat 2 tsp (10 mL) oil over high heat; brown pork in batches. Transfer to a plate. Add remaining oil to pan; reduce heat to medium. Add onions, garlic, chili powder, oregano, cumin, optional salt and hot pepper flakes; cook, stirring, for 2 minutes or until softened.

2. Sprinkle with flour; stir in stock and tomatoes with juice. Bring to a boil, stirring until thickened. Return pork and accumulated juices to pan; reduce heat, cover and simmer for 1 hour or until meat is tender.

3. Add bell peppers, corn and kidney beans; simmer, covered, for 15 minutes or until vegetables are tender. Garnish with chopped cilantro, if desired.

Choices Per Serving

2½ Carbohydrates

3½ Meat & Alternatives

Nutritional Analysis Per Serving

Calories	384		Fat, total	9 g
Carbohydrate	51 g		Fat, saturated	2 g
Fiber	10 g		Sodium	737 mg
Protein	30 g		Cholesterol	42 mg

Skillet Pork Stew

The apples in this super easy stew turn into a lovely sauce. Use pork shoulder, a leg steak, butt chops or a roast — whatever is on special.

This delicious pork stew is an excellent source of vitamins A and C, B vitamins and phosphorus, iron, magnesium and zinc.

1 lb	lean pork	500 g
2 tbsp	all-purpose flour	25 mL
¼ tsp	salt	1 mL
¼ tsp	pepper	1 mL
2 tbsp	vegetable oil (approx.)	25 mL
1	onion, coarsely chopped	1
1 cup	apple juice or water	250 mL
2 tsp	Dijon mustard	10 mL
2 tsp	vinegar	10 mL
½ tsp	dried thyme	2 mL
4	cloves garlic, halved	4
2	carrots, cut in 2-inch (5 cm) pieces	2
2	apples, peeled and quartered	2
5	small potatoes, quartered	4
1 cup	frozen peas	250 mL

1. Cut pork into 1-inch (2.5 cm) cubes. In bag, combine flour, salt and pepper; add pork and shake to coat. Set aside.

2. In large skillet, heat half of the oil over low heat; cook onion for 5 minutes. Transfer to bowl.

3. Heat remaining oil over medium-high heat; brown pork, in batches if necessary and adding more oil if needed. Add to bowl.

4. Pour apple juice into skillet; bring to boil, scraping up brown bits from bottom of pan. Stir in mustard, vinegar and thyme. Return pork and onion to skillet. Add garlic, carrots and apples; cover and bring to boil. Reduce heat and cook for 15 minutes, stirring occasionally.

5. Add potatoes; cook for 15 to 20 minutes or until meat and vegetables are tender. Stir in peas; cook for 5 minutes.

Nutritional Analysis Per Serving

Calories	424	Fat, total	14 g
Carbohydrate	47 g	Fat, saturated	3 g
Fiber	5 g	Sodium	250 mg
Protein	28 g	Cholesterol	68 mg

Tips

Ground pork or veal can replace chicken.

Sweet potatoes are a nice change from white potatoes.

Adjust spiciness by adding more cayenne.

Canned tomatoes and chicken stock are both sources of salt or sodium in this recipe. Reduce sodium by using low-sodium chicken stock.

Almost a "meal in a bowl," finish with fresh fruit and low-fat milk.

Make Ahead

Prepare soup up to a day ahead. Add pasta until 10 minutes before serving.

Chili, Chicken, Bean and Pasta Stew

2 tsp	vegetable oil	10 mL
2 tsp	crushed garlic	10 mL
1 cup	chopped onions	250 mL
8 oz	ground chicken	250 g
1	can (19 oz/540 mL) crushed tomatoes	1
2½ cups	chicken stock	625 mL
1½ cups	diced peeled potatoes	375 mL
½ cup	canned red kidney beans, drained	125 mL
½ cup	canned chick peas, drained	125 mL
2 tbsp	tomato paste	25 mL
1 tbsp	chili powder	15 mL
2 tsp	dried basil	10 mL
1 tsp	dried oregano	5 mL
Pinch	cayenne	Pinch
⅓ cup	macaroni	75 mL

1. In large nonstick saucepan, heat oil; sauté garlic and onions until softened, approximately 5 minutes.

2. Add chicken and cook, stirring to break up chunks, until no longer pink; pour off any fat.

3. Add tomatoes, stock, potatoes, kidney beans, chick peas, tomato paste, chili powder, basil, oregano and cayenne. Cover and reduce heat; simmer for 40 minutes, stirring occasionally.

4. Add pasta; cook until firm to the bite, approximately 10 minutes.

Choices Per Serving

2   Carbohydrates

1½   Meat & Alternatives

Nutritional Analysis Per Serving			
Calories	267	Fat, total	9 g
Carbohydrate	36 g	Fat, saturated	0 g
Fiber	3 g	Sodium	1001 mg
Protein	14 g	Cholesterol	0 mg

Salads

Salads can serve as a starter, act as a side dish or be a complete meal. The combination of ingredients can provide delicious taste, texture and variety.

　　People attempting to increase their intake of fresh vegetables may include traditional "salads" such as coleslaw more often, failing to consider commercial dressings, sweet sauces or brines used in their preparation. Choose salad ingredients wisely and pay attention to how they "fit" into your meal plan. Use some of the delicious salads that follow to increase your mealtime flexibility, provide great lunchtime alternatives and pack away plenty of good nutrition at the same time.

Tips

This is a lovely summer party dish.

To make this a complete meal, serve with whole grain bread, milk and low-fat cheese.

Avocado Melissa Sue Anderson

2 tbsp	lime juice	25 mL
2	ripe avocados	2
1	Granny Smith apple, peeled and thinly sliced	1
2	peaches, peeled and cut into chunks	2
5	green onions, cut into ½-inch (1 cm) pieces	5
3 cups	sliced mushrooms	750 mL
2	stalks celery, chopped	2
¾ cup	unpeeled, diced English cucumber	175 mL
2	tomatoes, cubed	2
⅓ cup	toasted cashew pieces	75 mL
3 tbsp	finely chopped fresh coriander	45 mL
2 tbsp	vegetable oil	25 mL
1 tbsp	sesame oil	15 mL
1 tbsp	raspberry (or white wine) vinegar	15 mL
1 tsp	salt	5 mL
1 tsp	cayenne (optional)	5 mL
	Alfalfa sprouts	

1. Put lime juice in a large bowl. Peel avocado and cut into slices (or scoop out with a small spoon) and add to the lime juice. Toss gently until well coated. Add apple slices and toss again. Add peaches, green onions, mushrooms, celery, cucumber, tomato and cashew pieces.

2. In a small bowl whisk together coriander, vegetable oil, sesame oil, vinegar, salt and optional cayenne until emulsified. Drizzle half of the dressing over the salad. Fold in the dressing, mixing the various ingredients of the salad. Do this gently but thoroughly. Add the rest of the dressing, and fold in 5 or 6 more times.

3. Transfer to a serving bowl and garnish with alfalfa sprouts for that final California touch. Serve immediately or keep up to 1 hour, covered and unrefrigerated.

Choices Per Serving

½	Carbohydrate
½	Meat & Alternative
2	Fats

Nutritional Analysis Per Serving			
Calories	159	Fat, total	13 g
Carbohydrate	12 g	Fat, saturated	2 g
Fiber	3 g	Sodium	276 mg
Protein	3 g	Cholesterol	0 mg

Tips
The vegetables and dried fruit give this salad a wonderful flavor and texture.

Substitute coriander, basil or parsley for the dill.

This recipe is an excellent source of vitamins A and C and folic acid.

Make Ahead
Prepare early in the day. Best served chilled.

Broccoli, Apricot and Red Pepper Salad in a Creamy Dressing

4 cups	broccoli florets	1 L
1 cup	chopped carrots	250 mL
1 cup	sliced red bell peppers	250 mL
¾ cup	sliced water chestnuts	175 mL
½ cup	chopped red onions	125 mL
½ cup	chopped dried apricots or dates	125 mL
⅓ cup	raisins	75 mL
2 oz	feta cheese, crumbled	50 g

DRESSING

¼ cup	chopped fresh dill	50 mL
¼ cup	light mayonnaise	50 mL
¼ cup	light sour cream	50 mL
2 tbsp	freshly squeezed lemon juice	25 mL
1½ tsp	minced garlic	7 mL
	Freshly ground black pepper, to taste	

1. Boil or steam broccoli 3 minutes or until tender-crisp; drain. Rinse under cold water; drain well.

2. In a large serving bowl, combine broccoli, carrots, red peppers, water chestnuts, red onions, apricots, raisins and feta cheese.

3. *Dressing:* In a small bowl, whisk together dill, mayonnaise, sour cream, lemon juice and garlic. Pour over salad; toss to coat. Season to taste with pepper.

Nutritional Analysis Per Serving

Calories	181	Fat, total	6 g
Carbohydrate	31 g	Fat, saturated	2 g
Fiber	5 g	Sodium	208 mg
Protein	5 g	Cholesterol	9 mg

Tips

Sweet fruit and a combination of lettuces make this a perfect salad.

If you don't care for the bitter flavor of curly endive and radicchio, use romaine or Bibb lettuce instead.

If you don't want the salad to wilt, use a larger amount of romaine lettuce.

Make Ahead

Prepare salad and dressing early in the day. Toss just before serving.

Pear, Lettuce and Feta Cheese Salad

DRESSING

2 tbsp	raspberry vinegar	25 mL
2½ tbsp	olive oil	35 mL
1 tsp	minced garlic	5 mL
1½ tsp	honey	7 mL
1 tsp	sesame oil	5 mL

SALAD

4 cups	red or green leaf lettuce, washed, dried and torn into pieces	1 L
1½ cups	curly endive or escarole, washed, dried and torn into pieces	375 mL
1½ cups	radicchio, washed, dried and torn into pieces	375 mL
1 cup	diced pears (about 1 pear)	250 mL
2 oz	feta cheese, crumbled	50 g
⅓ cup	sliced black olives	75 mL

1. *Prepare the dressing:* In a small bowl, whisk together vinegar, olive oil, garlic, honey and sesame oil; set aside.

2. *Make the salad:* In a serving bowl, combine leaf lettuce, curly endive, radicchio, pears, feta and olives. Pour dressing over; toss gently to coat. Serve immediately.

Choices Per Serving

½ Carbohydrate

2 Fats

Nutritional Analysis Per Serving			
Calories	128	Fat, total	9 g
Carbohydrate	10 g	Fat, saturated	2 g
Fiber	2 g	Sodium	144 mg
Protein	3 g	Cholesterol	9 mg

Tip

Toast sesame seeds in nonstick skillet over high heat for 2 to 3 minutes.

Make Ahead

Prepare salad and dressing earlier in the day. Keep separate in refrigerator until ready to serve.

Oriental Vegetable Salad

2½ cups	trimmed green beans	625 mL
2 cups	asparagus cut into 1-inch (2.5 cm) pieces	500 mL
1½ cups	halved snow peas	375 mL
1¾ cups	bean sprouts	425 mL
1½ cups	sliced red bell peppers	375 mL
1 cup	chopped baby corn cobs	250 mL
¾ cup	canned sliced water chestnuts, drained	175 mL
¾ cup	canned mandarin oranges, drained	175 mL

DRESSING

4 tsp	soya sauce	20 mL
4 tsp	rice wine vinegar	20 mL
1 tbsp	olive oil	15 mL
1 tbsp	honey	15 mL
2 tsp	sesame oil	10 mL
2 tsp	toasted sesame seeds	10 mL
1½ tsp	minced garlic	7 mL
1 tsp	minced gingerroot	5 mL

1. Boil or steam green beans and asparagus for 2 to 3 minutes or until tender-crisp; drain. Rinse under cold water and drain; transfer to a large serving bowl.

2. Boil or steam snow peas 45 seconds or until tender-crisp; drain. Rinse under cold water and drain; add to serving bowl along with bean sprouts, red peppers, corn cobs, water chestnuts and mandarin oranges. Toss to combine.

3. In a small bowl, whisk together soya sauce, vinegar, olive oil, honey, sesame oil, sesame seeds, garlic and ginger. Pour over salad; toss to coat.

Choices Per Serving

1½	Carbohydrates
½	Meat & Alternative
½	Fat

Nutritional Analysis Per Serving			
Calories	170	Fat, total	5 g
Carbohydrate	30 g	Fat, saturated	1 g
Fiber	4 g	Sodium	230 mg
Protein	6 g	Cholesterol	0 mg

Four-Tomato Salad

½ cup	sun-dried tomatoes	125 mL
2 cups	sliced field tomatoes	500 mL
2 cups	halved red or yellow cherry tomatoes	500 mL
2 cups	quartered plum tomatoes	500 mL
1 cup	sliced red onions	250 mL

DRESSING

3 tbsp	olive oil	45 mL
¼ cup	balsamic vinegar	50 mL
1½ tsp	minced garlic	7 mL
½ cup	chopped fresh basil (or 2 tsp/10 mL dried)	125 mL
⅛ tsp	ground black pepper	0.5 mL

1. Pour boiling water over sun-dried tomatoes. Let rest for 15 minutes until softened. Drain and slice.

2. Place sun-dried tomatoes, field tomatoes, cherry tomatoes, plum tomatoes, red onions and fresh basil in serving bowl or on platter.

3. Whisk together olive oil, balsamic vinegar, garlic and pepper; pour over tomatoes just before serving.

Make Ahead

Prepare dressing early in the day only if using dried basil. Salad portion can be prepared early in the day.

Choices Per Serving

1 Carbohydrate

1½ Fats

Nutritional Analysis Per Serving

Calories	134	Fat, total	8 g
Carbohydrate	17 g	Fat, saturated	1 g
Fiber	3 g	Sodium	116 mg
Protein	3 g	Cholesterol	0 mg

Tips

A combination of red and white cabbage is attractive.

For curry lovers, 1 tsp (5 mL) curry powder can be added to the dressing.

Make Ahead

Prepare and refrigerate early in day and stir well before serving.

Creamy Coleslaw with Apples and Raisins

1	medium carrot, diced	1
1/3 cup	finely chopped red onion	75 mL
1/2 cup	finely chopped sweet red or green pepper	125 mL
2	green onions, diced	2
3 cups	thinly sliced white or red cabbage	750 mL
1/3 cup	diced (unpeeled) apple	75 mL
1/3 cup	raisins	75 mL

DRESSING

1/4 cup	light mayonnaise	50 mL
2 tbsp	2% yogurt	25 mL
2 tbsp	lemon juice	25 mL
1 1/2 tsp	honey	7 mL
	Salt and pepper	

1. In serving bowl, combine carrot, red onion, red pepper, green onions, cabbage, apple and raisins.

2. *Dressing:* In small bowl, stir together mayonnaise, yogurt, lemon juice, honey, and salt and pepper to taste, mixing well. Pour over salad and toss gently to combine.

Choices Per Serving

1 1/2   Carbohydrates

1   Fat

Nutritional Analysis Per Serving			
Calories	147	Fat, total	5 g
Carbohydrate	26 g	Fat, saturated	1 g
Fiber	3 g	Sodium	179 mg
Protein	2 g	Cholesterol	3 mg

Tips

Here's a great twist on traditional coleslaw, with the sweet flavors of apricots, fennel and balsamic vinegar.

Toast nuts in a nonstick skillet over high heat until browned, about 2 to 3 minutes.

Make Ahead

Prepare up to 1 day in advance. Best if tossed just before serving.

Red-and-Green Coleslaw with Apricots and Fennel

SALAD

3 cups	thinly sliced green cabbage	750 mL
3 cups	thinly sliced red cabbage	750 mL
1½ cups	thinly sliced red bell peppers	375 mL
1 cup	chopped dried apricots	250 mL
1 cup	canned corn kernels, drained	250 mL
1 cup	thinly sliced fennel	250 mL
½ cup	chopped green onions	125 mL
¼ cup	toasted slivered almonds	50 mL
2 tbsp	toasted sesame seeds	25 mL

DRESSING

¼ cup	balsamic vinegar	50 mL
3 tbsp	olive oil	45 mL
1½ tsp	minced garlic	7 mL

1. *Salad:* In a large bowl, combine green cabbage, red cabbage, red peppers, apricots, corn, fennel, green onions, almonds and sesame seeds.

2. *Dressing:* In a small bowl, whisk together vinegar, oil and garlic.

3. Pour dressing over salad; toss to coat.

Choices Per Serving

1½	Carbohydrates
1	Meat & Alternative
1½	Fats

Nutritional Analysis Per Serving			
Calories	224	Fat, total	12 g
Carbohydrate	30 g	Fat, saturated	2 g
Fiber	5 g	Sodium	107 mg
Protein	5 g	Cholesterol	0 mg

Split peas and rice are a dynamic combination.

A nutrient-filled main dish salad, this is an excellent source of magnesium, phosphorus, zinc, vitamins A and C, thiamin and folate and a good source of iron, riboflavin, niacin and pantothenic acid.

Make Ahead

Prepare early in the day.

Split-Pea and Rice Greek Salad

4½ cups	basic vegetable stock (see recipe, page 55)	1.125 L
1 cup	dried green split peas	250 mL
1 cup	white or brown rice	250 mL
1½ cups	chopped tomatoes	375 mL
1 cup	chopped unpeeled cucumbers	250 mL
1 cup	chopped red bell peppers	250 mL
¾ cup	chopped red onions	175 mL
⅓ cup	sliced black olives	75 mL
3 oz	feta cheese, crumbled	75 g

DRESSING

2 tbsp	freshly squeezed lemon juice	25 mL
1½ tbsp	olive oil	20 mL
1 tbsp	balsamic vinegar	15 mL
1½ tsp	minced garlic	7 mL
1½ tsp	dried oregano	7 mL
½ tsp	coarsely ground black pepper	2 mL

1. In a saucepan bring 3 cups (750 mL) of the stock to a boil. Stir in split peas; reduce heat to medium and cook, covered, 25 to 35 minutes or until tender. Rinse under cold water and drain; set aside to cool.

2. Meanwhile, in a saucepan bring remaining 1½ cups (375 mL) stock to a boil. Stir in rice; reduce heat to low, cover and cook 20 minutes or until rice is tender and stock absorbed. (Brown rice will need 35 minutes and a little more stock.) Set aside to cool.

3. In a large serving bowl, combine tomatoes, cucumbers, red peppers, onions, olives, feta and cooled rice and split peas.

4. *Make the dressing:* In a small bowl, whisk together lemon juice, olive oil, balsamic vinegar, garlic, oregano and pepper. Pour over salad; toss to coat.

Choices Per Serving

3½ Carbohydrates
1   Meat & Alternative
½   Fat

Nutritional Analysis Per Serving			
Calories	351	Fat, total	9 g
Carbohydrate	57 g	Fat, saturated	3 g
Fiber	6 g	Sodium	246 mg
Protein	14 g	Cholesterol	13 mg

This recipe can be prepared using all wild rice or all white rice.

Great salad for brunch or picnic. Sits well for hours.

Make Ahead

Prepare up to a day ahead. Keep refrigerated and stir well before serving.

Polynesian Wild Rice Salad

2 cups	chicken stock	500 mL
½ cup	white rice	125 mL
½ cup	wild rice	125 mL
1 cup	halved snow peas	250 mL
1 cup	chopped red peppers	250 mL
¾ cup	chopped celery	175 mL
⅔ cup	sliced water chestnuts	150 mL
½ cup	canned mandarin oranges, drained	125 mL
2	medium green onions, chopped	2

DRESSING

2 tsp	orange juice concentrate, thawed	10 mL
2 tsp	honey	10 mL
1 tsp	soya sauce	5 mL
1 tsp	vegetable oil	5 mL
½ tsp	sesame oil	2 mL
½ tsp	lemon juice	2 mL
½ tsp	minced garlic	2 mL
¼ tsp	minced gingerroot	1 mL

1. Bring stock to boil in medium saucepan; add wild rice and white rice. Cover, reduce heat to medium low and simmer for 15 to 20 minutes, or until rice is tender and liquid is absorbed. Rinse with cold water. Put rice in serving bowl.

2. In a saucepan of boiling water or microwave, blanch snow peas for 1 or 2 minutes or until tender-crisp; refresh in cold water and drain. Add to serving bowl along with red peppers, celery, water chestnuts, mandarin oranges and green onions; toss well.

3. In small bowl, whisk together orange juice concentrate, honey, soya sauce, vegetable oil, sesame oil, lemon juice, garlic and ginger; pour over salad and toss well.

Choices Per Serving

2 Carbohydrates
½ Fat

Nutritional Analysis Per Serving			
Calories	157	Fat, total	2 g
Carbohydrate	32 g	Fat, saturated	0 g
Fiber	3 g	Sodium	552 mg
Protein	5 g	Cholesterol	0 mg

Southwest Barley Salad

3 cups	vegetable or chicken stock	750 mL
¾ cup	pearl barley	175 mL
1 cup	canned corn kernels, drained	250 mL
1 cup	canned black beans, rinsed and drained	250 mL
¾ cup	chopped red bell peppers	175 mL
½ cup	chopped green bell peppers	125 mL
½ cup	chopped green onions	125 mL

DRESSING

½ cup	medium salsa	125 mL
3 tbsp	low-fat sour cream	45 mL
2 tbsp	fresh lime or lemon juice	25 mL
½ cup	chopped fresh coriander	125 mL
1 tsp	minced garlic	5 mL

1. In a saucepan over high heat, bring stock to a boil. Add barley; reduce heat to medium-low. Simmer, covered, for 40 minutes or until barley is tender and liquid is absorbed. Transfer to a serving bowl; cool to room temperature. Add corn, black beans, red peppers, green peppers and green onions.

2. In a bowl combine salsa, sour cream, lime juice, coriander and garlic. Pour dressing over salad; toss to coat well.

Choices Per Serving

2 Carbohydrates
½ Meat & Alternative

Nutritional Analysis Per Serving

Calories	190	Fat, total	2 g
Carbohydrate	37 g	Fat, saturated	1 g
Fiber	6 g	Sodium	998 mg
Protein	8 g	Cholesterol	3 mg

Couscous Salad with Basil and Pine Nuts

Tips

Tender basil leaves bruise easily when chopped. Stack the leaves one on top of the other, roll up into a cigar shape and using a sharp knife, cut into fine thin shreds. To keep basil fresh like other fresh herbs (including parsley), wrap it in several layers of paper towel and place in a plastic bag; store in the warmest part of your fridge — in the butter keeper, for example, or the side door.

If you can't find fresh basil, substitute ¼ cup (50 mL) chopped fresh parsley and 1 tsp (5 mL) dried basil.

Pine nuts are the buttery edible seeds of the pine tree. To toast, place in a dry skillet over medium heat, stirring constantly, until lightly toasted. Watch carefully — pine nuts are high in oil and burn easily.

1 cup	low-sodium chicken stock or vegetable stock (see recipe, page 53)	250 mL
1 cup	couscous	250 mL
4	green onions, chopped	4
1	sweet red pepper, diced	1
1	medium zucchini, diced	1
¼ cup	raisins	50 mL
¼ cup	olive oil	50 mL
2 tbsp	red wine vinegar	25 mL
2 tbsp	orange juice	25 mL
1 tsp	grated orange rind	5 mL
1	large garlic clove, minced	1
½ tsp	salt, optional	2 mL
	Pepper to taste	
¼ cup	chopped fresh basil	50 mL
¼ cup	toasted pine nuts	50 mL

1. Place couscous in a large bowl; pour stock over. Cover with a dinner plate and let stand for 5 minutes. Fluff with a fork to break up any lumps. Let cool to room temperature. Add onions, pepper, zucchini and raisins.

2. In a small bowl, whisk together oil, vinegar, orange juice and rind, garlic, optional salt and pepper. Pour over salad; toss well. Just before serving, stir in basil and pine nuts. Serve salad at room temperature.

Choices Per Serving

3 Carbohydrates
1 Meat & Alternative
3 Fats

Nutritional Analysis Per Serving

Calories	406	Fat, total	19 g
Carbohydrate	51 g	Fat, saturated	3 g
Fiber	5 g	Sodium	132 mg
Protein	11 g	Cholesterol	0 mg

Old-Fashioned Beef Stew *page 80*
Overleaf: Make-Ahead Southwestern Pork Stew *page 82*

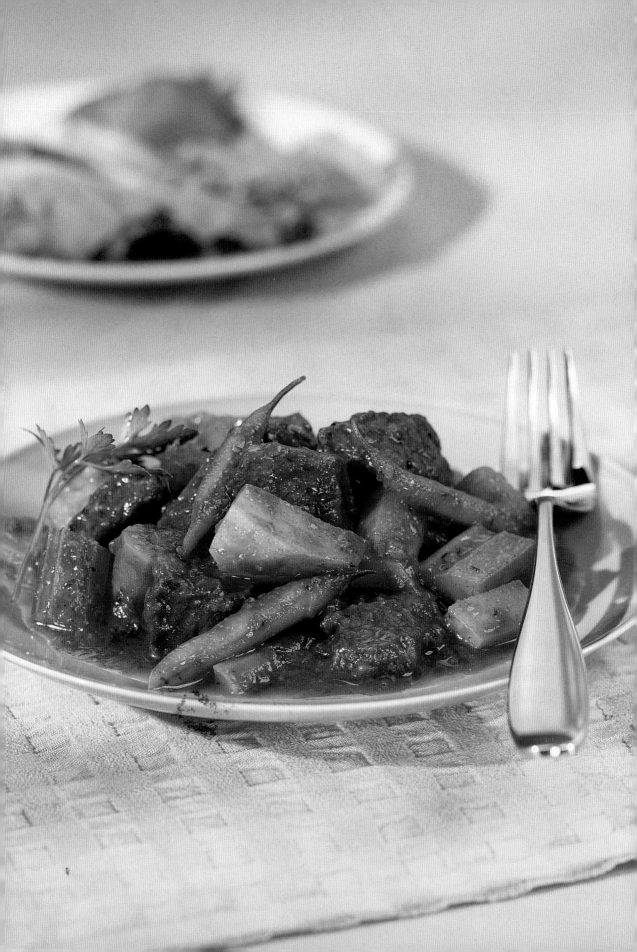

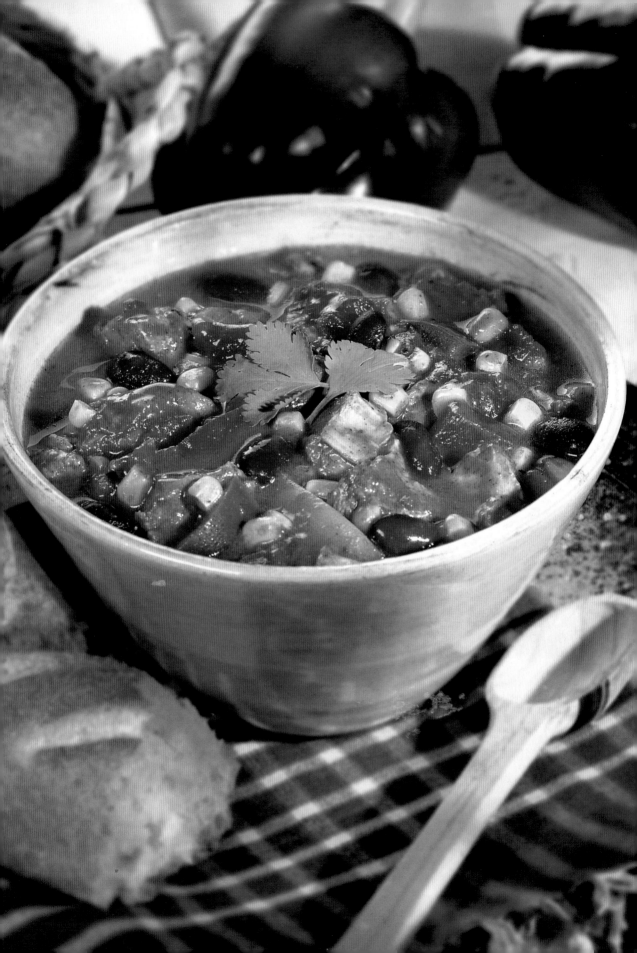

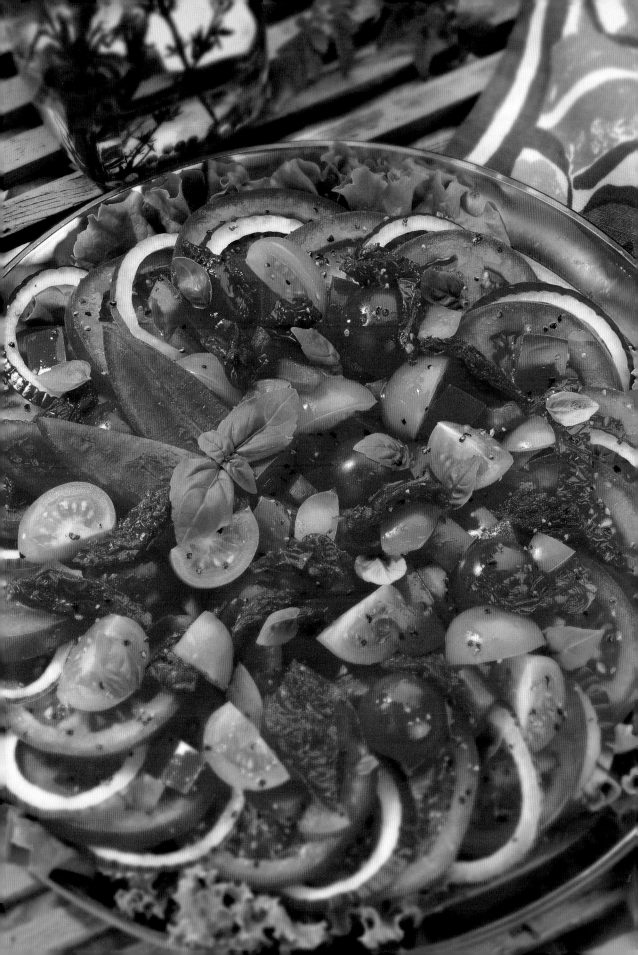

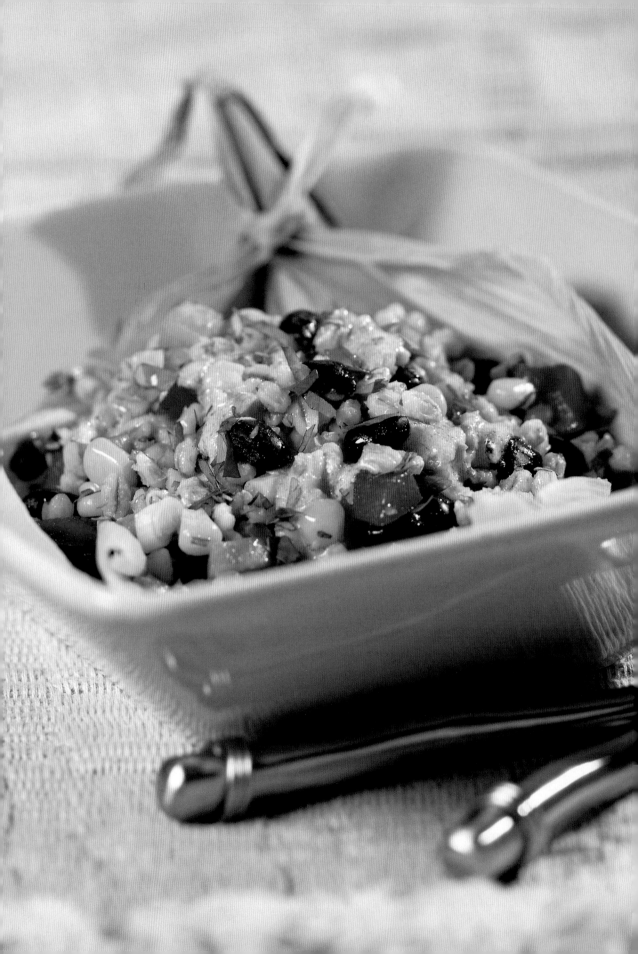

Tips

Bulgur wheat can often be found in grocery stores next to the rice and other grains. If not, health food stores always carry it.

A granular sugar substitute can replace the honey in this recipe and reduce the carbohydrate by about 5 g/serving.

Make Ahead

Prepare early in the day. Dressing can be poured over early, allowing salad to marinate.

Asian Tabbouleh Salad with Soya Orange Dressing

SALAD

2 cups	basic vegetable stock (see recipe, page 55) or water	500 mL
1½ cups	bulgur wheat	375 mL
1 cup	finely chopped red bell peppers	250 mL
1 cup	finely chopped water chestnuts	250 mL
½ cup	finely chopped green onions	125 mL
⅓ cup	chopped fresh coriander	75 mL
1 cup	broccoli florets	250 mL
1 cup	chopped snow peas	250 mL

DRESSING

4 tsp	orange juice concentrate	20 mL
4 tsp	honey	20 mL
2½ tsp	sesame oil	12 mL
2½ tsp	soya sauce	12 mL
1 tsp	minced garlic	5 mL
1 tsp	freshly squeezed lemon juice	5 mL
¾ tsp	minced gingerroot	4 mL

1. In a saucepan bring stock or water to a boil. Stir in bulgur, cover and turn heat off. Let stand 15 minutes; drain, rinse with cold water and place in a serving bowl. Stir in red peppers, water chestnuts, green onions and coriander.

2. Boil or steam broccoli florets and snow peas 2 minutes or until tender-crisp. Rinse under cold water, drain and add to bulgur mixture.

3. *Make the dressing:* In a small bowl, whisk together orange juice concentrate, honey, sesame oil, soya sauce, garlic, lemon juice and ginger. Pour over bulgur mixture and toss to coat. Serve chilled or at room temperature.

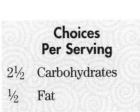

Choices Per Serving

2½ Carbohydrates

½ Fat

Nutritional Analysis Per Serving			
Calories	217	Fat, total	3 g
Carbohydrate	45 g	Fat, saturated	0 g
Fiber	6 g	Sodium	177 mg
Protein	7 g	Cholesterol	0 mg

Southwest Barley Salad *page 95*
Overleaf: Four-Tomato Salad *page 90*

Wheat berries are unprocessed whole kernels of wheat. They're tender, chewy and crunchy — great for salads and pilafs! Wheat berries are also extremely nutritious, and make a great high-fiber substitute in traditional meat loaf recipes.

This recipe is an excellent source of vitamins A and C.

Wheat Berry Salad with Sesame Dressing

DRESSING

1 tbsp	honey	15 mL
1 tbsp	rice wine vinegar	15 mL
1 tbsp	sesame oil	15 mL
1 tbsp	toasted sesame seeds	15 mL
1 tbsp	light soya sauce	15 mL
1 tbsp	tahini (sesame paste)	15 mL
1 tsp	minced garlic	5 mL
½ tsp	minced gingerroot	2 mL

SALAD

3½ cups	seafood stock or chicken stock	875 mL
1 cup	wheat berries	250 mL
½ cup	thinly sliced green onions	125 mL
½ cup	diced carrots	125 mL
½ cup	diced green bell peppers	125 mL
½ cup	diced red bell peppers	125 mL
½ cup	diced snow peas	125 mL
8 oz	scallops	250 g

1. *Dressing:* In a bowl combine honey, rice wine vinegar, sesame oil, sesame seeds, soya sauce, tahini, garlic and ginger; whisk well. Set aside.

2. *Salad:* In a saucepan over high heat, bring stock to a boil. Add wheat berries; reduce heat to low. Cook, covered, for approximately 45 minutes or until berries are tender but chewy. Drain any excess liquid; allow to cool. Add green onions, carrots, green peppers, red peppers and snow peas. Set aside.

3. In a nonstick frying pan sprayed with vegetable spray or on a preheated grill, cook scallops over medium-high heat for 3 minutes or until cooked through. Drain any excess liquid; dice scallops.

4. In a serving bowl, combine wheat berry mixture, scallops and dressing; toss to coat well. Serve.

Choices Per Serving

2 Carbohydrates

1½ Meat & Alternatives

Nutritional Analysis Per Serving			
Calories	255	Fat, total	6 g
Carbohydrate	31 g	Fat, saturated	1 g
Fiber	2 g	Sodium	366 mg
Protein	14 g	Cholesterol	19 mg

Tip

The beans in this salad, like most beans and legumes, are an excellent source of folic acid.

Variation

French Salad Dressing: In a bowl, stir together 2 tbsp (25 mL) red wine vinegar and 1½ tsp (7 mL) Dijon mustard. Add ⅓ cup (75 mL) olive oil (or use part vegetable oil), 1 minced clove garlic and 1 tsp (5 mL) dried fine herbs. Season with a pinch of granulated sugar, salt and pepper to taste. Store in covered jar in the refrigerator. Makes ½ cup (125 mL).

Bean Salad with Mustard-Dill Dressing

1 lb	green beans	500 g
1	can (19 oz/540 mL) chickpeas, rinsed and drained	1
⅓ cup	chopped red onions	75 mL
2 tbsp	finely chopped fresh dill	25 mL
2 tbsp	olive oil	25 mL
2 tbsp	red wine vinegar	25 mL
1 tbsp	Dijon mustard	15 mL
1 tbsp	granulated sugar	15 mL
¼ tsp	salt	1 mL
¼ tsp	pepper	1 mL

1. Trim ends of beans; cut into 1-inch (2.5 cm) lengths. In a large pot of boiling salted water, cook beans for 3 to 5 minutes (count from time water returns to boil) or until tender-crisp. Drain; rinse under cold water to chill. Drain well.

2. In a serving bowl, combine green beans, chickpeas, onions and dill.

3. In a small bowl, whisk together oil, vinegar, mustard, sugar, salt and pepper until smooth.

4. Pour over beans and toss well. Refrigerate until serving.

Choices Per Serving	
2	Carbohydrates
1	Meat & Alternative
½	Fat

Nutritional Analysis Per Serving			
Calories	219	Fat, total	7 g
Carbohydrate	32 g	Fat, saturated	1 g
Fiber	5 g	Sodium	324 mg
Protein	9 g	Cholesterol	0 mg

• • • • • • • • • • • • • • •

Tips

This recipe is high in fiber and is also an excellent source of vitamin A and folic acid.

Together with a fruit and a Milk & Alternatives choice, such as a low-fat no-sugar-added yogurt, this salad is a complete meal.

Pasta and Bean Salad with Creamy Basil Dressing

DRESSING

1½ cups	tightly packed fresh basil leaves	375 mL
3 tbsp	grated low-fat Parmesan cheese	45 mL
2 tbsp	toasted pine nuts	25 mL
1½ tsp	minced garlic	7 mL
⅓ cup	low-fat yogurt	75 mL
3 tbsp	fresh lemon juice	45 mL
3 tbsp	light mayonnaise	45 mL
3 tbsp	water	45 mL
1 tbsp	olive oil	15 mL
¼ tsp	freshly ground black pepper	1 mL

SALAD

12 oz	medium shell pasta	375 g
¾ cup	canned black beans, rinsed and drained	175 mL
¾ cup	canned chickpeas, rinsed and drained	175 mL
¾ cup	canned red kidney beans, rinsed and drained	175 mL
¾ cup	diced red onions	175 mL
½ cup	shredded carrots	125 mL
2 cups	diced ripe plum tomatoes	500 mL

1. *Dressing:* In a food processor or blender, combine basil, Parmesan cheese, pine nuts and garlic; process until finely chopped. Add yogurt, lemon juice, mayonnaise, water, olive oil and pepper; purée until smooth. Set aside.

2. *Salad:* In a large pot of boiling water, cook pasta for 8 to 10 minutes or until tender but firm; drain. Rinse under cold running water; drain.

3. In a serving bowl, combine pasta, black beans, chickpeas, kidney beans, red onions, carrots and plum tomatoes. Pour dressing over salad; toss to coat well. Serve immediately.

Choices Per Serving

3	Carbohydrates
½	Meat & Alternative
1	Fat

Nutritional Analysis Per Serving

Calories	289	Fat, total	7 g
Carbohydrate	49 g	Fat, saturated	1 g
Fiber	4 g	Sodium	34 mg
Protein	10 g	Cholesterol	0 mg

Tips

A delicious sweet pasta salad that goes well with a grilled fish or chicken entrée.

Prunes can replace apricots or dates or use in combination.

Make Ahead

Prepare salad and dressing early in day. Toss just before serving.

Pasta Salad with Apricots, Dates and Orange Dressing

12 oz	medium shell pasta	375 g
1½ cups	diced sweet red or green peppers	375 mL
¾ cup	diced dried apricots	175 mL
¾ cup	diced dried dates	175 mL
½ cup	chopped green onions	125 mL

DRESSING

3 tbsp	balsamic vinegar	45 mL
3 tbsp	frozen orange juice concentrate, thawed	45 mL
3 tbsp	olive oil	45 mL
2 tbsp	lemon juice	25 mL
2 tbsp	water	25 mL
1½ tsp	crushed garlic	7 mL
½ cup	chopped parsley	125 mL

1. Cook pasta in boiling water according to package instructions or until firm to the bite. Rinse with cold water. Drain and place in serving bowl.

2. Add sweet peppers, apricots, dates and green onions.

3. *Make the dressing:* In small bowl combine vinegar, orange juice concentrate, oil, lemon juice, water, garlic and parsley. Pour over salad, and toss.

Nutritional Analysis Per Serving			
Calories	302	Fat, total	6 g
Carbohydrate	57 g	Fat, saturated	1 g
Fiber	4 g	Sodium	8 mg
Protein	7 g	Cholesterol	0 mg

Tips

This recipe needs little oil because the tomatoes give it the necessary liquid. Use ripe juicy tomatoes.

Sweet Vidalia onions are great to use in season.

If your meal plan calls for extra protein add extra Brie.

Make Ahead

Prepare tomato dressing early in day and let marinate. Do not toss until ready to serve.

Penne with Brie Cheese, Tomatoes and Basil

12 oz	penne	375 g
1½ lb	chopped tomatoes	750 g
2 tsp	crushed garlic	10 mL
1 cup	chopped red onions	250 mL
3 oz	diced Brie cheese	75 g
⅓ cup	sliced black olives	75 mL
⅔ cup	chopped fresh basil (or 2 tsp/10 mL dried)	150 mL
3 tbsp	olive oil	45 mL
2 tbsp	lemon juice	25 mL
1 tbsp	red wine vinegar	15 mL
	Pepper	

1. Cook pasta in boiling water according to package instructions or until firm to the bite. Rinse with cold water. Drain and place in serving bowl.

2. Add tomatoes, garlic, onions, cheese, olives, basil, oil, lemon juice, vinegar and pepper. Mix well.

Choices Per Serving

2½ Carbohydrates

½ Meat & Alternative

1½ Fats

Nutritional Analysis Per Serving			
Calories	274	Fat, total	9 g
Carbohydrate	40 g	Fat, saturated	3 g
Fiber	3 g	Sodium	94 mg
Protein	9 g	Cholesterol	11 mg

● ● ● ● ● ● ● ● ● ● ● ● ● ● ● ●

Tip

Use a ripe sweet mango
for a more intense flavor.
If unripe, mangoes are
unpleasantly sour.

● ● ● ● ● ● ● ● ● ● ● ● ● ● ● ●

Make Ahead

Prepare salsa early in day
and refrigerate. (This will
also allow it to develop
more flavor.) Pour over
pasta just before serving.

Mango Salsa over Vermicelli

8 oz	vermicelli or other fine-strand pasta	250 g
1¾ cups	diced mangoes	425 mL
¾ cup	diced sweet red peppers	175 mL
½ cup	diced red onions	125 mL
½ cup	diced sweet green peppers	125 mL
3 tbsp	olive oil	45 mL
3 tbsp	lemon juice	45 mL
2 tsp	crushed garlic	10 mL
½ cup	chopped coriander or parsley	125 mL

1. Cook pasta in boiling water according to package instructions or until firm to the bite. Rinse with cold water. Drain and set aside.

2. In bowl of food processor, combine mangoes, red peppers, onions, green peppers, oil, lemon juice, garlic and coriander. Process on and off just until finely diced. Pour over pasta; serve at room temperature.

**Choices
Per Serving**

2½ Carbohydrates

1½ Fats

Nutritional Analysis Per Serving

Calories	255	Fat, total	8 g
Carbohydrate	42 g	Fat, saturated	1 g
Fiber	3 g	Sodium	8 mg
Protein	6 g	Cholesterol	0 mg

Warm Caesar Pasta Salad

SERVES 6

Tips

Sauce is wonderful served over cooked vegetables, fish, chicken or meat.

If prosciutto is not available, use sliced ham or smoked salmon.

Make Ahead

Prepare sauce up to a day ahead. Refrigerate. Toss just before serving.

SAUCE

1	egg	1
3	anchovies, chopped	3
3 tbsp	olive oil	45 mL
2 tbsp	grated Parmesan cheese	25 mL
1 tbsp	lemon juice	15 mL
1 tbsp	red wine vinegar	15 mL
2 tsp	Dijon mustard	10 mL
1½ tsp	minced garlic	7 mL
2 cups	washed, dried and torn romaine lettuce	500 mL
2 oz	prosciutto, shredded	50 g
12 oz	penne	375 g

1. Put egg, anchovies, olive oil, Parmesan, lemon juice, vinegar, mustard and garlic in food processor; process until smooth.

2. Put lettuce and prosciutto in large serving bowl. In large pot of boiling water, cook pasta according to package directions or until tender but firm; drain and add to serving bowl. Pour dressing over pasta and toss.

Choices Per Serving

3	Carbohydrates
1	Meat & Alternative
1	Fat

Nutritional Analysis Per Serving

Calories	344	Fat, total	11 g
Carbohydrate	48 g	Fat, saturated	2 g
Fiber	2 g	Sodium	228 mg
Protein	14 g	Cholesterol	50 mg

Tips

If basil is unavailable, try spinach or parsley leaves.

Roasted corn kernels (1 cob) make a delicious replacement for canned kernels. Broil or barbecue corn for 15 minutes or until charred.

Make Ahead

Prepare potatoes, pesto and vegetables up to a day ahead. Toss before serving. Tastes great the next day.

Pesto Potato Salad

2 lb	scrubbed whole red potatoes with skins on	1 kg

PESTO

1¼ cups	packed fresh basil leaves	300 mL
3 tbsp	olive oil	45 mL
2 tbsp	toasted pine nuts	25 mL
2 tbsp	grated Parmesan cheese	25 mL
1 tsp	minced garlic	5 mL
¼ tsp	salt	1 mL

¼ cup	chicken stock or water	50 mL
1 cup	halved snow peas	250 mL
¾ cup	chopped red onions	175 mL
¾ cup	chopped red peppers	175 mL
¾ cup	chopped green peppers	175 mL
½ cup	corn kernels	125 mL
2	medium green onions, chopped	2
2 tbsp	toasted pine nuts	25 mL
2 tbsp	lemon juice	25 mL

1. Put potatoes in saucepan with cold water to cover; bring to a boil and cook for 20 to 25 minutes, or until easily pierced with a sharp knife. Drain and set aside.

2. Meanwhile, put basil, olive oil, 2 tbsp (25 mL) pine nuts, Parmesan, garlic and salt in food processor; process until finely chopped. With the processor running, gradually add stock through the feed tube; process until smooth.

3. In saucepan of boiling water or microwave, blanch snow peas for 1 or 2 minutes, or until tender-crisp; refresh in cold water and drain. Place in large serving bowl, along with pesto, red onions, red and green peppers, corn, green onions, 2 tbsp (25 mL) pine nuts and lemon juice. When potatoes are cool enough to handle, cut into wedges and add to serving bowl; toss well to combine.

Choices Per Serving

1½ Carbohydrates

1 Fat

Nutritional Analysis Per Serving			
Calories	161	Fat, total	5 g
Carbohydrate	27 g	Fat, saturated	1 g
Fiber	3 g	Sodium	128 mg
Protein	4 g	Cholesterol	1 mg

Tips

If tarragon is unavailable, substitute ¼ cup (50 mL) chopped fresh dill.

Fresh tuna or swordfish are delicious substitutes for chicken.

Toast pecans in small skillet on medium heat until browned, 2 to 3 minutes.

Make Ahead

Prepare and refrigerate salad and dressing separately early in day, but do not mix until ready to serve.

Chicken Salad with Tarragon and Pecans

10 oz	boneless skinless chicken breast, cubed	300 g
¾ cup	chopped sweet red or green pepper	175 mL
¾ cup	chopped carrot	175 mL
¾ cup	chopped broccoli florets	175 mL
¾ cup	chopped snow peas	175 mL
¾ cup	chopped red onion	175 mL
1 tbsp	chopped pecans, toasted	15 mL

DRESSING

½ cup	2% yogurt	125 mL
2 tbsp	lemon juice	25 mL
2 tbsp	light mayonnaise	25 mL
1 tsp	crushed garlic	5 mL
1 tsp	Dijon mustard	5 mL
¼ cup	chopped fresh parsley	50 mL
2 tsp	dried tarragon (or 3 tbsp/45 mL chopped fresh)	10 mL
	Salt and pepper	

1. In small saucepan, bring 2 cups (500 mL) water to boil; reduce heat to simmer. Add chicken; cover and cook just until no longer pink inside, 2 to 4 minutes. Drain and place in serving bowl.

2. Add red pepper, carrot, broccoli, snow peas and onion; toss well.

3. *Dressing:* In small bowl, combine yogurt, lemon juice, mayonnaise, garlic, mustard, parsley, tarragon, and salt and pepper to taste; pour over chicken and mix well. Taste and adjust seasoning. Sprinkle with pecans.

Choices Per Serving

1   Carbohydrate
2   Meat & Alternatives

Nutritional Analysis Per Serving			
Calories	179	Fat, total	6 g
Carbohydrate	17 g	Fat, saturated	1 g
Fiber	4 g	Sodium	164 mg
Protein	17 g	Cholesterol	35 mg

Tips

Serve this salad with whole grain bread and complete the meal with ½ cup (125 mL) of no-sugar-added fruit yogurt served over sliced pears or orange sections.

Substitute broccoli or fresh green beans for the asparagus.

Chicken and Asparagus Salad with Lemon Dill Vinaigrette

12	baby red potatoes (or 4 small white)	12
8 oz	boneless skinless chicken breasts, cubed	250 g
¼ cup	water	50 mL
¼ cup	white wine	50 mL
8 oz	asparagus, trimmed and cut into small pieces	250 g
2	small heads Boston lettuce, torn into pieces	2

LEMON DILL VINAIGRETTE

3 tbsp	balsamic vinegar	45 mL
2 tbsp	lemon juice	25 mL
1 tbsp	water	15 mL
1	large green onion, minced	1
¾ tsp	garlic	4 mL
2 tbsp	chopped fresh dill (or 1 tsp/5 mL dried dillweed)	25 mL
3 tbsp	olive oil	45 mL

1. In saucepan of boiling water, cook potatoes until just tender. Peel and cut into cubes. Place in salad bowl and set aside.

2. In saucepan, bring chicken, water and wine to boil; reduce heat, cover and simmer for approximately 2 minutes or until chicken is no longer pink. Drain and add to potatoes in bowl.

3. Steam or microwave asparagus until just tender-crisp; drain and add to bowl. Add lettuce.

4. *Lemon Dill Vinaigrette:* In bowl, whisk together vinegar, lemon juice, water, onion, garlic and dill; whisk in oil until combined. Pour over chicken mixture; toss to coat well.

Choices Per Serving

1	Carbohydrate
1	Meat & Alternative
½	Fat

Nutritional Analysis Per Serving			
Calories	186	Fat, total	8 g
Carbohydrate	19 g	Fat, saturated	1 g
Fiber	2 g	Sodium	24 mg
Protein	10 g	Cholesterol	18 mg

Seafood Salad with Dill Dressing

4 oz	deveined peeled (uncooked) shrimp, chopped	125 g
4 oz	scallops, chopped	125 g
4 oz	squid, chopped	125 g
½ cup	chopped sweet red or yellow pepper	125 mL
½ cup	chopped sweet green pepper	125 mL
½ cup	chopped celery	125 mL
½ cup	chopped red onion	125 mL
1	large green onion, sliced	1
	Lettuce leaves	
	Parsley sprigs	

DRESSING

½ cup	2% yogurt	125 mL
2 tbsp	light mayonnaise	25 mL
3 tbsp	chopped fresh parsley	45 mL
¼ cup	chopped fresh dill (or 4 tsp/20 mL dried dillweed)	50 mL
1 tsp	Dijon mustard	5 mL
1 tsp	crushed garlic	5 mL
	Salt and pepper	

1. In shallow saucepan, bring 2 cups (500 mL) water to boil; reduce heat to simmer. Add shrimp, scallops and squid; cover and poach until shrimp are pink and squid and scallops opaque, approximately 2 minutes. Drain and rinse with cold water; drain well and place in bowl. Add red and green peppers, celery and red and green onions.

2. *Dressing:* In small bowl, combine yogurt, mayonnaise, parsley, dill, mustard, garlic, and salt and pepper to taste, mixing well. Pour over salad and toss well.

3. Line serving bowl with lettuce; top with salad and garnish with parsley.

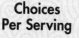

Nutritional Analysis Per Serving			
Calories	169	Fat, total	5 g
Carbohydrate	12 g	Fat, saturated	1 g
Fiber	2 g	Sodium	289 mg
Protein	19 g	Cholesterol	135 mg

Tips

Orzo is a rice-shaped pasta. If unavailable, substitute a small shell pasta.

Substitute squid or any firm white fish for part or all of the shrimp or scallops.

Definitely use fresh lemon juice — bottled will give too tart a taste. If a less intense lemon flavor is desired, use 3 tbsp (45 mL) instead of ¼ cup (50 mL).

Make Ahead

Prepare early in the day and keep refrigerated. This tastes fine the next day.

Greek Orzo Seafood Salad

1¾ cups	orzo	425 mL
8 oz	shrimp or scallops or a combination, chopped	250 g
1 cup	halved snow peas	250 mL
12 oz	tomatoes, chopped	375 g
3 oz	feta cheese, crumbled	75 g

DRESSING

¼ cup	olive oil	50 mL
¼ cup	freshly squeezed lemon juice	50 mL
1 tbsp	dried oregano (or ⅓ cup/75 mL chopped fresh)	15 mL
2 tsp	minced garlic	10 mL
2 tsp	grated lemon zest	10 mL
¼ tsp	ground black pepper	1 mL

1. In large pot of boiling water cook the orzo for 8 to 10 minutes or until tender but firm; rinse under cold water and drain. Put in large serving bowl.

2. In nonstick skillet sprayed with vegetable spray, cook shrimp or scallops over high heat for 2 minutes or until just done at center. Drain any excess liquid. Add to orzo in serving bowl.

3. In a saucepan of boiling water, blanch snow peas for 1 minute, or until tender-crisp; refresh in cold water and drain. Place in serving bowl, along with tomatoes and feta cheese.

4. In small bowl whisk together olive oil, lemon juice, oregano, garlic, lemon zest and pepper; pour over salad and toss well. Chill before serving.

Choices Per Serving

1½ Carbohydrates

1 Meat & Alternative

1 Fat

Nutritional Analysis Per Serving			
Calories	226	Fat, total	10 g
Carbohydrate	23 g	Fat, saturated	3 g
Fiber	2 g	Sodium	163 mg
Protein	11 g	Cholesterol	53 mg

Tip

To make your own croutons, mix 1 tsp (5 mL) each crushed garlic and melted margarine; brush on both sides of 1 slice whole wheat bread. Broil for 3 minutes until browned, then cut into cubes.

Make Ahead

Dressing can be prepared and refrigerated early in the day; toss with salad just before serving.

Caesar Salad with Baby Shrimp

2 oz	cooked baby shrimp	50 g
1	medium head romaine lettuce, torn into bite-sized pieces	1
1 tbsp	grated Parmesan cheese	15 mL
1 cup	croutons, preferably homemade	250 mL

DRESSING

1	egg	1
1 tsp	crushed garlic	5 mL
1	anchovy, minced	1
4 tsp	lemon juice	20 mL
1 tbsp	red wine vinegar	15 mL
1 tsp	Dijon mustard	5 mL
1 tbsp	grated Parmesan cheese	15 mL
2 tbsp	olive oil	25 mL

1. In large bowl, place shrimp, lettuce, cheese and croutons.

2. *Dressing:* In small bowl, combine egg, garlic, anchovy, lemon juice, vinegar, mustard and cheese; gradually whisk in oil until combined. Pour over salad and toss to coat.

Choices Per Serving

1   Meat & Alternative
½   Fat

Nutritional Analysis Per Serving

Calories	99	Fat, total	7 g
Carbohydrate	5 g	Fat, saturated	1 g
Fiber	1 g	Sodium	117 mg
Protein	5 g	Cholesterol	56 mg

Dressings, Marinades and Sauces

Many commercial sauces, marinades and dressings can wreak havoc on your attempts to control your fat and carbohydrate intake. When shopping for these, read the labels carefully, keeping in mind that 5 g of fat is the equivalent of 1 teaspoon (5 mL) oil and 4 g of carbohydrate is the same as 1 teaspoon (5 mL) sugar.

In most of these commercial products, if one nutrient is reduced the other is increased. Try some of these homemade favorites. In those where there is "added sugar," using a granulated sugar substitute of your choice can reduce the carbohydrate content and usually eliminate the Other Choices.

● ● ● ● ● ● ● ● ● ● ● ● ● ● ●

Tip

Serve over a variety
of mild-tasting lettuce
leaves (Boston,
red, leafy).

● ● ● ● ● ● ● ● ● ● ● ● ● ● ●

Make Ahead

Refrigerate for up to
3 weeks.

Herb Vinaigrette

1 tbsp	red wine vinegar	15 mL
4 tsp	water	20 mL
4 tsp	lemon juice	20 mL
½ tsp	Dijon mustard	2 mL
¾ tsp	crushed garlic	4 mL
2 tbsp	chopped fresh basil (or ½ tsp/2 mL dried)	25 mL
	Salt and pepper	
2 tbsp	vegetable oil	25 mL

1. In small bowl, whisk together vinegar, water, lemon
juice, mustard, garlic, basil, and salt and pepper to taste;
whisk in oil until combined.

Choices Per Serving

1	Fat

Nutritional Analysis Per Serving

Calories	51	Fat, total	6 g
Carbohydrate	1 g	Fat, saturated	0 g
Fiber	0 g	Sodium	289 mg
Protein	0 g	Cholesterol	0 mg

● ● ● ● ● ● ● ● ● ● ● ● ● ● ● ●

Tip

Use in a seafood salad,
or serve as a tartar sauce
with grilled fish.

● ● ● ● ● ● ● ● ● ● ● ● ● ● ● ●

Make Ahead

Refrigerate for up
to 1 day.

Light Creamy Dill Dressing

½ cup	2% yogurt	125 mL
2 tbsp	light mayonnaise	25 mL
3 tbsp	chopped fresh parsley	45 mL
¼ cup	chopped fresh dill (or 1½ tsp/7 mL dried dillweed)	50 mL
1 tsp	Dijon mustard	5 mL
¾ tsp	crushed garlic	4 mL
	Salt and pepper	

1. In bowl, combine yogurt, mayonnaise, parsley, dill, mustard, garlic, and salt and pepper to taste until well mixed.

Choices
Per Serving

1	Extra

Nutritional Analysis Per Serving			
Calories	11	Fat, total	1 g
Carbohydrate	1 g	Fat, saturated	0 g
Fiber	0 g	Sodium	20 mg
Protein	1 g	Cholesterol	1 mg

Balsamic Orange Vinaigrette

Tips

Great over leafy lettuce or spinach.

For a stronger orange flavor, add 1 tsp (5 mL) grated orange zest.

Balsamic vinegar is commonly found in the specialty section of most supermarkets, and it contributes to a wonderful flavor wherever it is added.

Make Ahead

Prepare up to 2 days in advance.

¼ cup	chopped fresh parsley	50 mL
3 tbsp	vegetable oil	45 mL
3 tbsp	balsamic vinegar	45 mL
3 tbsp	minced red onions	45 mL
2 tbsp	orange juice concentrate	25 mL
1 tbsp	packed brown sugar	15 mL
1 tsp	minced garlic	5 mL

1. In a small bowl, whisk together parsley, oil, vinegar, red onions, orange juice concentrate, sugar and garlic.

Choices Per Serving

1 Fat

Nutritional Analysis Per Serving

Calories	50	Fat, total	4 g
Carbohydrate	4 g	Fat, saturated	0 g
Fiber	0 g	Sodium	2 mg
Protein	0 g	Cholesterol	0 mg

. . . .

Tips

Serve as a dipping
sauce for fruit spears
or serve over a salad of
spinach, orange slices
and red onions.

This is a great recipe
for those who like sweet
dressings rather
than tart.

. . . .

Make Ahead

Prepare up to 2 days
in advance.

Creamy Poppy Seed Dressing

¼ cup	orange juice	50 mL
3 tbsp	light mayonnaise	45 mL
3 tbsp	light sour cream	45 mL
1 tbsp	honey	15 mL
2 tsp	poppy seeds	10 mL
1 tsp	grated orange zest	5 mL

1. In a small bowl, whisk together orange juice,
mayonnaise, sour cream, honey, poppy seeds and
orange zest.

Choices Per Serving

½   Fat

Nutritional Analysis Per Serving			
Calories	28	Fat, total	2 g
Carbohydrate	3 g	Fat, saturated	0 g
Fiber	0 g	Sodium	22 mg
Protein	0 g	Cholesterol	2 mg

● ● ● ● ● ● ● ● ● ● ● ● ● ● ●

Tip

Serve over salad,
stir-fried vegetables or
rice noodles. Also great
over steamed vegetables.

● ● ● ● ● ● ● ● ● ● ● ● ● ● ●

Make Ahead

Prepare up to 3 days
in advance. Stir
before using.

Thai Lime Dressing

3 tbsp	chopped fresh coriander	45 mL
2 tbsp	vegetable oil	25 mL
2 tbsp	freshly squeezed lime juice	25 mL
2 tbsp	peanut butter	25 mL
1 tbsp	rice wine vinegar	15 mL
1 tbsp	packed brown sugar	15 mL
1 tsp	sesame oil	5 mL
½ tsp	minced garlic	2 mL
½ tsp	minced gingerroot	2 mL
1	green onion, chopped	1

1. In a food processor combine coriander, oil, lime juice,
peanut butter, vinegar, brown sugar, sesame oil, garlic,
ginger and green onion; process until smooth.

Nutritional Analysis Per Serving

Calories	68	Fat, total	6 g
Carbohydrate	3 g	Fat, saturated	1 g
Fiber	0 g	Sodium	3 mg
Protein	1 g	Cholesterol	0 mg

**Choices
Per Serving**

1   Fat

Tips

Use to marinate chicken, fish or veal. Remove meat and boil marinade for 3 to 5 minutes until thickened. Brush over meat before cooking.

A granulated sugar substitute can replace the brown sugar in this recipe to reduce the carbohydrate to less than 1 g/serving.

Make Ahead

Prepare up to 2 days in advance and refrigerate.

Ginger Lemon Marinade

3 tbsp	lemon juice	45 mL
2 tbsp	water	25 mL
1 tbsp	vegetable oil	15 mL
1½ tsp	red wine vinegar	7 mL
4 tsp	brown sugar	20 mL
2 tsp	sesame oil	10 mL
1 tsp	minced gingerroot (or ¼ tsp/1 mL ground ginger)	5 mL
½ tsp	ground coriander	2 mL
½ tsp	ground fennel seeds (optional)	2 mL

1. In small bowl, combine lemon juice, water, vegetable oil, vinegar, sugar, sesame oil, ginger, coriander, and fennel seeds (if using); mix well.

Choices Per Serving

½ Fat

Nutritional Analysis Per Serving

Calories	36	Fat, total	3 g
Carbohydrate	3 g	Fat, saturated	0 g
Fiber	0 g	Sodium	1 mg
Protein	0 g	Cholesterol	0 mg

Pesto Sauce

½ cup	well-packed chopped fresh parsley	125 mL
½ cup	well-packed chopped fresh basil	125 mL
¼ cup	water or chicken stock	50 mL
1 tbsp	toasted pine nuts	15 mL
2 tbsp	grated Parmesan cheese	25 mL
3 tbsp	olive oil	45 mL
¾ tsp	crushed garlic	4 mL

1. In food processor, combine parsley, basil, water, pine nuts, Parmesan, oil and garlic; process until smooth.

Tips

You can be creative with pesto sauces by substituting different leaves such as spinach or coriander, or using a combination of different leaves.

Serve over ¾ lb (375 g) pasta.

Serve over cooked fish or chicken.

Make Ahead

Refrigerate for up to a week or freeze for up to 6 weeks.

Nutritional Analysis Per Serving

Calories	37	Fat, total	4 g
Carbohydrate	0 g	Fat, saturated	1 g
Fiber	0 g	Sodium	21 mg
Protein	1 g	Cholesterol	1 mg

Choices Per Serving

1   Fat

Tip

For a fast dinner
suggestion, toss this
pesto with cooked
pasta. (Remember,
½ cup/125 mL cooked
pasta equals 1 Grains
& Starches choice.)
Complete the meal with
low-fat, no-sugar-added
yogurt over fruit if your
meal plan permits.

Sun-Dried Tomato Pesto

½ cup	sun-dried tomatoes	125 mL
½ cup	lightly packed fresh basil	125 mL
½ cup	lightly packed fresh parsley	125 mL
1	large clove garlic	1
⅓ cup	vegetable stock (see recipe, page 53)	75 mL
2 tbsp	olive oil	25 mL
⅓ cup	freshly grated Parmesan cheese	75 mL
½ tsp	freshly ground black pepper	2 mL

1. In a bowl, cover sun-dried tomatoes with boiling water; let stand for 10 minutes or until softened. Drain and pat dry; chop coarsely.

2. In a food processor, combine rehydrated tomatoes, basil, parsley and garlic. With motor running, add stock and oil in a stream. Stir in Parmesan cheese and pepper.

**Choices
Per Serving**

½ Carbohydrate

1 Meat & Alternative

1½ Fats

Nutritional Analysis Per Serving			
Calories	170	Fat, total	13 g
Carbohydrate	8 g	Fat, saturated	3 g
Fiber	0 g	Sodium	465 mg
Protein	7 g	Cholesterol	9 mg

Tips

Toss with pasta or
serve over cooked fish
or chicken.

If sauce is too thick, add
a little water to thin.

This sauce makes enough
for 1½ lb (750 g) pasta.

This sauce is a good
source of vitamin C.
Tomatoes are also a good
source of lycopene, the
red pigment which gives
tomato products their
color. Lycopene is a
phytochemical which
some research indicates
may be associated with
reduced risk of some
kinds of cancers.

Sun-Dried Tomato Sauce

4 oz	sun-dried tomatoes	125 g
1 tsp	crushed garlic	5 mL
¾ cup	water or chicken stock	175 mL
½ cup	chopped fresh parsley	125 mL
2 tbsp	olive oil	25 mL
2 tbsp	toasted pine nuts	25 mL
1 tbsp	grated Parmesan cheese	15 mL

1. In bowl, pour enough boiling water over tomatoes to
cover; let sit for 15 minutes or until soft enough to cut.
Cut into smaller pieces.

2. In food processor, combine tomatoes, garlic, water,
parsley, oil, pine nuts and cheese; process until
well blended.

Choices
Per Serving

½	Carbohydrate
1	Fat

Nutritional Analysis Per Serving

Calories	73	Fat, total	4 g
Carbohydrate	8 g	Fat, saturated	1 g
Fiber	0 g	Sodium	314 mg
Protein	3 g	Cholesterol	1 mg

Sweet and mild or spicy and hot, sausages add a wonderful flavor to meat dishes. Although traditionally made from beef and/or pork, they're now made with other (often leaner) meats, including chicken and turkey. So experiment — and use whatever type of sausage you prefer. Just remember that all sausages have extra fat added, so use them in moderate quantities and be sure to drain the fat after sautéeing.

Rose's Hearty Pasta Sauce with Beef and Sausage

½ cup	chopped onions	125 mL
¼ cup	finely chopped carrots	50 mL
1 tsp	minced garlic	5 mL
6 oz	lean ground beef	175 g
4 oz	Italian sausage, casings removed	125 g
1½ lbs	ripe plum tomatoes, chopped	750 g
2 tbsp	tomato paste	25 mL
1	bay leaf	1
1½ tsp	dried basil	7 mL
1 tsp	chili powder	5 mL
¼ tsp	salt	1 mL
¼ tsp	freshly ground black pepper	1 mL
1 lb	rigatoni	500 g
¼ cup	grated low-fat Parmesan cheese	50 mL

1. In a nonstick saucepan sprayed with vegetable spray, cook onions, carrots and garlic over medium-high heat for 3 minutes or until onions are softened. Add beef and sausage; cook, stirring to break up meat, for 4 minutes or until no longer pink. Add tomatoes, tomato paste, bay leaf, basil and chili powder. Season to taste with salt and pepper. Reduce heat to medium; cook, covered, for 20 minutes or until thickened.

2. Meanwhile, in a large pot of boiling water, cook rigatoni for 8 to 10 minutes or until tender but firm; drain. In a serving bowl combine pasta and sauce; sprinkle with Parmesan cheese. Serve immediately.

Choices Per Serving

3	Carbohydrates
1	Meat & Alternative
1	Fat

Nutritional Analysis Per Serving

Calories	338	Fat, total	9 g
Carbohydrate	49 g	Fat, saturated	3 g
Fiber	3 g	Sodium	202 mg
Protein	15 g	Cholesterol	23 mg

Mushroom Sauce

1 tbsp	margarine	15 mL
1½ cups	sliced mushrooms	375 mL
2 tbsp	all-purpose flour	25 mL
½ cup	chicken or beef stock	125 mL
½ cup	2% milk	125 mL
1 tbsp	sherry (optional)	5 mL

Tips

If they're available, use wild mushrooms, such as chanterelle or oyster.

Serve over cooked beef, chicken or pork.

This flavorful mushroom sauce has much less fat than others that might be commercially available.

1. In small nonstick saucepan, melt margarine; sauté mushrooms until tender, approximately 3 minutes. Add flour and stir until combined.

2. Add stock and milk; cook on low heat, stirring constantly, until thickened, 4 to 5 minutes. Add sherry (if using). If too thick add more milk.

Make Ahead

Prepare and refrigerate up to a day before, then gently reheat.

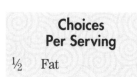

**Choices
Per Serving**

½ Fat

Nutritional Analysis Per Serving

Calories	32	Fat, total	2 g
Carbohydrate	3 g	Fat, saturated	0 g
Fiber	0 g	Sodium	112 mg
Protein	1 g	Cholesterol	1 mg

Pastas

All pasta sold in Canada is now fortified with folic acid, so most of the recipes containing pasta will be a good source of this nutrient. You can also increase the fiber content of the pasta recipes by looking for whole grain pastas in your supermarket.

Combined with fruits, vegetables and small amounts of Meat & Alternatives, many of these recipes are almost complete meals in themselves. Check your meal plan to include any missing choices.

continued on next page

Tips

When buying artichoke hearts for this recipe, be sure that they're packed in water, not oil. The oil-packed variety have double the calories and triple the fat — a huge difference!

This recipe is an excellent source of thiamin, niacin, calcium and magnesium.

Artichoke Cheese Dill Sauce over Rotini

12 oz	rotini	375 g
1	can (14 oz/398 mL) artichoke hearts, drained	1
⅔ cup	vegetable stock (see recipe, page 53) or chicken stock	150 mL
½ cup	chopped red onions	125 mL
½ cup	shredded low-fat mozzarella cheese	125 mL
⅓ cup	shredded low-fat Swiss cheese	75 mL
⅓ cup	chopped fresh dill (or 1 tsp/5 mL dried)	75 mL
⅓ cup	low-fat sour cream	75 mL
2 tbsp	light mayonnaise	25 mL
2 tbsp	fresh lemon juice	25 mL
1 tsp	minced garlic	5 mL
	Fresh chopped parsley	

1. In a large pot of boiling water, cook rotini for 8 to 10 minutes or until tender but firm; drain.

2. Meanwhile, in a food processor combine artichokes, stock, red onions, mozzarella cheese, Swiss cheese, dill, sour cream, mayonnaise, lemon juice and garlic; process until smooth. Transfer to a nonstick saucepan; cook over medium heat, stirring frequently, for 4 minutes or until heated through.

3. In a serving bowl, combine pasta and sauce; toss well. Garnish with fresh chopped parsley. Serve immediately.

Choices Per Serving

3½ Carbohydrates

2 Meat & Alternatives

Nutritional Analysis Per Serving			
Calories	381	Fat, total	9 g
Carbohydrate	55 g	Fat, saturated	4 g
Fiber	5 g	Sodium	434 mg
Protein	20 g	Cholesterol	19 mg

Tip

Unless you like your pesto with crunchy grit, remember to wash the leeks thoroughly. To make sure you get all the dirt, slice the leeks lengthwise, open the leaves and wash well. Then chop and use as directed.

Leek Pesto over Linguine

1 cup	chopped leeks	250 mL
1½ cups	tightly packed fresh basil leaves	375 mL
3 tbsp	grated low-fat Parmesan cheese	45 mL
3 tbsp	toasted pine nuts	45 mL
2 tsp	packed brown sugar	10 mL
1 tsp	minced garlic	5 mL
1 cup	vegetable stock (see recipe, page 53) or chicken stock	250 mL
3 tbsp	olive oil	45 mL
8 oz	linguine	250 g

1. In a nonstick frying pan sprayed with vegetable spray, cook leeks over medium heat for 4 minutes or until softened. In a food processor combine leeks, basil, Parmesan cheese, pine nuts, brown sugar, garlic, stock and olive oil; purée until smooth.

2. Meanwhile, in a large pot of boiling water, cook linguine for 8 to 10 minutes or until tender but firm; drain. In a serving bowl, combine pasta and pesto; toss well. Serve immediately.

Choices Per Serving

3½ Carbohydrates

3½ Fats

Nutritional Analysis Per Serving

Calories	391	Fat, total	18 g
Carbohydrate	52 g	Fat, saturated	3 g
Fiber	2 g	Sodium	28 mg
Protein	10 g	Cholesterol	0 mg

Penne with Wild Mushrooms

12 oz	penne	375 g
1 tsp	margarine or butter	5 mL
3 cups	sliced wild mushrooms (oyster, cremini, portobello)	750 mL
2 tsp	olive oil	10 mL
2 tsp	crushed garlic	10 mL
1 cup	diced onions	250 mL
1 lb	chopped tomatoes (about 3 cups/750 mL)	500 g
2 cups	2% milk	500 mL
4 tsp	all-purpose flour	20 mL
½ cup	fresh chopped basil (or 2 tsp/10 mL dried)	125 mL
	Pepper	

1. Cook pasta in boiling water according to package instructions or until firm to the bite. Drain and place in serving bowl.

2. In large nonstick skillet, melt margarine; sauté mushrooms for 5 minutes. Drain off excess liquid. Add oil; sauté garlic and onions just until tender, approximately 3 minutes. Add tomatoes; simmer on low heat for 10 minutes just until tomatoes become very soft.

3. Meanwhile, in small bowl, mix milk and flour until smooth; add to tomato mixture and simmer on medium heat for 3 minutes or until sauce thickens slightly. Pour over pasta. Sprinkle with basil and pepper, and toss.

Choices Per Serving

4 Carbohydrates

1 Meat & Alternative

Nutritional Analysis Per Serving			
Calories	346	Fat, total	5 g
Carbohydrate	62 g	Fat, saturated	2 g
Fiber	4 g	Sodium	63 mg
Protein	13 g	Cholesterol	6 mg

Preheat oven to
350°F (180°C)

9-inch (2.5 L) springform
pan lined with foil
and sprayed with
vegetable spray

Tips

To soften sun-dried
tomatoes, pour boiling
water over them and soak
15 minutes or until soft.
Drain and chop.

Any small, shaped pasta
works well in this recipe.
Try macaroni or orzo.

Make Ahead

Prepare up to 1 day in
advance. Reheat gently.

Sun-Dried Tomato and Leek Pasta Bake

1 cup	small shell pasta	250 mL
2 tsp	vegetable oil	10 mL
2 tsp	minced garlic	10 mL
1½ cups	chopped leeks	375 mL
1½ cups	sliced mushrooms	375 mL
1 cup	chopped red bell peppers	250 mL
½ cup	chopped softened sun-dried tomatoes (see Tip, at left)	125 mL
⅓ cup	sliced black olives	75 mL
2	eggs	2
2	egg whites	2
1 cup	2% evaporated milk	250 mL
½ cup	shredded part-skim mozzarella cheese (about 2 oz/50 g)	125 mL
2 tsp	dried basil	10 mL
3 oz	feta cheese, crumbled	75 g
2 tbsp	grated Parmesan cheese	25 mL

1. In a pot of boiling water, cook pasta 5 minutes or until tender but firm. Rinse under cold water, drain and set aside.

2. In a nonstick frying pan, heat oil over medium heat. Add garlic and leeks; cook 4 minutes or until softened. Stir in mushrooms and red peppers; cook 6 minutes or until vegetables are tender and moisture is absorbed. Stir in sun-dried tomatoes and black olives; remove from heat.

3. In a large bowl, whisk together whole eggs, egg whites, evaporated milk, mozzarella and basil. Stir in pasta, cooled vegetable mixture and feta. Pour into prepared pan. Sprinkle with Parmesan cheese.

4. Bake 30 to 35 minutes or until set.

Choices Per Serving

1½	Carbohydrates
1½	Meat & Alternatives
½	Fat

Nutritional Analysis Per Serving

Calories	227	Fat, total	10 g
Carbohydrate	22 g	Fat, saturated	5 g
Fiber	2 g	Sodium	399 mg
Protein	14 g	Cholesterol	77 mg

Mango Salsa over Vermicelli *page 103*
Overleaf: Pesto Potato Salad *page 105*

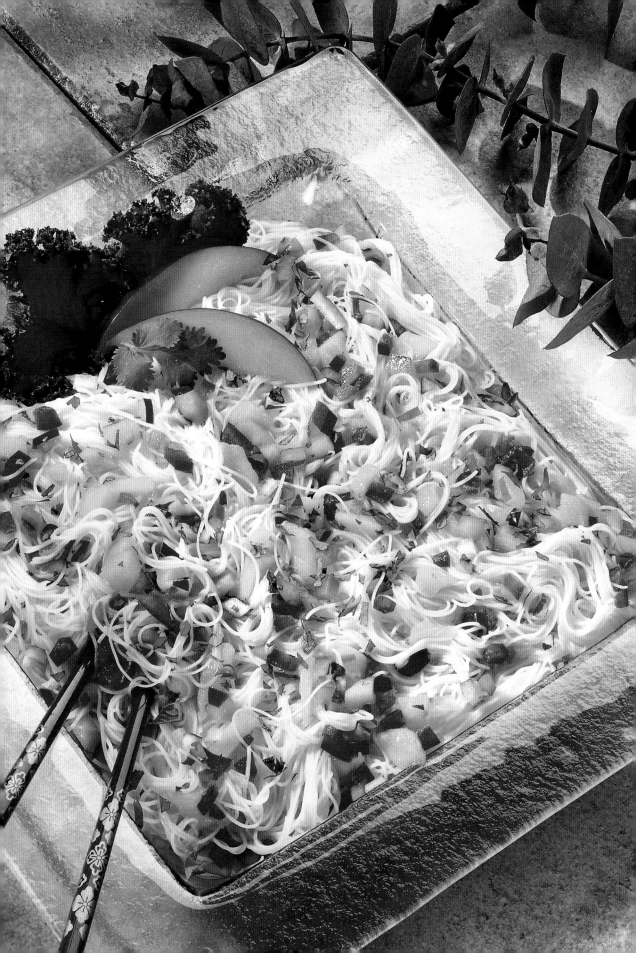

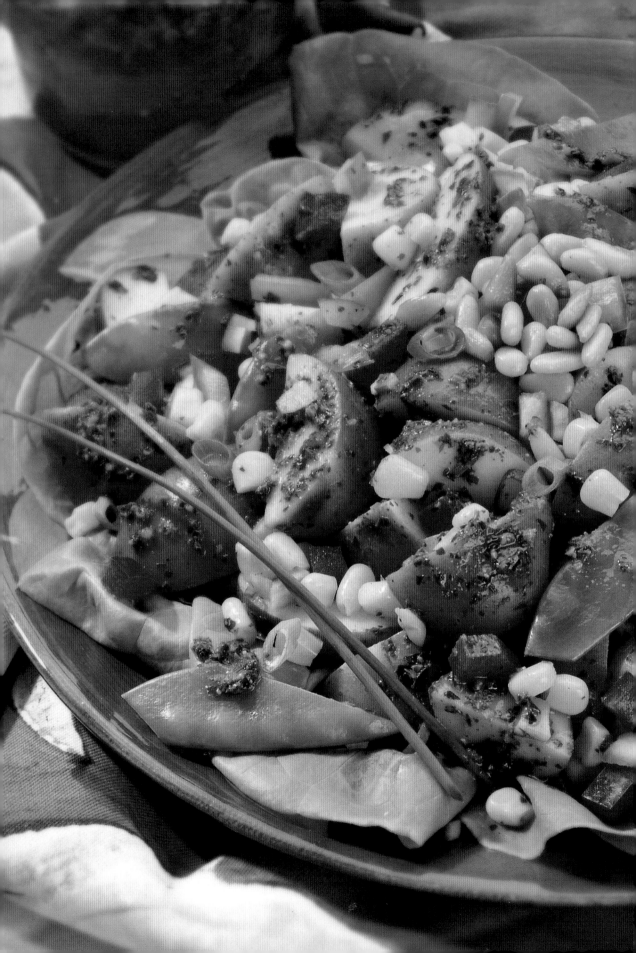

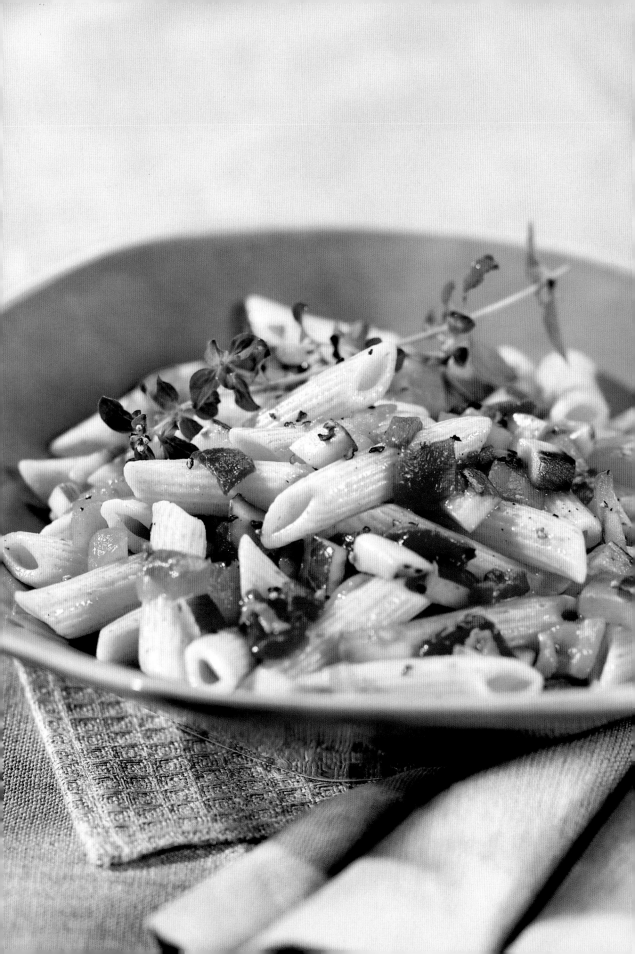

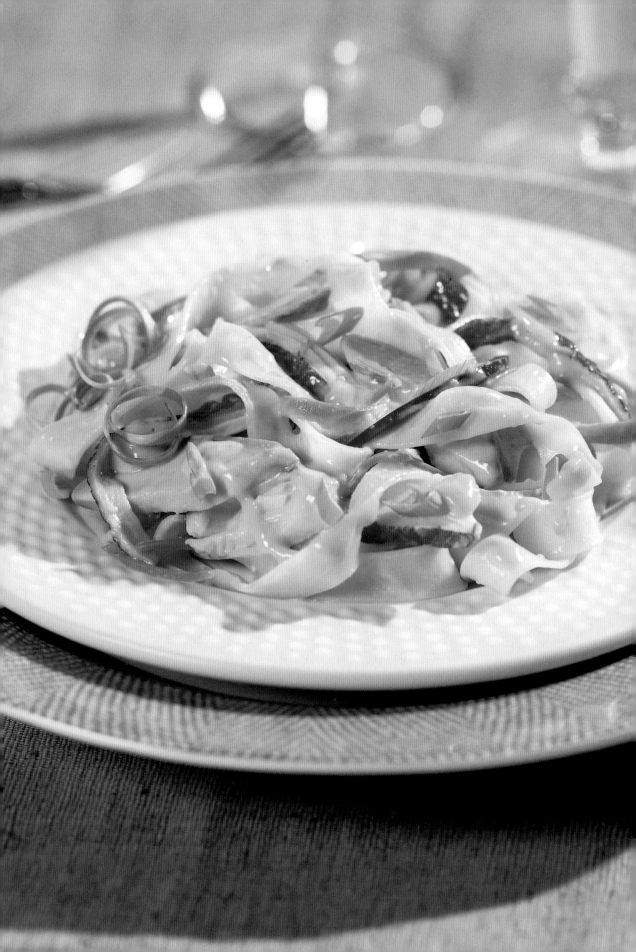

Tips

This is delicious served warm or cold.

The goat cheese can be substituted with feta cheese.

Make Ahead

If serving cold, prepare and refrigerate early in day and toss again prior to serving.

Rotini with Tomatoes, Black Olives and Goat Cheese

1 tbsp	vegetable oil	15 mL
1½ tsp	crushed garlic	7 mL
1 cup	chopped onions	250 mL
1	can (19 oz/540 mL) tomatoes, puréed	1
¼ cup	sliced pitted black olives	50 mL
1 tsp	dried basil (or 2 tbsp/25 mL chopped fresh)	5 mL
	Red pepper flakes	
2 oz	goat cheese	50 g
12 oz	rotini	375 g
1 tbsp	grated Parmesan cheese	15 mL
	Chopped fresh parsley	

1. In large nonstick saucepan, heat oil; sauté garlic and onions for 5 minutes. Add tomatoes, olives, basil, and red pepper flakes to taste; cover and simmer for 10 minutes, stirring often. Add goat cheese, stirring until melted.

2. Meanwhile, cook pasta according to package directions or until firm to the bite. Drain and place in serving bowl. Toss with sauce. Sprinkle with Parmesan cheese and garnish with parsley.

Choices Per Serving

3½ Carbohydrates
½ Meat & Alternative
1 Fat

Nutritional Analysis Per Serving

Calories	308	Fat, total	6 g
Carbohydrate	53 g	Fat, saturated	2 g
Fiber	4 g	Sodium	336 mg
Protein	11 g	Cholesterol	5 mg

Avocado Crab Meat over Rice Noodles *page 134*
Overleaf: Grilled Balsamic Vegetables over Penne *page 131*

●●●●●●●●●●●●●●●●

Tip

The sodium in this recipe comes from the cheese, canned tomatoes and salt. By eliminating the added salt you can reduce the sodium content to 800 mg/serving.

Tomato Macaroni and Cheese

2 cups	macaroni (8 oz/250 g)	500 mL
½ lb	low-fat Cheddar cheese, preferably old	250 g
1	can (19 oz/540 mL) tomatoes, chopped	1
1 tsp	granulated sugar	5 mL
1 tsp	Worcestershire sauce	5 mL
1 tsp	dry mustard	5 mL
½ tsp	salt	2 mL
½ tsp	dried thyme	2 mL
¼ tsp	pepper	1 mL
½ cup	dry bread crumbs	125 mL
2 tbsp	margarine or butter, melted	25 mL

1. In large pot of boiling salted water, cook macaroni until al dente, about 8 minutes. Drain well and transfer half to well-greased deep 12-cup (3 L) casserole.

2. Meanwhile, shred half of the cheese and dice remainder. Sprinkle half of each over macaroni in casserole. Top with remaining macaroni, then remaining cheese.

3. Stir together tomatoes, sugar, Worcestershire sauce, mustard, salt, thyme and pepper; pour over macaroni. Toss bread crumbs with butter; sprinkle evenly on top. (Casserole can be prepared to this point, covered and refrigerated for up to 1 day. Bring to room temperature.)

4. Bake, uncovered, in 350°F (190°C) oven for 40 to 50 minutes or until top is golden brown.

Choices Per Serving

3½	Carbohydrates
2½	Meat & Alternatives
3	Fats

Nutritional Analysis Per Serving			
Calories	490	Fat, total	17 g
Carbohydrate	61 g	Fat, saturated	7 g
Fiber	4 g	Sodium	1089 mg
Protein	24 g	Cholesterol	34 mg

**Preheat oven to broil
or start barbecue**

Tips

Try alternating different
vegetables such as
eggplant, yellow zucchini
or fennel.

If possible use one green,
one red and one yellow
or orange sweet pepper
for brilliant color.

Make Ahead

Grill vegetables early in
day. Chop before cooking
pasta.

Grilled Balsamic Vegetables over Penne

1	medium red onion, cut in half horizontally	1
1	medium zucchini, cut lengthwise into 4 strips	1
3	medium sweet peppers (green, red and/or yellow)	3
2	medium tomatoes, cut in half horizontally	2
1 lb	penne	500 g

DRESSING

3 tbsp	lemon juice	45 mL
3 tbsp	balsamic vinegar	45 mL
¼ cup	olive oil	50 mL
2 tsp	crushed garlic	10 mL

1. Place all vegetables on grill or barbecue. Grill onion for 25 minutes, turning until charred. Grill zucchini for 15 minutes until charred, turning as necessary. Grill sweet peppers for 15 minutes until charred. Grill tomatoes for 12 to 15 minutes until charred, rotating as necessary. Let vegetables cool for 10 minutes.

2. Remove top, skin and seeds of sweet peppers. Chop all vegetables into medium diced pieces, keeping juices. Set aside.

3. Meanwhile, cook pasta in boiling water according to package instructions or until firm to the bite. Drain and place in serving bowl. Add vegetables.

4. *Make the dressing:* Combine lemon juice, vinegar, oil and garlic. Pour over pasta, and toss.

Choices Per Serving

3½   Carbohydrates

1½   Fats

Nutritional Analysis Per Serving

Calories	324	Fat, total	9 g
Carbohydrate	54 g	Fat, saturated	1 g
Fiber	4 g	Sodium	9 mg
Protein	9 g	Cholesterol	0 mg

Roasted Vegetable Lasagna

Preheat oven to
425°F (220°C)

Baking sheet lined
with foil

9-inch (2.5 L) square
baking dish, sprayed
with vegetable spray

Tip

This lasagna is an
excellent source of
vitamins A and C,
B vitamins as well as
calcium, phosphorus,
magnesium and zinc.

1	medium sweet potato, peeled and cut crosswise into ½-inch (1 cm) slices	1
1	medium red bell pepper, quartered	1
1	medium yellow or green bell pepper, quartered	1
1	medium red onion, cut into wedges	1
1	medium zucchini, cut into half lengthwise	1
1 tbsp	olive oil	15 mL
1	medium head garlic, top ½ inch (1 cm) cut off, wrapped loosely in foil	1
9	lasagna noodles	9
1½ cups	5% ricotta cheese	375 mL
¾ cup	shredded low-fat mozzarella cheese	175 mL
⅓ cup	low-fat milk	75 mL
⅓ cup	prepared pesto	75 mL
¼ cup	grated low-fat Parmesan cheese	50 mL
1½ cups	tomato pasta sauce	375 mL
¼ cup	low-fat milk	50 mL

1. In a bowl combine sweet potato, red pepper, yellow pepper, red onion, zucchini and olive oil; toss well. Spread mixture over prepared baking sheet; add garlic. Bake in preheated oven for 45 minutes or until vegetables are tender; remove from oven. Squeeze garlic from skins; mash. Chop roasted vegetables; mix well with accumulated juices and mashed garlic. Set aside. Reduce oven temperature to 350°F (180°C).

2. Meanwhile, in a large pot of boiling water, cook lasagna noodles for 12 to 14 minutes or until tender; drain. Rinse under cold running water; drain. Set aside.

**Choices
Per Serving**

4	Carbohydrates
2½	Meat & Alternatives
1½	Fats

Nutritional Analysis Per Serving

Calories	528	Fat, total	21 g
Carbohydrate	60 g	Fat, saturated	8 g
Fiber	4 g	Sodium	569 mg
Protein	26 g	Cholesterol	39 mg

3. In a bowl combine ricotta cheese, mozzarella cheese, ⅓ cup (75 mL) milk, pesto and half the Parmesan cheese; set aside. In another bowl combine tomato sauce and milk; set aside.

4. Spread half the tomato sauce over bottom of prepared baking pan. Top with three lasagna noodles; trim to fit pan (discard trimmings). Add half the vegetable mixture, then half the cheese mixture; spread evenly. Top with three more lasagna noodles; repeat layers. Top with remaining tomato sauce; sprinkle with remaining Parmesan cheese. Bake, uncovered, in preheated oven for 30 minutes or until heated through. Serve.

● ● ● ● ● ● ● ● ● ● ● ● ● ●

Tips

A granulated sugar substitute can replace the honey in this recipe and reduce the carbohydrate by about 10 g/serving.

If you've heard that avocados are high in fat, you've heard right. In fact, one medium California avocado has 30 g of the stuff. The good news is that most of the fat is monounsaturated and does not raise blood lipid levels. If you want less fat, try a Florida avocado, which contains only 20 g fat per fruit.

Using low-sodium soya sauce rather than regular will reduce the sodium to 734 mg/serving.

Avocado Crab Meat over Rice Noodles

8 oz	crabmeat or surimi (imitation crab), diced	250 g
1 cup	julienned carrots	250 mL
1 cup	julienned red bell peppers	250 mL
⅓ cup	sliced green onions	75 mL
½ cup	diced ripe avocado	125 mL
¼ cup	light mayonnaise	50 mL
3 tbsp	light soya sauce	45 mL
2 tbsp	water	25 mL
2 tbsp	honey	25 mL
1 tbsp	sesame oil	15 mL
1½ tsp	minced garlic	7 mL
1½ tsp	minced gingerroot	7 mL
½ tsp	wasabi (Japanese horseradish), optional	2 mL
8 oz	wide rice noodles	250 g

1. In a serving bowl, combine crabmeat, carrots, red peppers and green onions; set aside.

2. In a food processor combine avocado, mayonnaise, soya sauce, water, honey, sesame oil, garlic, gingerroot and wasabi; process until smooth. Add to crab mixture.

3. In a large pot of boiling water, cook rice noodles for 5 minutes or until tender; drain well. Add to crab mixture; toss well. Garnish with 2 thin slices avocado. Serve immediately.

Choices Per Serving

4½	Carbohydrates
1	Meat & Alternative
2	Fats

Nutritional Analysis Per Serving

Calories	469	Fat, total	14 g
Carbohydrate	71 g	Fat, saturated	2 g
Fiber	4 g	Sodium	1171 mg
Protein	17 g	Cholesterol	53 mg

Tip

Mango and leeks make
this an excellent source
of vitamins A and C,
niacin and thiamin.

Mango-Leek Sauce over Halibut and Spaghettini

1 cup	chopped leeks	250 mL
1	ripe mango, peeled and chopped	1
1 tsp	minced garlic	5 mL
¾ cup	seafood stock (see fish stock, page 54) or chicken stock	175 mL
3 tbsp	fresh lemon juice	45 mL
2 tbsp	low-fat sour cream	25 mL
1 tsp	Dijon mustard	5 mL
8 oz	halibut	250 g
8 oz	spaghettini or bean noodles	250 g
1 cup	thinly sliced red bell peppers	250 mL
½ cup	chopped green onions	125 mL
⅓ cup	chopped fresh dill (or 1 tsp/5 mL dried)	75 mL

1. In a nonstick saucepan sprayed with vegetable spray, cook leeks over medium-high heat for 3 minutes or until softened. Add mango, garlic and stock; bring mixture to a boil. Reduce heat to medium-low; cook, covered, for 5 minutes or until leeks are tender. Transfer to a food processor. Add lemon juice, sour cream and Dijon mustard; process until smooth.

2. Broil or grill halibut, turning once, for 10 minutes per 1-inch (2.5 cm) thickness or until cooked through. Flake fish with a fork. Meanwhile, in a large pot of boiling water, cook spaghettini for 8 to 10 minutes or until tender but firm; drain.

3. In a large serving bowl, combine spaghettini, fish, red peppers, green onions, dill and dressing; toss to coat well.

Choices Per Serving

3½ Carbohydrates

2 Meat & Alternatives

Nutritional Analysis Per Serving			
Calories	351	Fat, total	3 g
Carbohydrate	60 g	Fat, saturated	0 g
Fiber	4 g	Sodium	67 mg
Protein	21 g	Cholesterol	19 mg

Tip

Here's a wonderful way to use fresh salmon and not have too much protein. Fresh tuna or swordfish is a great substitute.

Make Ahead

The white sauce can be prepared early in day or up to day before, but add a little extra milk when reheating before continuing with recipe.

Fettuccine with Fresh Salmon, Dill and Leeks

4 tsp	margarine	20 mL
4 tsp	all-purpose flour	20 mL
2 cups	2% milk	500 mL
¼ cup	grated Parmesan cheese	50 mL
¼ cup	white wine	50 mL
2 tbsp	chopped onion	25 mL
1 tsp	crushed garlic	5 mL
2	leeks, washed and sliced in thin rounds	2
12 oz	fresh salmon, boned and cubed	375 g
3 tbsp	chopped fresh dill (or 1 tsp/5 mL dried dillweed)	45 mL
10 oz	fettuccine noodles	300 g

1. In small saucepan, melt margarine; add flour and cook, stirring, for 30 seconds. Add milk and cook, stirring constantly, until thickened, 4 to 5 minutes. Stir in cheese until melted; set aside.

2. In large skillet, combine wine, onion, garlic and leeks; cook over medium heat for approximately 10 minutes or until leeks are softened. Add white sauce along with salmon. Cook for 2 to 3 minutes or until salmon is almost opaque, stirring gently. Stir in dill.

3. Meanwhile, cook fettuccine according to package directions or until firm to the bite. Drain and place in serving bowl. Toss with sauce.

Choices Per Serving

3	Carbohydrates
2½	Meat & Alternatives

Nutritional Analysis Per Serving			
Calories	410	Fat, total	11 g
Carbohydrate	52 g	Fat, saturated	3 g
Fiber	3 g	Sodium	197 mg
Protein	25 g	Cholesterol	43 mg

This recipe comes from Cal-A-Vie Spa in California.

Linguine with Salmon, Leeks and Dill

WHITE SAUCE

2 cups	low-fat milk	500 mL
¼ tsp	nutmeg	1 mL
Pinch	cayenne pepper	Pinch
4 tsp	flour, preferably whole wheat	20 mL
1 tbsp	olive oil	15 mL
¼ cup	grated Parmesan cheese	50 mL
2	leeks, thinly sliced	2
¼ cup	white wine	50 mL
2 tbsp	chopped shallots or onions	25 mL
2	cloves garlic, crushed	2
10 oz	linguine, preferably spinach pasta	300 g
12 oz	salmon fillets, skinned, boned and cubed	375 g
3 tbsp	minced fresh dill (or 1 tsp/5 mL dried)	45 mL
Pinch	freshly crushed peppercorns, preferably pink peppercorns	Pinch

1. *White Sauce:* In a saucepan bring milk, nutmeg and cayenne to a boil; remove from heat. In another saucepan, combine flour and olive oil over medium heat; cook, stirring, until blended. Gradually add hot milk mixture, whisking constantly; cook, whisking, until thickened, about 5 minutes. Stir in Parmesan; set aside.

2. In a saucepan combine leeks, wine, shallots and garlic; bring to a boil, reduce heat and cook until vegetables soft, about 10 minutes. Meanwhile, cook the pasta.

3. In a large pot of boiling salted water, cook linguine 8 to 10 minutes or until al dente. Stir white sauce and salmon into leek mixture; cook just until salmon is barely done, about 3 minutes. Toss drained pasta with sauce, dill and pepper. Serve immediately.

Choices Per Serving

3 Carbohydrates

2½ Meat & Alternatives

Nutritional Analysis Per Serving			
Calories	378	Fat, total	10 g
Carbohydrate	48 g	Fat, saturated	3 g
Fiber	5 g	Sodium	161 mg
Protein	23 g	Cholesterol	41 mg

Preheat oven to 350°F (180°C)

13- by 9-inch (3 L) baking dish

Tips

As an alternative to manicotti, use 24 jumbo shells.

Sprinkle ¼ cup (50 mL) shredded mozzarella cheese over pasta shells just before serving.

Replace the tomato sauce with ¾ cup (175 mL) tomato paste and ¾ cup (175 mL) water to reduce the sodium to 351 mg/serving.

Make Ahead

Prepare stuffed pasta shells up to a day ahead, with sauce poured over. Bake just before serving.

Manicotti Shells Filled with Cheese and Smoked Salmon Bits

12	manicotti shells	12
1½ cups	ricotta cheese	375 mL
1	egg	1
2½ oz	chopped smoked salmon	60 g
¼ cup	finely chopped green onions	50 mL
3 tbsp	fresh chopped dill (or 1 tsp/5 mL dried)	45 mL
2 tbsp	2% milk	25 mL
2 tbsp	grated Parmesan cheese	25 mL
1½ cups	prepared tomato sauce	375 mL

1. Cook pasta in boiling water according to package instructions or until firm to the bite. Drain, cover and set aside.

2. In bowl, combine ricotta cheese, egg, salmon, green onions, dill, milk and Parmesan cheese; mix until smooth. Fill pasta shells.

3. Pour half tomato sauce in bottom of large baking dish. Place pasta shells over sauce and pour other half tomato sauce over pasta. Cover and bake for 15 to 20 minutes or until hot.

Choices Per Serving

2 Carbohydrates

2½ Meat & Alternatives

Nutritional Analysis Per Serving			
Calories	331	Fat, total	11 g
Carbohydrate	36 g	Fat, saturated	6 g
Fiber	2 g	Sodium	848 mg
Protein	22 g	Cholesterol	90 mg

Tips

Other pasta such as angel hair can be substituted. Cook noodles according to package directions before adding to recipe.

This recipe is a complete source of vitamin C, and is an excellent source of iron, niacin and B$_{12}$.

Singapore Noodles

6 oz	rice vermicelli	175 g
3 tbsp	reduced-sodium soya sauce	45 mL
2 tsp	mild curry paste or powder	10 mL
2 tbsp	vegetable oil, divided	25 mL
1	red or green bell pepper, cut into thin strips	1
5	green onions, sliced	5
2	large cloves garlic, minced	2
3 cups	bean sprouts, rinsed and dried	375 mL
12 oz	cooked, peeled baby shrimp	375 g

1. In a large pot of lightly salted boiling water, cook noodles for 3 minutes. Drain; chill under cold water and drain well. Cut noodles using scissors into 3-inch (8 cm) lengths; set aside.

2. In a small bowl, combine soya sauce and curry paste; set aside.

3. Heat a wok or large nonstick skillet over high heat until very hot; add 1 tbsp (15 mL) oil, tilting wok to coat sides. Stir-fry pepper strips, green onions and garlic for 1 minute. Add bean sprouts and shrimp; stir-fry for 1 to 2 minutes or until vegetables are tender-crisp. Transfer to a bowl.

4. Add remaining oil to wok; when very hot, add noodles and soya sauce mixture. Stir-fry for 1 minute or until heated through. Return vegetable-shrimp mixture to wok and stir-fry for 1 minute more. Serve immediately.

Choices Per Serving

3 Carbohydrates

2½ Meat & Alternatives

Nutritional Analysis Per Serving			
Calories	347	Fat, total	8 g
Carbohydrate	45 g	Fat, saturated	1 g
Fiber	3 g	Sodium	606 mg
Protein	23 g	Cholesterol	166 mg

Tip

This recipe is an excellent source of vitamin C, B vitamins, iron and magnesium.

This recipe comes from Cal-A-Vie Spa in California.

Angel Hair Pasta with Shrimp in a Tomato Pesto Sauce

½ cup	white wine	125 mL
1 lb	shrimp, peeled and deveined	500 g

SAUCE

1 tbsp	olive oil	15 mL
1	green pepper, chopped	1
1 cup	chopped onions	250 mL
1 lb	mushrooms, chopped	500 g
½ cup	white wine	125 mL
2 lbs	plum tomatoes, finely chopped	1 kg
4 tsp	dried oregano	20 mL
1 tbsp	dried basil	15 mL
1 tsp	honey	5 mL
1	bay leaf	1
1 tbsp	tomato paste	15 mL

PESTO

2½ cups	packed fresh basil leaves	625 mL
¼ cup	walnuts	50 mL
2 tbsp	grated Parmesan cheese	25 mL
1 tbsp	olive oil	15 mL
3	cloves garlic, crushed	3
10 oz	angel hair pasta or capellini	300 g

1. In a small saucepan, bring wine to a simmer. Add shrimp; cook just until pink. Remove from heat; drain, reserving liquid.

Nutritional Analysis Per Serving			
Calories	460	Fat, total	12 g
Carbohydrate	56 g	Fat, saturated	2 g
Fiber	6 g	Sodium	261 mg
Protein	29 g	Cholesterol	151 mg

Choices Per Serving

3½	Carbohydrates
3	Meat & Alternatives

2. *Sauce:* In a large saucepan, heat oil over medium-high heat. Add green peppers and onions; cook for 5 minutes. Stir in mushrooms, wine and shrimp cooking liquid; cook for 2 minutes. Stir in tomatoes, oregano, basil, honey and bay leaf; bring to a boil, reduce heat to medium and cook until thickened, about 20 minutes. Stir in tomato paste; cook for another 10 minutes. Meanwhile, make the pesto.

3. *Pesto:* In food processor, purée basil, walnuts, Parmesan, olive oil and garlic until smooth. Measure out $\frac{1}{4}$ cup (50 mL) of pesto for dish; refrigerate or freeze remainder for later use.

4. In a large pot of boiling salted water, cook angel hair pasta for 6 to 8 minutes or until al dente; drain. Toss with shrimp, tomato sauce and pesto. Serve immediately.

Tips
Shrimp can be replaced with scallops, squid or firm fish fillets such as orange roughy or halibut.

Chicken can be substituted for fish.

Goat cheese can replace feta cheese.

Walnuts, pecans or cashews can replace pine nuts.

Both the fish or chicken stock and the feta cheese contribute sodium to this recipe. Using low-sodium chicken stock can reduce the sodium to 546 mg/serving.

Make Ahead
Prepare sauce in Steps 3 and 4 early in day. Do not add cheese. Reheat gently. Add cheese and continue with recipe.

Linguine with Shrimp, Red Peppers and Pine Nuts

8 oz	linguine	250 g
8 oz	shrimp, shelled, deveined and cut into pieces	250 g
2 tsp	vegetable oil	10 mL
2 tsp	crushed garlic	10 mL
2 cups	chopped sweet red peppers	500 mL
⅓ cup	chopped green onions	75 mL
½ cup	chopped fresh basil (or 2 tsp/10 mL dried)	125 mL
1½ tsp	dried oregano	7 mL
1¼ cups	cold fish or chicken stock	300 mL
3½ tsp	all-purpose flour	17 mL
3½ oz	feta cheese, crumbled	90 g
2 tbsp	toasted pine nuts	25 mL

1. Cook pasta in boiling water according to package instructions or until firm to the bite. Drain and place in serving bowl.

2. In medium nonstick skillet sprayed with nonstick vegetable spray, sauté shrimp just until pink and just cooked, approximately 3 minutes. Drain and add to pasta.

3. In large nonstick skillet, heat oil; sauté garlic and red peppers for 3 minutes. Add onions, basil and oregano; sauté for 3 minutes.

4. Meanwhile, in small bowl, combine stock and flour until smooth. Add to red pepper mixture; simmer, stirring constantly until thickened, approximately 3 minutes. Add cheese and allow to melt. Pour over pasta. Add pine nuts, and toss.

Choices Per Serving

3½ Carbohydrates

2½ Meat & Alternatives

Nutritional Analysis Per Serving

Calories	430	Fat, total	11 g
Carbohydrate	57 g	Fat, saturated	5 g
Fiber	3 g	Sodium	807 mg
Protein	26 g	Cholesterol	118 mg

Tips

Replace squid with shrimp, scallops or lobster.

For a spicier version, add ¼ tsp (1 mL) cayenne pepper.

Complete the meal with a vegetable salad and low-fat dressing.

Make Ahead

Prepare sauce a day ahead up to point where seafood is added. Reheat gently, then continue with recipe.

Pasta with Squid and Clams in a Spicy Tomato Sauce

12 oz	spaghetti	375 g
2 tsp	vegetable oil	10 mL
1½ tsp	crushed garlic	7 mL
1 cup	chopped onions	250 mL
1 cup	chopped sweet green peppers	250 mL
1	can (19 oz/540 mL) crushed tomatoes	1
2	cans (5 oz/142 mL) baby clams, liquid reserved from 1 can	2
1 tbsp	tomato paste	15 mL
2 tsp	capers	10 mL
1½ tsp	dried basil	7 mL
¾ tsp	dried oregano	4 mL
2 tsp	chili powder	10 mL
12 oz	squid, cleaned and sliced	375 g
3 tbsp	grated Parmesan cheese	45 mL
	Parsley	

1. Cook pasta in boiling water according to package instructions or until firm to the bite. Drain and place in serving bowl.

2. In large nonstick saucepan, heat oil; sauté garlic, onions and green peppers until soft, approximately 5 minutes. Add crushed tomatoes, liquid from 1 can of clams, tomato paste, capers, basil, oregano and chili powder. Cover and simmer on low heat until thick, for 15 to 20 minutes, stirring occasionally. Add clams and squid; simmer just until squid is cooked, approximately 3 minutes. Pour over pasta. Sprinkle with cheese, and toss. Garnish with parsley.

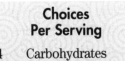

Choices Per Serving	
4	Carbohydrates
3½	Meat & Alternatives

Nutritional Analysis Per Serving			
Calories	445	Fat, total	6 g
Carbohydrate	65 g	Fat, saturated	1 g
Fiber	4 g	Sodium	439 mg
Protein	33 g	Cholesterol	180 mg

Tips

You can find dried cranberries — as well as dried cherries, blueberries and a whole range of other dried fruits — at bulk food stores, where they are reasonably inexpensive. (But they're not exactly cheap, either.) I buy large quantities and keep them in airtight containers in my freezer until needed. Use them as a delicious alternative to raisins in salads, pastas, rice pilafs and desserts.

Watch portion sizes with dried fruits when you are including them in your meal plan. Fifteen fresh grapes and ¼ cup (50 mL) raisins contain the same amount of carbohydrate.

Curried Chicken Coconut Pasta with Apricots and Cranberries

12 oz	skinless boneless chicken breast, cut into ½-inch (1 cm) cubes	375 g
2 tbsp	all-purpose flour	25 mL
1 cup	light coconut milk	250 mL
½ cup	chicken stock	125 mL
1 tsp	minced garlic	5 mL
1 tsp	curry powder	5 mL
2 tsp	all-purpose flour	10 mL
12 oz	penne or rotini	375 g
½ cup	chopped red bell peppers	125 mL
½ cup	chopped dried apricots	125 mL
½ cup	dried cranberries or raisins	125 mL
½ cup	chopped green onions	125 mL
⅓ cup	chopped fresh coriander or parsley	75 mL

1. In a bowl coat chicken with 2 tbsp (25 mL) flour; shake off excess. In a large nonstick frying pan sprayed with vegetable spray, cook chicken over medium-high heat for 4 minutes or until cooked through. Remove from pan; set aside.

2. In a bowl combine coconut milk, stock, garlic, curry powder and 2 tsp (10 mL) flour; set aside.

3. In a large pot of boiling water, cook penne for 8 to 10 minutes or until tender but firm; drain. Meanwhile, respray frying pan; return to medium-high heat. Cook red peppers for 2 minutes or until softened. Add apricots, cranberries, coconut milk mixture and chicken; cook for 4 minutes or until thickened and bubbly.

4. In a serving bowl, combine pasta, sauce, green onions and coriander; toss well. Serve immediately.

Choices Per Serving

4   Carbohydrates

2   Meat & Alternatives

Nutritional Analysis Per Serving

Calories	432	Fat, total	10 g
Carbohydrate	63 g	Fat, saturated	8 g
Fiber	3 g	Sodium	102 mg
Protein	22 g	Cholesterol	32 mg

Variation

It's easy to transform this recipe into a vegetarian dish: just substitute firm tofu for the chicken (grill or sauté it for 5 minutes or just until lightly browned); use a no-sugar-added soya milk instead of dairy milk; and replace chicken stock with vegetable stock (see recipe, page 53).

Curried Vegetable Chicken Fettuccine

8 oz	skinless boneless chicken breast	250 g
8 oz	fettuccine	250 g
¾ cup	chopped onions	175 mL
¾ cup	chopped green bell peppers	175 mL
½ cup	finely chopped carrots	125 mL
1 tsp	minced garlic	5 mL
1½ tbsp	all-purpose flour	20 mL
2 tsp	curry powder	10 mL
1 cup	chicken stock	250 mL
¾ cup	low-fat milk	175 mL
1½ tsp	packed brown sugar	7 mL
¼ tsp	freshly ground black pepper	1 mL

1. In a nonstick frying pan sprayed with vegetable spray or on a preheated grill, cook chicken over medium-high heat, turning once, for 12 minutes or until cooked through. Cut into thin slices; set aside.

2. In a large pot of boiling water, cook fettuccine for 8 to 10 minutes or until tender but firm; drain. Meanwhile, in a large nonstick frying pan sprayed with vegetable spray, cook onions, green peppers, carrots and garlic over medium-high heat for 5 minutes or until softened. Add flour and curry powder; cook for 30 seconds. Add stock, milk, brown sugar and pepper; reduce heat to medium. Cook for 2 minutes or until thickened.

3. In a serving bowl, combine pasta, sauce and chicken; toss well. Serve immediately.

Choices Per Serving

3½ Carbohydrates

2½ Meat & Alternatives

Nutritional Analysis Per Serving			
Calories	361	Fat, total	3 g
Carbohydrate	59 g	Fat, saturated	1 g
Fiber	4 g	Sodium	43 mg
Protein	24 g	Cholesterol	39 mg

Cajun Chicken over Fettuccine

12 oz	fettuccine	375 g
12 oz	skinless, boneless chicken breast cut into 2-inch (5-cm) strips	375 g

SPICE MIXTURE

1 tsp	cayenne	5 mL
1¾ tsp	onion powder	8 mL
1¼ tsp	garlic powder	6 mL
1 tsp	paprika	5 mL
1 tsp	dried basil	5 mL
¾ tsp	dried oregano	4 mL
2½ tbsp	unseasoned bread crumbs	35 mL

SAUCE

2 tsp	vegetable oil	10 mL
1 tsp	crushed garlic	5 mL
¾ cup	chopped onions	175 mL
¾ cup	chopped sweet green peppers	175 mL
4 cups	canned or fresh tomatoes, crushed	1 L
1½ tsp	dried basil	7 mL
1 tsp	dried oregano	5 mL
¼ tsp	cayenne	1 mL

1. Cook pasta in boiling water according to package instructions or until firm to the bite. Drain and place in serving bowl.

2. *Prepare the spices:* In small bowl combine cayenne, onion and garlic powders, paprika, basil, oregano and bread crumbs. Coat chicken in mixture.

Nutritional Analysis Per Serving

Calories	379	Fat, total	4 g
Carbohydrate	66 g	Fat, saturated	1 g
Fiber	5 g	Sodium	462 mg
Protein	21 g	Cholesterol	26 mg

3. In medium nonstick skillet sprayed with vegetable spray, sauté chicken on medium heat until no longer pink, approximately 4 minutes. Add to pasta.

4. *Make the sauce:* In same skillet, heat oil; sauté garlic, onions and green peppers for 5 minutes, until tender. Add tomatoes, basil, oregano and cayenne. Simmer for 20 to 25 minutes. Pour over pasta, and toss.

Tips

For a less distinct basil flavor, use half parsley and half basil.

Toast pine nuts on top of stove in skillet until brown, for 2 to 3 minutes.

Make Ahead

Refrigerate sauce for up to 5 days or up to 3 weeks in freezer.

Linguine with Pesto Chicken

| 12 oz | linguine | 375 g |
| 12 oz | skinless, boneless chicken breasts, thinly sliced | 375 g |

SAUCE

2 cups	fresh basil, packed down	500 mL
⅓ cup	chicken stock	75 mL
3 tbsp	olive oil	45 mL
2 tbsp	grated Parmesan cheese	25 mL
2 tbsp	toasted pine nuts or walnuts	25 mL
1½ tsp	crushed garlic	7 mL

1. Cook pasta in boiling water according to package instructions or until firm to the bite. Drain and place in serving bowl.

2. In medium nonstick skillet sprayed with vegetable spray, sauté chicken until no longer pink, approximately 3 minutes. Add to pasta.

3. *Make the sauce:* In food processor, purée basil, stock, oil, cheese, nuts and garlic until smooth. Pour over pasta, and toss.

Choices Per Serving

3 Carbohydrates

2 Meat & Alternatives

Nutritional Analysis Per Serving			
Calories	373	Fat, total	11 g
Carbohydrate	48 g	Fat, saturated	2 g
Fiber	2 g	Sodium	121 mg
Protein	20 g	Cholesterol	27 mg

●●●●●●●●●●●●●●●●

Parmesan cheese can replace Asiago or Romano.

Although this recipe contains 12 g of fat, the olive oil adds flavor, as well as a being a source of monounsaturated fat in the diet.

Toast pine nuts in a skillet until golden brown, approximately 3 minutes.

●●●●●●●●●●●●●●●●

Make Ahead

Prepare sauce up to 4 days ahead or freeze up to 4 weeks. If sauce thickens, thin with stock or water.

Rotini with Chicken, Sweet Peppers and Sun-Dried Tomato Sauce

12 oz	rotini	375 g
12 oz	skinless, boneless chicken breasts cut into 1-inch (2.5 cm) strips	375 g
1½ cups	thinly sliced yellow or green sweet peppers	375 mL
¼ cup	grated Asiago or Romano cheese	50 mL

SAUCE

4 oz	sun-dried tomatoes	100 g
2 tsp	crushed garlic	10 mL
1 cup	chicken stock or water	250 mL
½ cup	chopped parsley	125 mL
2 tbsp	toasted pine nuts	25 mL
3 tbsp	olive oil	45 mL
3 tbsp	grated Parmesan cheese	45 mL

1. Cover sun-dried tomatoes with boiling water; let soak for 15 minutes. Drain and chop. Set aside.

2. Cook pasta in boiling water according to package instructions or until firm to the bite. Drain and place in serving bowl.

3. In large nonstick skillet sprayed with nonstick vegetable spray, sauté chicken until no longer pink, approximately 5 minutes. Add to pasta.

4. Respray skillet and sauté sweet peppers just until tender, approximately 4 minutes. Add to pasta with Asiago cheese.

5. *Make the sauce:* In food processor, combine sun-dried tomatoes, garlic, stock, parsley, nuts, oil and cheese. Purée until smooth. Pour over pasta, and toss.

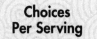

Choices Per Serving

4	Carbohydrates
2½	Meat & Alternatives

Nutritional Analysis Per Serving			
Calories	452	Fat, total	12 g
Carbohydrate	62 g	Fat, saturated	3 g
Fiber	3 g	Sodium	768 mg
Protein	25 g	Cholesterol	35 mg

Tips

Large shell pasta can replace rigatoni.

Chicken livers make this recipe an excellent source of iron, zinc, vitamin A and three B vitamins: riboflavin, niacin and pyridoxine.

Make Ahead

Prepare entire sauce early in day. Reheat gently, adding a little water or chicken stock if sauce thickens.

Rigatoni with Sautéed Chicken Livers in Basil Tomato Sauce

12 oz	rigatoni	375 g
1 tbsp	margarine or butter	15 mL
1½ tsp	crushed garlic	7 mL
¾ cup	diced onions	175 mL
8	medium chicken livers, cubed	8
2½ cups	canned or fresh tomatoes, crushed	625 mL
½ cup	chopped fresh basil (or 2 tsp/10 mL dried)	125 mL
¼ cup	grated Parmesan cheese	50 mL

1. Cook pasta in boiling water according to package instructions or until firm to the bite. Drain and place in serving bowl.

2. In large nonstick skillet, melt half the margarine; sauté garlic and onions until soft, approximately 5 minutes. Sauté livers in remaining margarine just until no longer pink, approximately 5 minutes. Add tomatoes and basil; simmer on low heat for 10 minutes, stirring occasionally. Pour over pasta. Sprinkle with cheese, and toss.

Choices Per Serving

3½ Carbohydrates

1½ Meat & Alternatives

Nutritional Analysis Per Serving			
Calories	361	Fat, total	6 g
Carbohydrate	58 g	Fat, saturated	2 g
Fiber	3 g	Sodium	391 mg
Protein	19 g	Cholesterol	191 mg

Tips

As a substitute for the turkey, try using ground veal, beef or chicken.

This meal is an excellent source of vitamins C and B$_6$, niacin, folate and magnesium, and a good source of phosphorus, iron, zinc and vitamin A.

• • • • • • • • • • • • • • • • •

Make Ahead

Sauce can be prepared up to 2 days before and gently reheated before serving. Do not add coriander or parsley until ready to serve.

Pasta with Spicy Turkey Tomato Sauce

12 oz	rotini	375 g
2 tsp	vegetable oil	10 mL
2 tsp	crushed garlic	10 mL
1 cup	diced red onions	250 mL
1 cup	diced red or green peppers	250 mL
12 oz	ground turkey	375 g
3 cups	crushed tomatoes (canned or fresh)	750 mL
1½ tsp	dried basil	7 mL
1 tsp	dried oregano	5 mL
2 tsp	chili powder	10 mL
Pinch	cayenne pepper	Pinch
½ cup	coriander leaves or parsley, chopped	125 mL

1. Cook pasta in boiling water according to package instructions or until firm to the bite. Drain and place in serving bowl.

2. In large nonstick saucepan sprayed with vegetable spray, heat oil; sauté garlic, onions and red peppers until soft, approximately 5 minutes. Add turkey and sauté on medium heat until cooked, approximately 5 minutes.

3. Add tomatoes, basil, oregano, chili powder and cayenne. Cover and simmer on low heat for 15 minutes, stirring occasionally. Add coriander. Pour over pasta, and toss.

Choices Per Serving

3½ Carbohydrates

2 Meat & Alternatives

Nutritional Analysis Per Serving			
Calories	342	Fat, total	5 g
Carbohydrate	54 g	Fat, saturated	1 g
Fiber	4 g	Sodium	63 mg
Protein	22 g	Cholesterol	37 mg

Preheat oven to
350°F (180°C)

9-inch (2.5 L) baking dish

● ● ● ● ● ● ● ● ● ● ● ● ●

Tips

This recipe is a sure-fire
hit with kids of all ages.
And why not? It
combines macaroni and
cheese, "beefaroni"
and pasta and meatballs
— all into one dish!
The mini-meatballs are
also unusual, appetizing
and just plain fun.

Although many foods
contain iron, the type
found in grains and
vegetables is not as
available to the body as
the iron found in meat,
poultry and fish. In fact,
a 3-oz (75 g) serving of
lean beef provides as
much useable iron as
4 cups (1 L) raw spinach.

Pasta Casserole with Mini Meatballs and Tomato Cheese Sauce

MEATBALLS

8 oz	lean ground beef	250 g
1	large egg white	1
3 tbsp	minced onions	45 mL
3 tbsp	plain dry bread crumbs	45 mL
1 tbsp	barbecue sauce	15 mL
1 tsp	minced garlic	5 mL

SAUCE

1/3 cup	mild salsa	75 mL
1/4 cup	tomato pasta sauce	50 mL
1/4 cup	water	50 mL

CHEESE SAUCE

1 cup	low-fat milk	250 mL
1 cup	beef stock or chicken stock	250 mL
2 1/2 tbsp	all-purpose flour	35 mL
1/2 cup	shredded low-fat Cheddar cheese	125 mL
3 tbsp	grated low-fat Parmesan cheese	45 mL
8 oz	small shell pasta	250 g

1. *Meatballs:* In a bowl combine ground beef, egg white, onions, bread crumbs, barbecue sauce and garlic. Form 1 1/2 tsp (7 mL) of mixture into a round meatball. Repeat to make about 36 balls; set aside.

2. *Sauce:* In a nonstick saucepan over medium-high heat, combine salsa, tomato sauce and water. Bring to a boil; add meatballs. Reduce heat to low; cook, covered, for 20 minutes, gently stirring occasionally. Set aside.

Nutritional Analysis Per Serving

Calories	518	Fat, total	17 g
Carbohydrate	58 g	Fat, saturated	8 g
Fiber	3 g	Sodium	469 mg
Protein	32 g	Cholesterol	56 mg

**Choices
Per Serving**

3 1/2   Carbohydrates

3 1/2   Meat & Alternatives

3. *Cheese Sauce:* In a saucepan over medium-high heat, whisk together milk, stock and flour. Bring to a boil, stirring constantly; reduce heat to low. Cook for 4 minutes or until thickened and bubbly. Add Cheddar cheese and 2 tbsp (25 mL) Parmesan cheese; set aside.

4. In a pot of boiling water, cook pasta for 8 to 10 minutes or until tender but firm; drain. In a bowl combine pasta and cheese sauce; pour into casserole dish. Top with meatball mixture; sprinkle with remaining 1 tbsp (15 mL) Parmesan cheese. Bake, covered, for 20 minutes or until heated through.

Tip

Look for naturally brewed soya sauce — it has a better flavor.

This recipe was developed at King Ranch in Toronto.

Fusilli with Stir-fried Beef and Vegetables

1 cup + 2 tbsp	water	275 mL
½ cup	reduced-sodium soya sauce	125 mL
1½ tsp	grated gingerroot	7 mL
1	clove garlic, crushed	1
8 oz	fusilli	250 g
1 tsp	oil, preferably sesame oil	5 mL
8 oz	good quality steak, cut in thin strips	250 g
1 cup	broccoli florets	250 mL
1 cup	finely chopped carrots	250 mL
1 cup	sliced mushrooms, preferably oyster	250 mL
1 cup	thinly sliced onions	250 mL
1 cup	snow peas	250 mL
2 cups	bean sprouts	500 mL
¼ tsp	pepper	1 mL
	Hot pepper flakes to taste	

1. In a saucepan bring water to a boil. Remove from heat; stir in soya sauce, ginger and garlic. Set aside.

2. In a large pot of boiling salted water, cook fusilli 8 to 10 minutes or until al dente. Meanwhile, in a wok or large saucepan, heat oil over high heat. Stir-fry beef until brown. Stir in sauce, broccoli, carrots, mushrooms, onions and snow peas; reduce heat to a simmer and cook for 5 minutes, stirring occasionally. Stir in bean sprouts, pepper, hot pepper flakes and drained pasta; cook for 3 minutes longer. Serve immediately.

Choices Per Serving

3 Carbohydrates
2 Meat & Alternatives

Nutritional Analysis Per Serving			
Calories	315	Fat, total	4 g
Carbohydrate	51 g	Fat, saturated	1 g
Fiber	4 g	Sodium	789 mg
Protein	21 g	Cholesterol	22 mg

Tips

A granulated sugar substitute can replace the brown sugar in this recipe and reduce the carbohydrate by about 5 g/serving.

The sodium or salt content of this recipe can be reduced to 413 mg by using a low-sodium soya sauce.

Make Ahead

Make sauce early in day and add steak to marinate in refrigerator until cooking time.

Rotini with Stir-fried Steak and Crisp Vegetables

½ lb	rotini	250 g
1½ tsp	vegetable oil	7 mL
1 cup	diced onions	250 mL
1 cup	chopped broccoli	250 mL
1 cup	snow peas	250 mL
½ cup	diced carrots	125 mL
8 oz	steak, sliced thinly	250 g
½ cup	sliced water chestnuts	125 mL

SAUCE

½ cup	hot water	125 mL
¼ cup	soya sauce	50 mL
2 tbsp	brown sugar	25 mL
2½ tsp	cornstarch	12 mL
1½ tsp	grated gingerroot (or ½ tsp/2 mL ground ginger)	7 mL
1 tsp	crushed garlic	5 mL

1. *Sauce:* In small bowl, combine water, soya sauce, sugar, cornstarch, ginger and garlic; set aside.

2. Cook rotini according to package directions or until firm to the bite. Drain and place in serving bowl.

3. Meanwhile, in nonstick skillet, heat oil; sauté onions, broccoli, snow peas and carrots almost until tendercrisp, approximately 5 minutes.

4. Add steak and water chestnuts; sauté for 1 minute. Add sauce; cook, stirring, just until beef is cooked, approximately 2 minutes. Pour over pasta and mix well.

Choices Per Serving

3½	Carbohydrates
2	Meat & Alternatives

Nutritional Analysis Per Serving

Calories	343	Fat, total	3 g
Carbohydrate	57 g	Fat, saturated	1 g
Fiber	4 g	Sodium	828 mg
Protein	20 g	Cholesterol	20 mg

Tips

Hoisin sauce can be found in Chinese food section of the grocery store.

Use any lean steak, such as rib-eye, porterhouse or filet tenderloin.

Hoisin sauce is a sweet sauce made from flour, soybeans, chili, red beans and vegetables. Although it adds ½ Carbohydrate choice to each portion, the wonderful flavor it lends is well worth it.

Make Ahead

Prepare sauce up to a day ahead, stirring before use.

Hoisin Beef, Red Peppers and Snow Peas over Fettuccine

12 oz	fettuccine	375 g
2 tsp	crushed garlic	10 mL
12 oz	sirloin steak cut into ½-inch (1 cm) strips	375 g
2 tsp	vegetable oil	10 mL
1 cup	thinly sliced sweet red peppers	250 mL
1 cup	snow peas, cut in half	250 mL
6 oz	sliced mushrooms	150 g
⅓ cup	chopped green onions	75 mL
¼ cup	sliced water chestnuts	50 mL

SAUCE

¾ cup	cold beef stock	175 mL
¼ cup	hoisin sauce	50 mL
2 tbsp	soya sauce	25 mL
1 tbsp	rice wine vinegar	15 mL
1 tbsp	cornstarch	15 mL
2 tsp	sesame oil	10 mL
2 tsp	minced gingerroot	10 mL

1. Cook pasta in boiling water according to package instructions or until firm to the bite. Drain and place in serving bowl.

2. *Make the sauce:* In small bowl, combine stock, hoisin sauce, soya sauce, rice wine vinegar, cornstarch, oil and gingerroot. Stir until smooth. Set aside.

3. In large nonstick skillet sprayed with vegetable spray, sauté garlic and steak just until beef is barely cooked, approximately 3 minutes. Drain and set beef aside.

Choices Per Serving

4 Carbohydrates

2 Meat & Alternatives

Nutritional Analysis Per Serving			
Calories	382	Fat, total	6 g
Carbohydrate	61 g	Fat, saturated	1 g
Fiber	3 g	Sodium	657 mg
Protein	20 g	Cholesterol	21 mg

4. In same skillet, heat oil; add red peppers and snow peas; sauté for 2 minutes. Add mushrooms, green onions and water chestnuts; sauté for 3 minutes. Add sauce and beef and simmer on medium heat until sauce thickens slightly, for 3 or 4 minutes, stirring constantly. Pour over pasta, and toss.

●●●●●●●●●●●●●●●

Tip

The good news about pork tenderloin is that it's very low in fat. The bad news is that its low fat content makes it susceptible to drying out when cooked. That's why you should always cook tenderloin quickly over high heat. Use it whole, sliced into medallions and pounded for scallopini, or cut into strips or cubes for stir-fries or kebabs. Keep in mind when shopping that the smaller the tenderloin, the more tender the meat.

Pork Tenderloin with Apricots and Bok Choy over Fettuccine

SAUCE

1 cup	beef stock or chicken stock	250 mL
¼ cup	Asian plum sauce	50 mL
3 tbsp	sweet tomato chili sauce	45 mL
1½ tbsp	light soya sauce	20 mL
2 tsp	cornstarch	10 mL
8 oz	pork tenderloin	250 g
1 cup	chopped onions	250 mL
1½ tsp	minced garlic	7 mL
1 tsp	minced gingerroot	5 mL
5 cups	sliced bok choy	1.25 L
¾ cup	chopped dried apricots	175 mL
12 oz	fettuccine	375 g

1. *Sauce:* In a bowl combine stock, plum sauce, chili sauce, soya sauce and cornstarch. Set aside.

2. In a nonstick frying pan sprayed with vegetable spray or on a preheated grill, cook pork tenderloin over medium-high heat, turning once, for 15 minutes or until cooked through.

3. Meanwhile, in a large nonstick frying pan sprayed with vegetable spray, cook onions, garlic and ginger over medium-high heat for 5 minutes or until softened. Add bok choy and apricots; cook for 3 minutes or until bok choy wilts. Add sauce; reduce heat to medium-low. Cook for 2 minutes or until thickened; remove from heat.

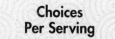

Choices Per Serving

4   Carbohydrates

1½ Meat & Alternatives

Nutritional Analysis Per Serving

Calories	344	Fat, total	2 g
Carbohydrate	62 g	Fat, saturated	1 g
Fiber	5 g	Sodium	276 mg
Protein	19 g	Cholesterol	23 mg

4. In a large pot of boiling water, cook fettuccine for 8 to 10 minutes or until tender but firm; drain. Slice pork tenderloin thinly crosswise. In a large serving bowl, combine pasta, sauce and pork; toss well. Serve immediately.

Tips

This recipe can be parceled into smaller portions that can be frozen for individual meals — just reheat in the microwave!

Whole wheat pasta is used here, but any type of pasta, such as vermicelli or spaghettini, can be substituted.

Speedy Singapore Noodles with Pork and Peppers

1 lb	pork tenderloin	500 g
1 tbsp	vegetable oil	15 mL
1	leek, white and light green part only, cut into thin strips	1
2	large cloves garlic, minced	2
1	red bell pepper, cut into thin strips	1
1	yellow bell pepper, cut into thin strips	1
1	green bell pepper, cut into thin strips	1
¾ cup	chicken stock	175 mL
1 tbsp	curry powder	15 mL
¼ cup	bottled oyster sauce	50 mL
2 tsp	cornstarch	10 mL
12 oz	whole-wheat spaghetti	375 g
¼ cup	chopped fresh coriander or parsley	50 mL

1. Cut pork into thin 2- by ¼-inch (5 cm by 5 mm) strips. In a wok or large nonstick skillet, heat oil over high heat. Brown meat on all sides; remove to a plate and set aside. Add leek, garlic, pepper strips, chicken stock and curry powder to skillet; cover and cook for 2 minutes. Stir in oyster sauce.

2. In a small dish, dissolve cornstarch in 1 tbsp (15 mL) water; add to skillet along with pork. Bring sauce to boil; cook, stirring, for 1 to 2 minutes or until pork is heated through.

3. Cook pasta in a large pot of boiling water until tender but firm. Drain well. Return to pot; stir in meat mixture and coriander. Toss to coat well in sauce.

Choices Per Serving

3½ Carbohydrates

3 Meat & Alternatives

Nutritional Analysis Per Serving

Calories	389	Fat, total	6 g
Carbohydrate	58 g	Fat, saturated	1 g
Fiber	6 g	Sodium	324 mg
Protein	29 g	Cholesterol	45 mg

Manicotti Shells Filled with Cheese and Smoked Salmon Bits *page 138*
Overleaf: Curried Chicken Coconut Pasta with Apricots and Cranberries *page 144*

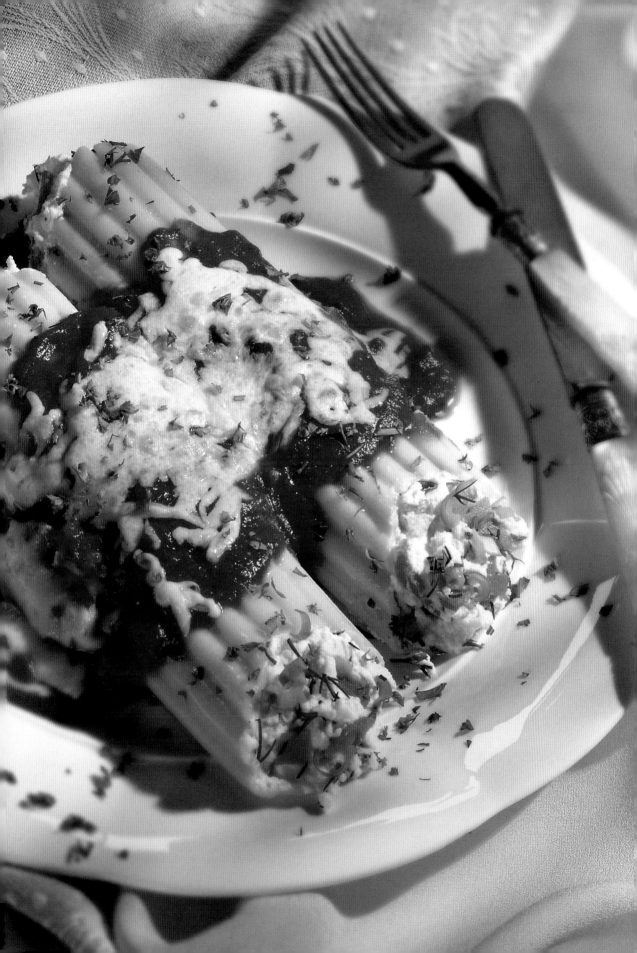

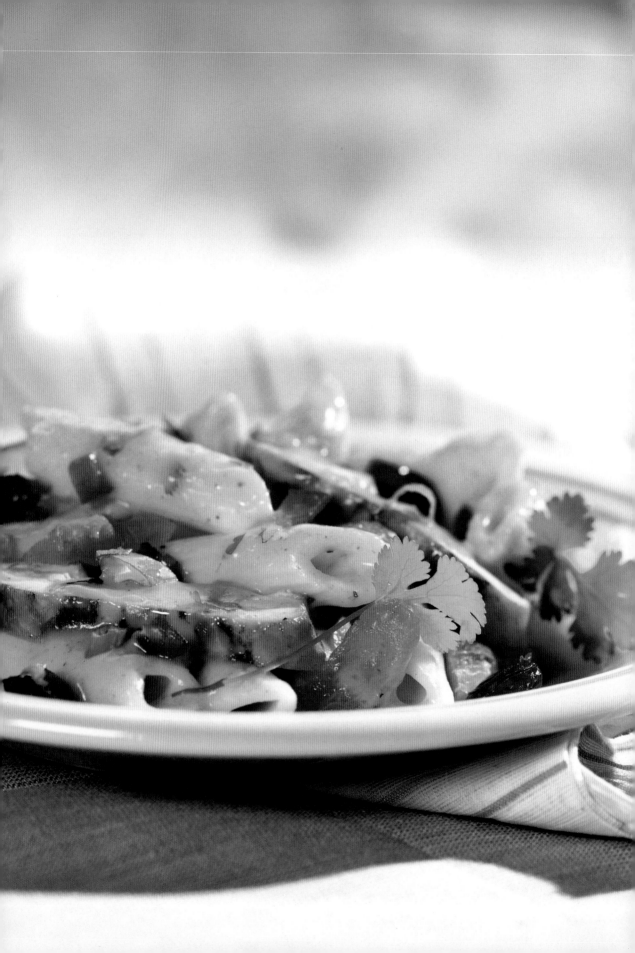

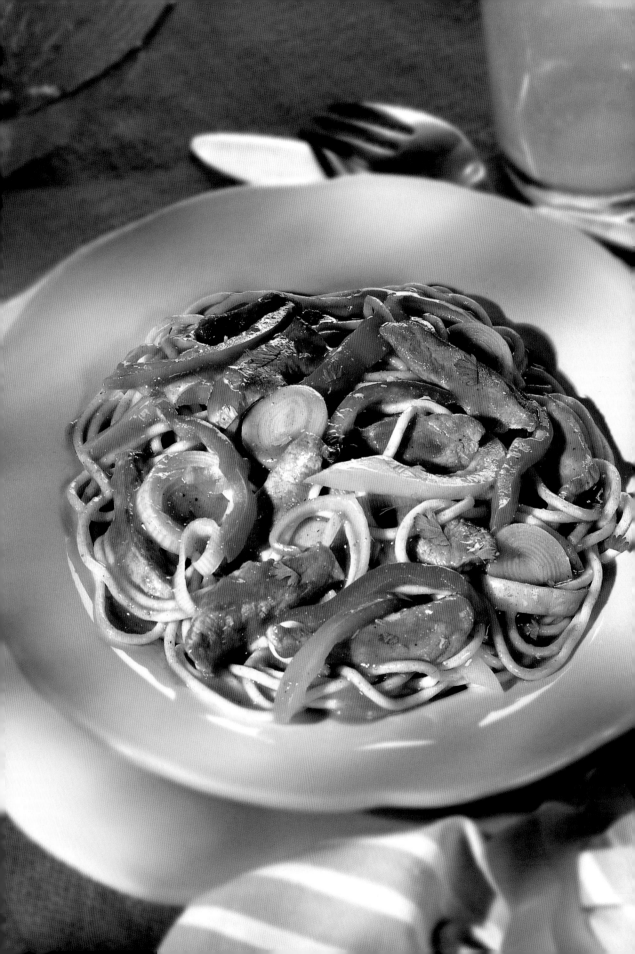

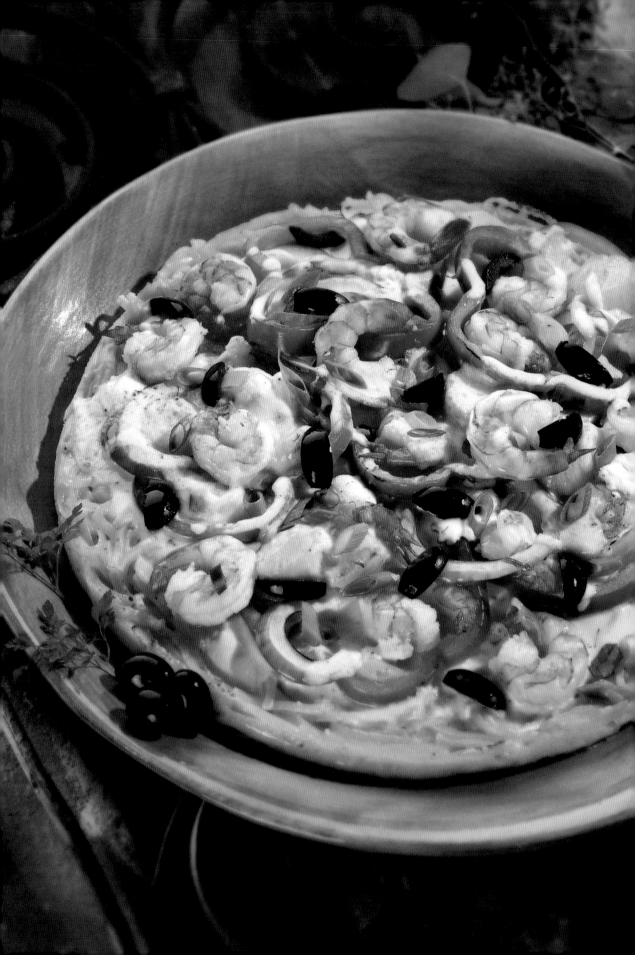

Preheat oven to
375°F (190°C)

9-inch (2.5 L) springform
pan sprayed with
vegetable spray

Tip

What's a pasta pizza?
Simple — a pizza with a
crust of pasta, not bread!
The success of this dish
depends on using the
sweetest onions you can
find. Try varieties such as
Spanish, Bermuda or
Vidalia. They're all
perfect — strong in flavor
but not as pungent as
standard yellow onions,
and sweet enough to be
eaten raw. Remember to
store onions in a dry, dark
and cool place; avoid
using plastic bags.

Pasta Pizza with Goat Cheese and Caramelized Onions

2	large sweet white onions (such as Spanish, Vidalia or Bermuda), sliced	2
2 tsp	minced garlic	10 mL
2 tbsp	packed brown sugar	25 mL
1 tbsp	balsamic vinegar	15 mL
6 oz	wide rice noodles, broken	175 g
1	large egg	1
⅓ cup	low-fat milk	75 mL
3 tbsp	grated low-fat Parmesan cheese	45 mL
2 oz	goat cheese	50 g

1. In a large nonstick saucepan sprayed with vegetable spray, cook onions and garlic over medium heat for 10 minutes. Add brown sugar and balsamic vinegar; reduce heat to medium-low. Cook, stirring occasionally, for 25 minutes or until golden brown and tender.

2. Meanwhile, in a large pot of boiling water, cook rice noodles for 5 minutes or until tender; drain. Rinse with cold water; drain well. In a bowl combine noodles, egg, milk and Parmesan cheese; stir well. Pour into prepared springform pan. Bake in preheated oven for 20 minutes; remove from oven. Set oven heat to broil.

3. Spread onion mixture over baked noodles; dot with goat cheese. Broil for 8 minutes or until cheese is melted.

**Choices
Per Serving**

2 Carbohydrates

½ Fat

Nutritional Analysis Per Serving			
Calories	180	Fat, total	3 g
Carbohydrate	32 g	Fat, saturated	2 g
Fiber	1 g	Sodium	101 mg
Protein	5 g	Cholesterol	42 mg

Seafood Pasta Pizza with Dill and Goat Cheese page 162
Overleaf: Speedy Singapore Noodles with Pork and Peppers page 160

Preheat oven to
350°F (180°C)

10- to 11-inch (3L)
springform pan sprayed
with vegetable spray

Tips

Small shell pasta or
broken spaghetti can be
substituted for linguine.

Instead of seafood, any
firm white fish fillets can
be used, such as orange
roughy, swordfish or
grouper.

Make Ahead

Crust can be made a
day ahead and covered.
Filling can be made
ahead; add more stock
if too thick.

Seafood Pasta Pizza with Dill and Goat Cheese

6 oz	broken linguine	150 g
1	egg	1
⅓ cup	2% milk	75 mL
3 tbsp	grated Parmesan cheese	45 mL
8 oz	seafood, cut in pieces or left whole (shrimp, scallops, squid)	250 g
1 tsp	vegetable oil	5 mL
1½ tsp	crushed garlic	7 mL
¾ cup	diced sweet red peppers	175 mL
¼ cup	chopped green onions	50 mL
¼ cup	sliced red onions	50 mL
1 cup	cold seafood or chicken stock	250 mL
1 cup	2% milk	250 mL
3 tbsp	all-purpose flour	45 mL
⅓ cup	chopped fresh dill (or 1 tbsp/15 mL dried)	75 mL
½ cup	shredded mozzarella cheese	125 mL
2 oz	goat cheese, crumbled	50 g

1. Cook pasta in boiling water according to package instructions or until firm to the bite. Drain and place in mixing bowl. Add egg, milk and cheese. Mix well. Pour into pan and bake for 20 minutes.

2. In large nonstick skillet sprayed with vegetable spray, sauté seafood just until cooked, approximately 3 minutes. Drain and set seafood aside.

3. In same skillet, heat oil; sauté garlic, red peppers and green and red onions for 4 minutes.

4. Meanwhile, in small bowl combine stock, milk and flour until smooth. Add to skillet and simmer on low heat until thickened, approximately 2 minutes, stirring constantly. Add dill and seafood. Pour into pan. Sprinkle with mozzarella and goat cheese; bake for 10 minutes. Let rest for 10 minutes before serving.

Nutritional Analysis Per Serving			
Calories	309	Fat, total	11 g
Carbohydrate	28 g	Fat, saturated	6 g
Fiber	1 g	Sodium	521 mg
Protein	24 g	Cholesterol	123 mg

Choices Per Serving

2	Carbohydrates
3	Meat & Alternatives

Fish and Seafood

Fish and seafood are excellent low-fat Meat & Alternatives servings. Research has shown that eating fish on a regular basis can be protective against cardiovascular disease. Fatty fish such as salmon and halibut are a good source of essential fatty acids.

What about seafood and cholesterol? Many people have expressed concern about the cholesterol content of shrimp, lobster, crab and other seafood. While some of these do contain cholesterol, we need to be more concerned about the intake of saturated fat in the diet. This means eating less processed meat.

My recommendation to people with diabetes is to choose fish and seafood regularly, as they are delicious and low in fat.

Preheat oven to
425°F (220°C)

Baking dish sprayed with
nonstick vegetable spray

Tips

This tasty recipe is higher
in carbohydrate than most
fish dishes. A granulated
sugar substitute can
replace the brown
sugar to reduce the
carbohydrate by about
5 g/serving.

Any white fish is suitable.
Try grouper, cod, halibut
or haddock.

Fish Fillets with Apples, Raisins and Pecans

1 lb	firm white fish fillets	500 g
1 tbsp	margarine	15 mL
1 cup	chopped peeled apples	250 mL
⅓ cup	raisins	75 mL
¼ cup	chopped pecans or walnuts	50 mL
4 tsp	brown sugar	20 mL
½ tsp	cinnamon	2 mL
1 tbsp	all-purpose flour	15 mL
1 cup	apple juice	250 mL

1. Place fish in single layer in baking dish.

2. In nonstick skillet, melt margarine; sauté apples,
raisins, pecans, sugar and cinnamon for 3 minutes
or until apples are tender.

3. Mix flour with apple juice until dissolved; add to pan and
cook until thickened, stirring constantly, 2 to 3 minutes.

4. Pour sauce over fish; cover and bake for approximately
15 minutes or until fish flakes easily when tested
with fork.

Choices
Per Serving

2	Carbohydrates
3	Meat & Alternatives

Nutritional Analysis Per Serving			
Calories	298	Fat, total	12 g
Carbohydrate	33 g	Fat, saturated	1 g
Fiber	2 g	Sodium	98 mg
Protein	23 g	Cholesterol	42 mg

Preheat broiler

Baking dish sprayed with vegetable spray

Tips

After broiling pepper, put in small bowl and cover tightly with plastic wrap; this allows the skin to be removed easily.

The fresh pepper can be replaced with 4 oz (125 g) sweet pepper packed in water in a jar.

Roasted corn gives an exceptional flavor in this recipe. Either barbecue or broil until just cooked and charred, along with pepper. Remove kernels with a sharp knife.

Make Ahead

Prepare salsa earlier in the day and refrigerate.

Fish Fillets with Corn and Red Pepper Salsa

SALSA

1	large red pepper	1
1½ cups	corn kernels	375 mL
⅓ cup	chopped red onions	75 mL
¼ cup	chopped fresh coriander	50 mL
2 tbsp	fresh lime or lemon juice	25 mL
3 tsp	olive oil	15 mL
2 tsp	minced garlic	7 mL
1 lb	fish fillets	500 g

1. *Salsa:* Broil red pepper for 15 to 20 minutes, turning occasionally, until charred on all sides. Remove pepper and set oven at 425°F (220°C). When pepper is cool, remove skin, seeds and stem. Chop and put in small bowl along with corn, onions, coriander, lime juice, 2 tsp (10 mL) of olive oil and 1 tsp (5 mL) of the garlic; mix well.

2. Put fish in single layer in prepared baking dish and brush with remaining 1 tsp (5 mL) garlic and 1 tsp (5 mL) oil. Bake uncovered for 10 minutes per inch (2.5 cm) thickness of fish or until fish flakes easily when pierced with a fork. Serve with salsa.

Choices Per Serving

1	Carbohydrate
3½	Meat & Alternatives

Nutritional Analysis Per Serving

Calories	218	Fat, total	5 g
Carbohydrate	21 g	Fat, saturated	1 g
Fiber	3 g	Sodium	87 mg
Protein	24 g	Cholesterol	65 mg

Preheat oven to
400°F (200°C)

8-inch (2 L) square
baking dish sprayed with
vegetable spray

Tips

Salmon, trout or
whitefish is ideal. Ask
to have fish butterflied,
scaled and deboned.

At 5½ Meat & Alternatives
choices, this recipe may
be more than the regular
amount of protein you
would choose at meal
time. To compensate,
you may choose to
reduce the amount of
Meat & Alternatives
servings at another meal
to maintain the same
total energy intake.

This cornbread stuffing
is also ideal for chicken
or turkey.

Make Ahead

Prepare entire stuffing
with vegetables up to
one day in advance.

Fish with Cornbread and Dill Stuffing

CORNBREAD

½ cup	cornmeal	125 mL
½ cup	all-purpose flour	125 mL
1½ tbsp	granulated sugar	20 mL
1½ tsp	baking powder	7 mL
¾ cup	2% yogurt	175 mL
¾ cup	corn kernels	175 mL
1	egg	1
1½ tbsp	melted margarine or butter	20 mL
2 tsp	vegetable oil	10 mL
1½ tsp	minced garlic	7 mL
1 cup	chopped onions	250 mL
1 cup	sliced mushrooms	250 mL
1 cup	chopped green or red peppers	250 mL
¼ cup	chopped fresh dill (or 2 tsp/10 mL dried)	50 mL
1	whole 2-lb (1 kg) fish, rinsed under cold water	1
1 tsp	vegetable oil	5 mL
1 tsp	minced garlic	5 mL
⅓ cup	chicken stock or water	75 mL
⅓ cup	white wine	75 mL

1. In large bowl stir together cornmeal, flour, sugar and
baking powder. In another bowl combine yogurt, corn,
egg and margarine. Add the wet ingredients to the dry
ingredients and stir just until combined. Pour batter
into prepared pan and bake for 15 to 18 minutes or until
cake tester inserted in center comes out clean.

Choices Per Serving

2½ Carbohydrates

5½ Meat & Alternatives

Nutritional Analysis Per Serving			
Calories	471	Fat, total	13 g
Carbohydrate	40 g	Fat, saturated	2 g
Fiber	2 g	Sodium	249 mg
Protein	45 g	Cholesterol	104 mg

2. In nonstick skillet sprayed with vegetable spray, heat oil over medium heat. Add garlic and onion and cook for 4 minutes or until softened. Add mushrooms and peppers and cook for 5 minutes or until vegetables are tender. Stir in dill and remove from heat.

3. Crumble the cooled cornbread into a large bowl. Add vegetable mixture and combine thoroughly. Stuff half of the mixture into fish. Place remaining mixture in dish and serve warmed with fish. Place fish in baking pan sprayed with vegetable spray and brush fish with oil and garlic. Pour stock and wine into pan. Cover and bake for 35 to 45 minutes or until fish flakes easily when pierced with a fork.

Tips

Try to make the relish as close to the time of serving as possible; otherwise the cucumber will make the sauce too watery.

Use cod, snapper or haddock.

Use 1½ tsp (7 mL) dried dill if fresh is unavailable.

The flatter the fish, the faster it cooks.

• • • • • • • • • • • • • • •

Make Ahead

Prepare fish early in the day and keep refrigerated until ready to bake.

Crunchy Fish with Cucumber Dill Relish

RELISH

2 cups	finely chopped cucumbers	500 mL
⅓ cup	chopped fresh dill	75 mL
⅓ cup	2% yogurt	75 mL
¼ cup	finely diced green onions (about 2 medium)	50 mL
¼ cup	finely diced green peppers	50 mL
3 tbsp	light mayonnaise	45 mL
1 tsp	minced garlic	5 mL

CRUNCHY FISH

2 cups	corn flakes	500 mL
1 tbsp	grated Parmesan cheese	15 mL
1 tsp	minced garlic	5 mL
½ tsp	dried basil	2 mL
1	egg	1
3 tbsp	2% milk	45 mL
3 tbsp	all-purpose flour	45 mL
1 lb	firm white fish fillets	500 g
1 tbsp	margarine or butter	15 mL

1. *Relish:* In bowl, combine cucumbers, dill, yogurt, green onions, green peppers, mayonnaise and garlic; mix to combine and set aside.

2. Put corn flakes, Parmesan, garlic and basil in food processor; process until fine and put on a plate. In shallow bowl whisk together egg and milk. Dust fish with flour.

3. Dip fish fillets in egg wash, then coat with crumb mixture. In large nonstick skillet sprayed with vegetable spray, melt margarine over medium heat. Add fillets and cook for 5 minutes or until browned, turn and cook for 2 minutes longer, or until fish is browned and flakes easily when pierced with a fork. Serve topped with cucumber dill relish.

Choices Per Serving

1½ Carbohydrates

3½ Meat & Alternatives

Nutritional Analysis Per Serving			
Calories	305	Fat, total	10 g
Carbohydrate	23 g	Fat, saturated	2 g
Fiber	2 g	Sodium	354 mg
Protein	30 g	Cholesterol	131 mg

Tips

Don't overcook the vegetables in this main course dish; they should still retain their bright color and texture.

Saffron makes this stew special; you can, however, eliminate the saffron and substitute chopped fresh dill for the parsley.

Leek and Halibut Ragout

2 tbsp	olive oil	25 mL
2	medium leeks, white and light green part only, chopped	2
2	cloves garlic, finely chopped	2
2 tbsp	all-purpose flour	25 mL
2½ cups	fish stock (see recipe, page 54) or chicken stock	625 mL
½ cup	white wine or additional stock	125 mL
¼ tsp	saffron threads, crushed	1 mL
2 cups	diced peeled potatoes	500 mL
2	medium carrots, peeled and diagonally sliced	2
2	small zucchini, halved lengthwise and sliced	2
1	small sweet red pepper, diced	1
1½ lbs	halibut, trimmed and cut into 1-inch (2.5 cm) cubes	750 g
	Salt and pepper	
¼ cup	chopped fresh parsley	50 mL

1. In a large saucepan, heat oil over medium heat; add leeks and garlic; cook, stirring often, for 5 minutes or until tender. (Do not let leeks brown.)

2. Stir in flour; add stock, wine and saffron. Bring to a boil, stirring, until thickened. Add potatoes and carrots; reduce heat to medium-low and simmer, covered, for 15 minutes. Stir in zucchini and red pepper; cook 5 minutes more or until vegetables are just tender.

3. Add halibut; cook for 3 to 5 minutes more or until fish is opaque. Adjust seasoning with salt and pepper to taste. Sprinkle with parsley; ladle into warmed wide shallow bowls.

Choices Per Serving

1½ Carbohydrates
3½ Meat & Alternatives

Nutritional Analysis Per Serving

Calories	310	Fat, total	8 g
Carbohydrate	27 g	Fat, saturated	1 g
Fiber	3 g	Sodium	388 mg
Protein	29 g	Cholesterol	36 mg

Preheat oven to
400°F (200°C)

Baking dish sprayed with
nonstick vegetable spray

Tips

Other white fish, such as
sole, flounder or turbot,
can be substituted.

If using a thin piece of
fish, you can probably
skip the baking time.
The fish will cook
through in the skillet.

Toast pecans either in
400°F (200°C) oven or in
skillet on top of stove for
2 minutes or until brown.

Halibut with Lemon and Pecans

½ cup	bread crumbs	125 mL
1 tsp	dried parsley	5 mL
½ tsp	dried basil	2 mL
½ tsp	crushed garlic	2 mL
1½ tsp	grated Parmesan cheese	7 mL
1 lb	halibut, cut into 4 serving-sized pieces	500 g
1	egg white	1
2 tbsp	margarine	25 mL
2 tbsp	white wine	25 mL
4 tsp	lemon juice	20 mL
1 tbsp	chopped fresh parsley	15 mL
1	green onion, chopped	1
1 tbsp	chopped pecans, toasted	15 mL

1. In shallow dish, combine bread crumbs, dried parsley, basil, garlic and cheese. Dip fish pieces into egg white, then into bread crumb mixture.

2. In large nonstick skillet, melt 1 tbsp (15 mL) of the margarine; add fish and cook just until browned on both sides. Transfer fish to baking dish and bake for 5 to 10 minutes or until fish flakes easily when tested with fork. Remove to serving platter and keep warm.

3. To skillet, add remaining margarine, wine, lemon juice, parsley, onions and pecans; cook for 1 minute. Pour over fish.

Choices Per Serving

1   Carbohydrate
4   Meat & Alternatives

Nutritional Analysis Per Serving			
Calories	275	Fat, total	11 g
Carbohydrate	13 g	Fat, saturated	2 g
Fiber	1 g	Sodium	274 mg
Protein	29 g	Cholesterol	41 mg

Preheat oven to
425°F (220°C)

Baking sheet sprayed
with nonstick
vegetable spray

Tips

When making the pesto,
use only parsley or only
coriander leaves for
an unusual taste.

Salmon is a good source
of Omega-3 fatty acids.
Eating fatty fish high
in Omega-3's weekly is
recommended.

This nutrient packed
recipe provides an
excellent source of
Vitamin D, phosphorus,
and the B vitamins
niacin, B_6 and B_{12}. It
is also a good source of
magnesium, vitamin C
and pantothenic acid.

Salmon with Pesto

1 lb	salmon steaks or fillet, cut into 4 serving-sized portions	500 g
1 tsp	vegetable oil	5 mL
1 tsp	lemon juice	5 mL
1 tsp	crushed garlic	5 mL
¼ cup	Pesto Sauce (recipe, page 118)	50 mL

1. Place salmon on baking sheet; brush with oil, lemon
juice and garlic. Bake approximately 10 minutes or just
until fish flakes easily when tested with fork.

2. Top each serving with 1 tbsp (15 mL) Pesto Sauce.

Choices Per Serving

4 Meat & Alternatives

Nutritional Analysis Per Serving

Calories	231	Fat, total	14 g
Carbohydrate	1 g	Fat, saturated	3 g
Fiber	0 g	Sodium	103 mg
Protein	26 g	Cholesterol	67 mg

Tips

To store gingerroot, peel it, place in glass jar and add white wine or sherry to cover. As an added bonus, you can use the ginger-infused wine or sherry to flavor other fish or chicken dishes, or stir-fries.

One of the best uses for the microwave in my kitchen is for quickly cooking fish such as this salmon. Arrange fish and sauce in a shallow baking dish and cover with microwave-safe plastic wrap; turn back one corner to vent. Microwave at Medium for 4 minutes. Turn fish over and re-cover; microwave at Medium for 3 to 5 minutes more or until salmon turns opaque.

This fish dish is also great to cook on the barbecue.

Salmon with Lemon-Ginger Sauce

MARINADE

2	green onions	2
1½ tsp	minced fresh gingerroot	7 mL
1	clove garlic, minced	1
2 tbsp	low-sodium soya sauce	25 mL
1 tbsp	fresh lemon juice	15 mL
1 tsp	grated lemon rind	5 mL
1 tsp	granulated sugar	5 mL
1 tsp	sesame oil	5 mL
4	salmon fillets, 5 oz (150 g) each	4

1. *Marinade:* Chop green onions; set aside chopped green tops for garnish. In a bowl combine white part of onions, gingerroot, garlic, soya sauce, lemon juice and rind, sugar and sesame oil.

2. Place salmon fillets in a single layer in a shallow baking dish. Pour marinade over; let stand at room temperature for 15 minutes or in the refrigerator for up to 1 hour.

3. Bake, uncovered, in preheated oven for 13 to 15 minutes or until salmon turns opaque. Arrange on serving plates, spoon sauce over and sprinkle with green onion tops.

Choices Per Serving

4   Meat & Alternatives

Nutritional Analysis Per Serving

Calories	237	Fat, total	11 g
Carbohydrate	3 g	Fat, saturated	2 g
Fiber	0 g	Sodium	293 mg
Protein	31 g	Cholesterol	83 mg

Salmon and Potato Strata

Tips

Potato slices replace the usual bread in this homey and economical main dish.

Canned salmon with the bones makes this dish an excellent source of calcium. It is also an excellent source of vitamins A, D, B$_6$ and B$_{12}$, as well as phosphorus, iron, magnesium and zinc.

1	can (7½ oz/213 g) red sockeye salmon	1
2	stalks celery, sliced	2
1	onion, chopped	1
4	eggs	4
1⅓ cups	milk	325 mL
¾ tsp	paprika	4 mL
¾ tsp	salt, optional	4 mL
½ tsp	pepper	2 mL
½ tsp	dried tarragon	2 mL
4	potatoes, peeled and thinly sliced	4
½ cup	dry bread crumbs	125 mL
¼ cup	chopped fresh parsley	50 mL
2 tbsp	margarine or butter, cut in bits	25 mL

1. In large bowl, mash salmon with juices and bones; stir in celery, onion, eggs, milk, paprika, optional ½ tsp (2 mL) salt, pepper and tarragon until well mixed.

2. In greased 8-cup (2 L) casserole, arrange half of the potato slices; sprinkle with optional remaining salt. Pour salmon mixture over top; layer with remaining potato slices.

3. Stir together crumbs and parsley, sprinkle on potatoes. Dot with butter. Bake, uncovered, in 350°F (180°C) oven for 1 hour and 15 minutes or until potatoes are tender.

Choices Per Serving

2	Carbohydrates
2½	Meat & Alternatives
1	Fat

Nutritional Analysis Per Serving			
Calories	397	Fat, total	17 g
Carbohydrate	38 g	Fat, saturated	4 g
Fiber	3 g	Sodium	500 mg
Protein	23 g	Cholesterol	230 mg

Preheat oven to
425°F (220°C)

Tips

Serve with boiled new
potatoes, leaving the
skin on.

Select broccoli with tight
green heads on numerous
firm stalks, rather than
one or two stalks.

Fresh cauliflower can
replace the broccoli.

Red Snapper with Broccoli and Dill Cheese Sauce

2 cups	chopped broccoli florets	500 mL
1 lb	red snapper (or any firm fish fillets)	500 g
1 tbsp	margarine	15 mL
1 tbsp	all-purpose flour	15 mL
1 cup	2% milk	250 mL
1/3 cup	shredded Cheddar cheese	75 mL
2 tbsp	chopped fresh dill (or 1/2 tsp/2 mL dried dillweed)	25 mL
	Salt and pepper	

1. In boiling water, blanch broccoli until still crisp and color brightens; drain and place in baking dish. Place fish in single layer over top.

2. In small saucepan, melt margarine; add flour and cook, stirring, for 1 minute. Add milk and cook, stirring constantly, until thickened, approximately 3 minutes. Stir in cheese, dill, and salt and pepper to taste until cheese has melted; pour over fish.

3. Bake, uncovered, for 15 to 20 minutes or until fish flakes easily when tested with fork.

Choices Per Serving

1/2   Carbohydrate

4 1/2   Meat & Alternatives

Nutritional Analysis Per Serving

Calories	306	Fat, total	15 g
Carbohydrate	7 g	Fat, saturated	6 g
Fiber	1 g	Sodium	303 mg
Protein	34 g	Cholesterol	100 mg

Start barbecue or
preheat oven to
425°F (220°C)

Tips

Any firm fish can be
substituted.

Try tuna or shark. Parsley
or dill can be substituted
for coriander.

This salsa can be used
over chicken or pork.

Make Ahead

Make salsa early in the
day and refrigerate.

Swordfish with Mango Coriander Salsa

1½ lbs	swordfish steaks	750 g
1 tsp	vegetable oil	5 mL

SALSA

1½ cups	finely diced mango or peach	375 mL
¾ cup	finely diced red peppers	175 mL
½ cup	finely diced green peppers	125 mL
½ cup	finely diced red onions	125 mL
¼ cup	chopped fresh coriander	50 mL
2 tbsp	lemon juice	25 mL
2 tsp	olive oil	10 mL
1 tsp	minced garlic	5 mL

1. Brush fish with 1 tsp (5 mL) of oil on both sides.
   Barbecue or bake fish for 10 minutes per inch (2.5 cm)
   thickness, or until it flakes easily when pierced with
   a fork.

2. Meanwhile, in bowl combine mango, red peppers, green
   peppers, red onions, coriander, lemon juice, olive oil
   and garlic; mix thoroughly. Serve over fish.

Choices Per Serving

½ Carbohydrate

3½ Meat & Alternatives

Nutritional Analysis Per Serving			
Calories	219	Fat, total	8 g
Carbohydrate	12 g	Fat, saturated	2 g
Fiber	2 g	Sodium	111 mg
Protein	26 g	Cholesterol	49 mg

Tips

Imitation crab is less expensive than real crab meat. However, real crab (or cooked, chopped shrimp) can also be used. This dish can be served as an appetizer or as an entrée.

Both the imitation crab and seasoned dried bread crumbs are significant sources of sodium in this recipe. You can reduce this by using plain dry bread crumbs.

Make Ahead

Prepare crab mixture and sauce earlier in the day. They can also be cooked in advance and gently reheated.

Sautéed Crab Cakes with Chunky Dill Tartar Sauce

½ tsp	vegetable oil	2 tsp
1 tsp	minced garlic	5 mL
½ cup	chopped onions	125 mL
12 oz	imitation crab (sea legs, Krab legs or Krab flakes)	375 g
⅔ cup	seasoned bread crumbs	150 mL
¼ cup	chopped fresh dill (or 2 tsp/10 mL dried)	50 mL
1	whole egg	1
1	egg white	1
2 tbsp	light mayonnaise	25 mL
2 tsp	lemon juice	10 mL
1 tbsp	margarine or butter	15 mL

CHUNKY DILL TARTAR SAUCE

3 tbsp	light mayonnaise	45 mL
3 tbsp	light sour cream	45 mL
2 tbsp	finely chopped green peppers	25 mL
2 tbsp	finely chopped red onions	25 mL
2 tbsp	chopped fresh dill (or ½ tsp/2 mL dried)	25 mL
2 tsp	lemon juice	10 mL

1. Heat oil in small nonstick skillet over medium heat; add garlic and onions and cook for 5 minutes or until softened. Put in food processor along with crab, bread crumbs, dill, whole egg, egg white, mayonnaise and lemon juice. Pulse on and off until finely chopped. Form each ⅓ cup (75 mL) into a patty.

Choices Per Serving

1½ Carbohydrates

2½ Meat & Alternatives

Nutritional Analysis Per Serving

Calories	272	Fat, total	11 g
Carbohydrate	20 g	Fat, saturated	2 g
Fiber	1 g	Sodium	1336 mg
Protein	22 g	Cholesterol	98 mg

2. *Sauce:* In small bowl combine mayonnaise, sour cream, green peppers, onions, dill and lemon juice; set aside.

3. Melt margarine in large nonstick skillet sprayed with vegetable spray over medium heat. Add crab cakes and cook for 6 minutes, or until golden; turn and cook for 6 minutes longer, or until golden and hot. Serve with chunky dill tartar sauce.

Mussels with Tomatoes, Basil and Garlic

SERVES 4

Tips

When you're buying mussels, the shells should be tightly closed.

Fresh juicy tomatoes are excellent when in season.

Substitute clams for the mussels.

An excellent source of vitamin B$_{12}$, this recipe also is a good source of iron and vitamin C. The body will absorb more iron when vitamin C is present.

2 lb	mussels	1 kg
1½ tsp	vegetable oil	7 mL
½ cup	finely diced onions	125 mL
2 tsp	crushed garlic	10 mL
1	can (14 oz/398 mL) tomatoes, drained and chopped	1
⅓ cup	dry white wine	75 mL
1 tbsp	chopped fresh basil (or ½ tsp/2 mL dried)	15 mL
1½ tsp	chopped fresh oregano (or ¼ tsp/1 mL dried)	7 mL

1. Scrub mussels under cold water; pull off hairy beards. Discard any that do not close when tapped. Set aside.

2. In large nonstick saucepan, heat oil; sauté onions and garlic for 2 minutes. Add tomatoes, wine, basil and oregano; cook for 3 minutes, stirring constantly.

3. Add mussels; cover and cook until mussels fully open, 4 to 5 minutes. Discard any that do not open. Arrange mussels in bowls; pour sauce over top.

Choices Per Serving

½   Carbohydrate

1   Meat & Alternative

Nutritional Analysis Per Serving

Calories	117	Fat, total	3 g
Carbohydrate	12 g	Fat, saturated	0 g
Fiber	2 g	Sodium	421 mg
Protein	8 g	Cholesterol	15 mg

Shrimp or squid can
be used in place of
the scallops, or try a
combination of the two.

Serve on a bed of
wild rice or couscous.
Complete the meal with
a dessert of sliced kiwi
or ½ cup (125 mL) of
blueberries topped with
a low-fat no-sugar-added
vanilla yogurt.

Scallops with Basil Tomato Sauce

1 tbsp	margarine	15 mL
3/4 cup	chopped onions	175 mL
1 tsp	crushed garlic	5 mL
3/4 cup	diced sweet green pepper	175 mL
3/4 cup	sliced mushrooms	175 mL
2 tsp	all-purpose flour	10 mL
1 cup	2% milk	250 mL
2 tbsp	tomato paste	25 mL
1¼ tsp	dried basil (or 2 tbsp/25 mL chopped fresh)	6 mL
1 lb	scallops, sliced in half if large	500 g
1 tbsp	grated Parmesan cheese	15 mL

1. In large nonstick skillet, melt margarine; sauté onions, garlic, green pepper and mushrooms until softened, approximately 5 minutes. Stir in flour and cook for 1 minute, stirring.

2. Add milk, tomato paste and basil; cook, stirring continuously, until thickened, 2 to 3 minutes.

3. Add scallops; cook just until opaque, 2 to 3 minutes. Place on serving dish; sprinkle with Parmesan cheese.

Choices
Per Serving

1   Carbohydrate

2½ Meat & Alternatives

Nutritional Analysis Per Serving

Calories	216	Fat, total	6 g
Carbohydrate	16 g	Fat, saturated	2 g
Fiber	2 g	Sodium	290 mg
Protein	25 g	Cholesterol	47 mg

· · · · · · · · · · · · · · · · · ·

Tips

There are many combinations of seafood that can be used. A more economical version can be made by combining a firm white fish such as cod, grouper or halibut with some of the seafood.

Freeze shrimp with their shells to preserve the best taste.

Shrimp and Scallops with Cheesy Cream Sauce

1 tbsp	margarine	15 mL
1 tsp	crushed garlic	5 mL
⅓ cup	chopped green onions	75 mL
1 lb	seafood (shrimp, scallops or combination)	500 g
¼ cup	chopped fresh parsley	50 mL
2 oz	goat or feta cheese, crumbled	50 g

SAUCE

1 tbsp	margarine	15 mL
2½ tsp	all-purpose flour	12 mL
⅓ cup	dry white wine	75 mL
½ cup	2% milk	125 mL

1. *Sauce:* In small saucepan, melt margarine; stir in flour and cook, stirring, for 1 minute. Add wine and milk; cook, stirring, until thickened and smooth, approximately 2 minutes. Set aside and keep warm.

2. In nonstick skillet, melt margarine; sauté garlic, green onions and seafood just until seafood is opaque. Remove from stove; add sauce and mix well.

3. Pour into serving dish; sprinkle parsley and cheese over top.

Choices Per Serving

4   Meat & Alternatives

Nutritional Analysis Per Serving			
Calories	260	Fat, total	12 g
Carbohydrate	5 g	Fat, saturated	4 g
Fiber	0 g	Sodium	316 mg
Protein	30 g	Cholesterol	199 mg

Tip

If you haven't got the time or ingredients necessary to make seafood stock from scratch, you can buy it canned or in powdered form (1 tsp/ 5 mL in 1 cup/250 mL boiling water yields 1 cup/250 mL stock). Keep in mind, however, that these stocks are often loaded with sodium. To cut back on the sodium, try using only ½ tsp (2 mL) powder.

Shrimp Risotto with Artichoke Hearts and Parmesan

3 cups	seafood stock (see fish stock, page 54) or chicken stock	750 mL
½ cup	chopped onions	125 mL
2 tsp	minced garlic	10 mL
1 cup	Arborio rice (risotto rice)	250 mL
1 tsp	dried basil	5 mL
Half	can (14 oz/398 mL) artichoke hearts, drained and chopped	Half
8 oz	raw shrimp, shelled and chopped	250 g
¼ cup	chopped green onions	50 mL
¼ cup	grated low-fat Parmesan cheese	50 mL
¼ tsp	freshly ground black pepper	1 mL

1. In a saucepan over medium-high heat, bring stock to a boil; reduce heat to low. In another nonstick saucepan sprayed with vegetable spray, cook onions and garlic over medium-high heat for 3 minutes or until softened. Add rice and basil; cook for 1 minute.

2. Using a ladle, add ½ cup (125 mL) stock to rice; stir to keep rice from sticking to pan. When liquid is absorbed, add another ½ cup (125 mL) stock. Reduce heat if necessary to maintain a slow, steady simmer. Repeat this process, ladling in hot stock and stirring constantly, for 15 minutes, reducing amount of stock added to ¼ cup (50 mL) near end of cooking time.

3. Add artichokes and shrimp; cook, adding more stock as necessary, for 3 minutes or until shrimp turn pink and rice is tender but firm. Add green onions, Parmesan cheese and pepper. Serve immediately.

Choices Per Serving

3 Carbohydrates

2 Meat & Alternatives

Nutritional Analysis Per Serving			
Calories	288	Fat, total	2 g
Carbohydrate	49 g	Fat, saturated	0 g
Fiber	2 g	Sodium	254 mg
Protein	19 g	Cholesterol	91 mg

Tips

The shrimp can be replaced with scallops or a combination of both.

This delicious recipe is chock full of nutrients too. It is an excellent source of magnesium, phosphorus, iron, niacin, and vitamins A, B_{12} and C and a good source of zinc, vitamin B_6 and folic acid.

Chinese Shrimp Sauté with Green Onions and Pecans

1½ cups	chopped broccoli florets	375 mL
1½ cups	snow peas, trimmed	375 mL
⅔ cup	chicken stock	150 mL
2 tbsp	hoisin sauce	25 mL
1 tbsp	cornstarch	15 mL
1 tsp	minced gingerroot (or ½ tsp/2 mL ground)	5 mL
1 tbsp	olive oil	15 mL
1½ tsp	crushed garlic	7 mL
¾ cup	chopped sweet red pepper	175 mL
1 lb	medium shrimp, peeled and deveined	500 g
1 tbsp	chopped pecans	15 mL
1	green onion, finely chopped	1

1. Blanch broccoli and snow peas in boiling water just until color brightens; drain and set aside.

2. Combine chicken stock, hoisin sauce, cornstarch and ginger until mixed. Set aside.

3. In large skillet, heat oil; sauté garlic and red pepper for 2 minutes. Add shrimp and hoisin mixture; sauté just until shrimp turns pink and sauce thickens. Add broccoli, snow peas and pecans; toss well. Sprinkle with green onions.

Choices Per Serving

1 Carbohydrate

4 Meat & Alternatives

Nutritional Analysis Per Serving

Calories	245	Fat, total	8 g
Carbohydrate	15 g	Fat, saturated	1 g
Fiber	3 g	Sodium	535 mg
Protein	29 g	Cholesterol	190 mg

Poultry

Chicken is a lean meat that goes well with a variety of vegetables and tastes. A low-fat Meat & Alternatives choice, boneless skinless chicken breasts are the basis for the majority of the recipes. In fact, one roasted 3 oz (100 g) boneless skinless chicken breast contains only 2.1 g of fat (or less than $\frac{1}{2}$ tsp/2 mL) and is a source of more than 10 vitamins and minerals. The mouth-watering recipes which follow provide some new alternatives to "traditional" chicken meals and are sure to become some of your family favorites.

Tips

Tender beef or veal can replace the chicken.

Serve over a bed of rice and with a low-fat Milk & Alternative choice to make this a complete meal.

An excellent source of vitamin C, niacin and vitamin B_6.

Chicken, Red Pepper and Snow Pea Stir-fry

SAUCE

½ cup	chicken stock	125 mL
1 tbsp	soya sauce	15 mL
1 tbsp	hoisin sauce	15 mL
2 tsp	cornstarch	10 mL
1 tsp	minced gingerroot	5 mL
8 oz	boneless skinless chicken breasts, cubed	250 g
	All-purpose flour for dusting	
1 tbsp	vegetable oil	15 mL
1 tsp	sesame oil	5 mL
1 tsp	crushed garlic	5 mL
1 cup	thinly sliced sweet red pepper	250 mL
1 cup	sliced water chestnuts	250 mL
1 cup	snow peas, cut in half	250 mL
¼ cup	cashews, coarsely chopped	50 mL
1	large green onion, chopped	1

1. *Sauce:* In small bowl, mix together stock, soya sauce, hoisin sauce, cornstarch and ginger; set aside.

2. Dust chicken cubes with flour. In nonstick skillet, heat vegetable and sesame oils; sauté garlic, chicken, red pepper, water chestnuts and snow peas over high heat just until vegetables are tender-crisp, approximately 2 minutes.

3. Add sauce to skillet; cook for 2 minutes or just until chicken is no longer pink inside and sauce has thickened. Garnish with cashews and green onions.

Choices Per Serving

1 Carbohydrate

2 Meat & Alternatives

Nutritional Analysis Per Serving			
Calories	240	Fat, total	10 g
Carbohydrate	21 g	Fat, saturated	2 g
Fiber	2 g	Sodium	430 mg
Protein	17 g	Cholesterol	32 mg

Tip

If you have time, let
the chicken marinate
for several hours or
overnight in the
refrigerator to intensify
the flavors. To avoid
bacterial contamination,
baste the chicken only
once, halfway through
cooking, then discard
any leftover marinade.

Indian-Style Grilled Chicken Breasts

½ cup	plain low-fat yogurt	125 mL
1 tbsp	tomato paste	15 mL
2	green onions, coarsely chopped	2
2	cloves garlic, quartered	2
1	piece (1-inch/2.5 cm) peeled ginger root, coarsely chopped (or 1 tsp/5 mL ground ginger)	1
½ tsp	ground cumin	2 mL
½ tsp	ground coriander	2 mL
½ tsp	salt	2 mL
¼ tsp	cayenne pepper	1 mL
4	chicken breasts (bone-in)	4
2 tbsp	chopped fresh coriander or parsley	25 mL

1. In a food processor, combine yogurt, tomato paste, green onions, garlic, ginger, cumin, coriander, salt and cayenne pepper; purée until smooth.

2. Arrange chicken in a shallow dish; coat with yogurt mixture. Cover and refrigerate for 1 hour or up to 1 day ahead. Remove from refrigerator 30 minutes before cooking.

3. Place chicken skin-side down on greased grill over medium-high heat; cook for 15 minutes. Brush with marinade; turn and cook for 10 to 15 minutes longer or until golden and juices run clear. (Or place chicken on rack set on baking sheet; roast, basting after 30 minutes with marinade, for 50 to 55 minutes or until juices run clear.) Serve garnished with chopped coriander.

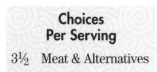

**Choices
Per Serving**

3½   Meat & Alternatives

Nutritional Analysis Per Serving			
Calories	133	Fat, total	2 g
Carbohydrate	4 g	Fat, saturated	1 g
Fiber	0 g	Sodium	300 mg
Protein	24 g	Cholesterol	59 mg

Preheat oven to
400°F (200°C)

9-inch (2 L) springform
pan sprayed with
vegetable spray

Tip

Soluble fiber can help to
control blood glucose and
lower blood cholesterol
levels. Insoluble fibers
in wheat bran and whole
grains help prevent
bowel disorders.

Chicken Cacciatore over Crisp Barley Crust

CRUST

3 cups	chicken stock	750 mL
¾ cup	pearl barley	175 mL
3 tbsp	low-fat milk	45 mL
2	large egg whites	2
1 tbsp	grated low-fat Parmesan cheese	15 mL
½ tsp	dried basil	2 mL

TOPPING

1 cup	chopped onions	250 mL
1	clove garlic, minced	1
1 cup	chopped mushrooms	250 mL
1 cup	chopped green bell peppers	250 mL
1	can (19 oz/540 mL) tomatoes, crushed	1
½ cup	chicken stock	125 mL
2 tbsp	tomato paste	25 mL
1	bay leaf	1
2 tsp	packed brown sugar	10 mL
½ tsp	chili powder	2 mL
1 tsp	dried Italian seasoning	5 mL
4 oz	boneless skinless chicken breast, cut into ½-inch (1 cm) cubes	125 g
2 tbsp	grated low-fat Parmesan cheese	25 mL

1. *Crust:* In a nonstick saucepan over high heat, bring stock to a boil. Add barley; reduce heat to medium-low. Cook, covered, for 45 to 50 minutes or until grain is tender and liquid absorbed; cool for 10 minutes. Add milk, egg whites, Parmesan cheese and basil. Press mixture into bottom of prepared springform pan. Bake in preheated oven for 25 minutes or until golden at edges and firm on top; remove from oven.

**Choices
Per Serving**

2   Carbohydrates

1   Meat & Alternative

Nutritional Analysis Per Serving			
Calories	190	Fat, total	1 g
Carbohydrate	35 g	Fat, saturated	0 g
Fiber	5 g	Sodium	278 mg
Protein	12 g	Cholesterol	15 mg

2. *Topping:* In a nonstick saucepan sprayed with vegetable spray, cook onions and garlic over medium-high heat for 3 minutes or until softened and lightly browned. Add mushrooms and green peppers; cook for 3 minutes or until softened. Add crushed tomatoes, stock, tomato paste, bay leaf, brown sugar, chili powder and Italian seasoning. Bring to a boil; reduce heat to medium. Cook, uncovered, for 20 minutes, stirring occasionally. Add chicken; cook for 3 minutes or until cooked through. Spread mixture over baked crust. Sprinkle with Parmesan cheese. Bake in preheated oven for 10 minutes.

• • • • • • • • • • • • • •

Preheat oven to
400°F (200°C)

• • • • • • • • • • • • • •

Tips

If leeks are unavailable,
use the same measurement
of sliced onions.

Dried apricots or raisins
can replace the dates,
or use a combination.

If using a food processor
to chop the dates, oil
the blade first to avoid
sticking.

To complete this meal,
serve with a garden or
spinach salad and low-fat
dressing such as Herb
Viniagrette (page 112).

Sweet potatoes make
this recipe an excellent
source of vitamins A
and E.

Chicken with Leeks, Sweet Potatoes and Dates

4	chicken breasts or legs	4
	All-purpose flour for dusting	
1 tbsp	margarine	15 mL
2 tsp	crushed garlic	10 mL
2 cups	chopped leeks	500 mL
2 cups	chopped peeled sweet potatoes	500 mL
1½ cups	chicken stock	375 mL
⅓ cup	white wine	75 mL
½ tsp	cinnamon	2 mL
½ tsp	ground ginger	2 mL
½ cup	chopped dates	125 mL

1. Dust chicken with flour. In nonstick skillet sprayed with nonstick vegetable spray, brown chicken on both sides, approximately 10 minutes. Place in baking dish.

2. In same skillet, melt margarine; sauté garlic, leeks and potatoes until softened, approximately 10 minutes, stirring constantly. Add chicken stock, wine, cinnamon and ginger; cover and simmer for 10 minutes. Stir in dates.

3. Pour sauce over chicken; bake for 20 to 30 minutes, basting occasionally, or until chicken is no longer pink inside and juices run clear when chicken is pierced. Remove skin before eating.

Choices Per Serving

3   Carbohydrates

2½   Meat & Alternatives

Nutritional Analysis Per Serving

Calories	362	Fat, total	5 g
Carbohydrate	55 g	Fat, saturated	1 g
Fiber	7 g	Sodium	591 mg
Protein	22 g	Cholesterol	46 mg

Preheat oven to
375°F (190°C)

8- by 4-inch (20 by
10 cm) loaf pan sprayed
with vegetable spray

Tip

This is a wonderful
alternative to traditional
meatloaf. The peppers
help make this recipe
an excellent source
of vitamin C.

Chicken and Bulgur Loaf

¾ cup	chicken stock or vegetable stock (see recipe, page 53)	175 mL
½ cup	bulgur	125 mL
1 cup	chopped red bell peppers	250 mL
1 cup	chopped onions	250 mL
12 oz	ground chicken	375 g
1	large egg	1
1	large egg white	1
¼ cup	ketchup	50 mL
¼ cup	dry seasoned bread crumbs	50 mL
1½ tsp	minced garlic	7 mL
½ tsp	dried basil	2 mL
⅛ tsp	salt	0.5 mL
⅛ tsp	freshly ground black pepper	0.5 mL
¼ cup	barbecue sauce	50 mL

1. In a saucepan over medium-high heat, bring stock to a boil. Add bulgur; remove from heat. Let stand, covered, for 20 minutes or until liquid is absorbed and grain is tender. Set aside to cool.

2. In a nonstick frying pan sprayed with vegetable spray, cook red peppers and onions over medium-high heat for 10 minutes or until golden and tender; set aside to cool.

3. In a bowl combine bulgur, ground chicken, egg, egg white, ketchup, bread crumbs, garlic, basil, salt and pepper. On a piece of waxed paper, pat mixture into an 8-inch (20 cm) square. Spread cooled red peppers and onions over surface. Using waxed paper as an aid, roll up mixture from bottom. Lifting waxed paper, gently drop loaf seam-side down into prepared loaf pan. Spread barbecue sauce over top. Bake in preheated oven, uncovered, for 30 minutes.

Choices
Per Serving

1	Carbohydrate
2	Meat & Alternatives

Nutritional Analysis Per Serving

Calories	218	Fat, total	9 g
Carbohydrate	20 g	Fat, saturated	0 g
Fiber	3 g	Sodium	262 mg
Protein	15 g	Cholesterol	37 mg

Chicken Bulgur Niçoise

Tips

Bulgar is made of wheat kernels that have been steamed, dried and crushed.

This recipe is an excellent source of vitamin C, magnesium, niacin and vitamin B$_6$.

DRESSING

¼ cup	water	50 mL
3 tbsp	fresh lemon juice	45 mL
2 tbsp	balsamic or red wine vinegar	25 mL
2 tbsp	olive oil	25 mL
4	anchovy fillets, drained and chopped	4
1½ tsp	minced garlic	7 mL

SALAD

1⅓ cups	chicken stock or vegetable stock (see recipe, page 53)	325 mL
1 cup	bulgur	250 mL
2	medium red potatoes, scrubbed and quartered	2
8 oz	boneless skinless chicken breast	250 g
8 oz	green beans, trimmed and halved	250 g
1 cup	ripe cherry tomatoes, cut into halves	250 mL
⅓ cup	diced red onions	75 mL
⅓ cup	sliced black olives	75 mL
	Freshly ground black pepper	

1. *Dressing:* In a food processor or blender, combine water, lemon juice, vinegar, olive oil, anchovies and garlic; purée until smooth. Set aside.

2. *Salad:* In a saucepan over high heat, bring stock to a boil. Add bulgur; remove from heat. Let stand, covered, for 15 minutes or until tender and liquid is absorbed. Set aside to cool.

3. Meanwhile, in a saucepan over high heat, cover potatoes with cold water. Cover saucepan; bring to a boil. Reduce heat to medium; cook for 15 minutes or until tender when pierced with a knife. Drain; let cool. Cut potatoes into cubes.

Choices Per Serving

3   Carbohydrates

2½   Meat & Alternatives

Nutritional Analysis Per Serving

Calories	363	Fat, total	10 g
Carbohydrate	50 g	Fat, saturated	2 g
Fiber	7 g	Sodium	286 mg
Protein	22 g	Cholesterol	38 mg

4. In a nonstick frying pan sprayed with vegetable spray or on a preheated grill, cook chicken over medium-high heat, turning once, for 12 minutes or until cooked through. Cut chicken into chunks.

5. In a pot of boiling water, cook green beans for 2 minutes or until tender-crisp; drain. Rinse under cold running water; drain.

6. In a serving bowl, combine bulgur, potatoes, chicken, green beans, cherry tomatoes, red onions and black olives. Pour dressing over; season to taste with pepper. Toss to coat well. Serve.

Tips

This tart yet sweet marinade complements veal and firm white fish, too.

For a change, try a combination of red or yellow pepper instead of the green pepper.

Serve over a bed of brown rice.

Chicken Kabobs with Ginger Lemon Marinade

8 oz	boneless skinless chicken breasts, cut into 2-inch (5 cm) cubes	250 g
16	squares sweet green pepper	16
16	pineapple chunks (fresh or canned)	16
16	cherry tomatoes	16

GINGER LEMON MARINADE

3 tbsp	lemon juice	45 mL
2 tbsp	water	25 mL
1 tbsp	vegetable oil	15 mL
2 tsp	sesame oil	10 mL
1½ tsp	red wine vinegar	7 mL
4 tsp	brown sugar	20 mL
1 tsp	minced gingerroot (or ¼ tsp/1 mL ground)	5 mL
½ tsp	ground coriander	2 mL
½ tsp	ground fennel seeds (optional)	2 mL

1. *Ginger Lemon Marinade:* In small bowl, combine lemon juice, water, vegetable oil, sesame oil, vinegar, brown sugar, ginger, coriander, and fennel seeds (if using); mix well. Add chicken and mix well; marinate for 20 minutes.

2. Alternately thread chicken cubes, green pepper, pineapple and tomatoes onto 4 long or 8 short barbecue skewers. Barbecue for 15 to 20 minutes or just until chicken is no longer pink inside, brushing often with marinade and rotating every 5 minutes.

Choices Per Serving

1   Carbohydrate

1½   Meat & Alternatives

Nutritional Analysis Per Serving			
Calories	165	Fat, total	7 g
Carbohydrate	16 g	Fat, saturated	1 g
Fiber	2 g	Sodium	31 mg
Protein	11 g	Cholesterol	26 mg

Swordfish with Mango Coriander Salsa page 175

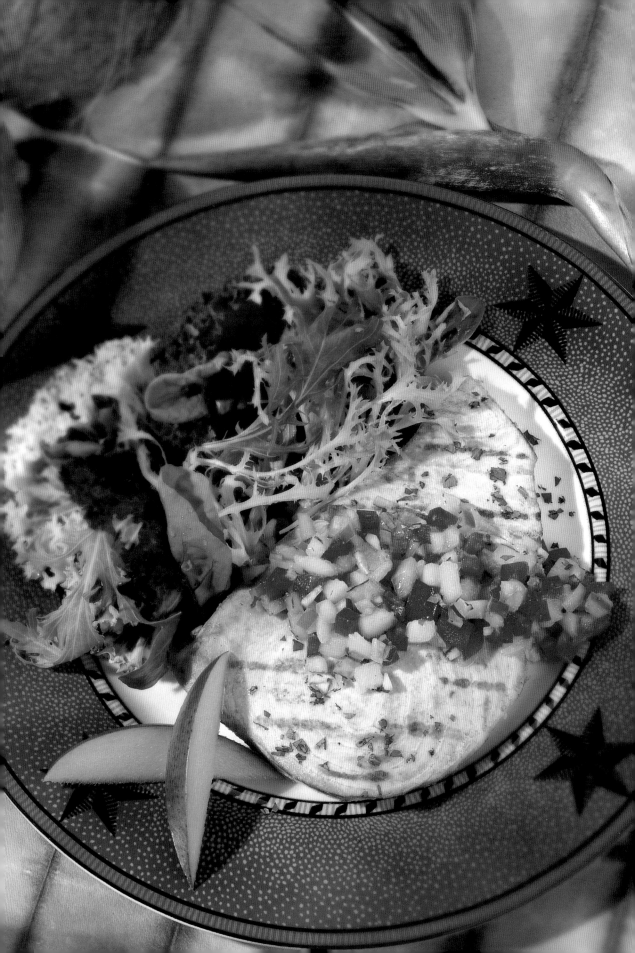

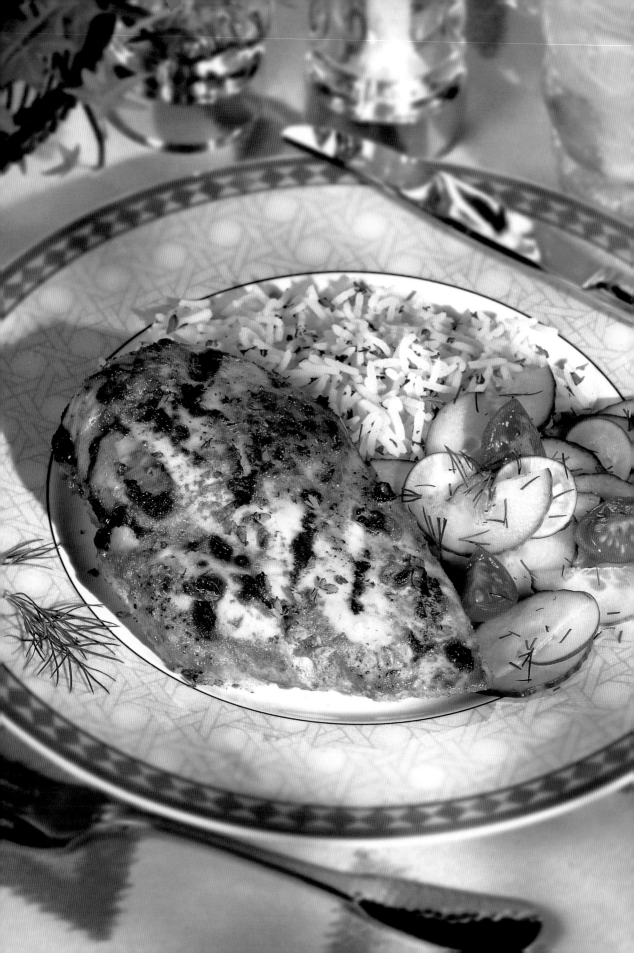

Preheat oven to
425°F (220°C)

Baking dish sprayed with
nonstick vegetable spray

Tips

Chicken quarters or
breasts with the bone in
can also be used. Bake for
20 to 30 minutes or until
no longer pink inside.

The 3 tbsp (45 mL)
brown sugar contributes
15 g of carbohydrate to
this recipe. Substituting
a low-calorie sugar
substitute can eliminate
the Carbohydrate choice,
altering the taste slightly.

Chicken with Teriyaki Vegetables

4	boneless skinless chicken breasts	4
1 tsp	vegetable oil	5 mL
1 tsp	crushed garlic	5 mL
1	large sweet red pepper, sliced thinly	1
1 cup	snow peas, trimmed	250 mL

MARINADE

3 tbsp	sherry	45 mL
3 tbsp	brown sugar	45 mL
2 tbsp	water	25 mL
2 tbsp	soya sauce	25 mL
2 tbsp	vegetable oil	25 mL
1½ tsp	minced gingerroot	7 mL

1. *Marinade:* In medium bowl, combine sherry, sugar, water, soya sauce, oil and ginger. Set aside.

2. Place chicken between 2 sheets of waxed paper; pound until thin and flattened. Add to bowl and marinate for 30 minutes.

3. Remove chicken and place in baking dish. Pour marinade into saucepan; cook for 3 to 4 minutes or until thickened and syrupy. Set 2 tbsp (25 mL) aside; brush remainder over chicken. Cover and bake for 10 to 15 minutes or until no longer pink inside.

4. Meanwhile, in large nonstick skillet, heat oil; sauté garlic, red pepper and snow peas for 2 minutes. Add reserved marinade; cook for 2 minutes, stirring constantly. Serve over chicken.

Choices Per Serving

1 Carbohydrate

3 Meat & Alternatives

Nutritional Analysis Per Serving			
Calories	243	Fat, total	10 g
Carbohydrate	17 g	Fat, saturated	1 g
Fiber	1 g	Sodium	536 mg
Protein	21 g	Cholesterol	48 mg

● ● ● ● ● ● ● ● ● ● ● ● ● ● ●

Preheat oven to
375°F (190°C)

Baking dish sprayed with
nonstick vegetable spray

● ● ● ● ● ● ● ● ● ● ● ● ● ● ●

Tips

Try yellow pepper
instead of the red.

Fresh herbs will last
longer if placed in a glass
with some water covering
the stems and plastic
wrap to cover the glass.
Store in the refrigerator.

● ● ● ● ● ● ● ● ● ● ● ● ● ● ●

Make Ahead

Assemble stuffed
breasts early in day and
refrigerate. Bake just
before serving. Prepare
sauce early in day and
reheat gently, adding
a little more milk if
too thick.

Chicken Breasts Stuffed with Red Pepper Purée in Creamy Sauce

4	boneless skinless chicken breasts	4
1 tbsp	vegetable oil	15 mL
½ tsp	crushed garlic	2 mL
¾ cup	diced sweet red pepper	175 mL
1 tbsp	water	15 mL
2 tbsp	chopped fresh dill (or ½ tsp/2 mL dried dillweed)	25 mL
2 tbsp	dry bread crumbs	25 mL
1½ tsp	grated Parmesan cheese	7 mL
1 tbsp	toasted pine nuts	15 mL
	Salt and pepper	
¼ cup	chicken stock or water	50 mL

SAUCE

1½ tsp	margarine	7 mL
1½ tsp	all-purpose flour	7 mL
¾ cup	2% milk	175 mL
1 tbsp	grated Parmesan cheese	15 mL
1 tbsp	chopped fresh dill (or ¼ tsp/1 mL dried dillweed)	15 mL
Pinch	paprika	Pinch

1. Place chicken between 2 sheets of waxed paper; pound until flattened. Set aside.

2. In nonstick skillet, heat oil; sauté garlic and red pepper for 3 minutes; stir in water. Transfer to food processor and purée; pour into bowl. Stir in dill, bread crumbs, cheese, pine nuts, and salt and pepper to taste, mixing well and adding a little water if too dry.

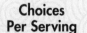

Choices Per Serving

½	Carbohydrate
3	Meat & Alternatives

Nutritional Analysis Per Serving

Calories	193	Fat, total	8 g
Carbohydrate	8 g	Fat, saturated	2 g
Fiber	1 g	Sodium	266 mg
Protein	21 g	Cholesterol	51 mg

3. Divide purée among chicken breasts; roll up and fasten with toothpicks. Place in baking dish; pour in stock. Cover and bake for about 15 minutes or until chicken is no longer pink inside. Transfer to serving dish.

4. *Sauce:* Meanwhile, in saucepan, melt margarine; add flour and cook, stirring, for 1 minute. Gradually add milk and cook, stirring, until thickened, approximately 3 minutes. Stir in cheese, dill and paprika. Pour over chicken.

Tips

Use 4 oz (125 g) of bottled roasted red peppers packed in water rather than roasting your own.

Serve chicken breasts whole or slice crosswise into medallions and fan out on the plate for a pretty presentation.

Reduce the sodium content of the recipe by substituting plain dry crumbs for the seasoned ones.

If prosciutto is unavailable, use thin slices of smoked ham.

If a more intense flavor is desired, use a stronger tasting cheese.

Make Ahead

Assemble chicken breasts early in the day, and refrigerate before baking. Bake 5 minutes longer due to refrigeration.

Chicken with Roasted Pepper and Prosciutto

1	small red pepper	1
1 lb	skinless, boneless chicken breasts (about 4)	500 g
1 oz	sliced prosciutto (4 thin slices)	25 g
2 oz	mozzarella cheese, cut into 4 equal-sized pieces	50 g
1	egg white	1
2 tbsp	water	25 mL
⅔ cup	seasoned bread crumbs	150 mL
2 tsp	vegetable oil	10 mL

1. Broil red pepper for 15 to 20 minutes, turning often until charred on all sides. Preheat oven to 425°F (220°C). Put pepper in bowl and cover tightly with plastic wrap. When cool enough to handle, remove stem, skin and seeds, and cut into thin strips.

2. Pound chicken breasts between sheets of waxed paper to ¼-inch (5 mm) thickness. Divide prosciutto slices among flattened chicken breasts. Place a piece of cheese at the short end of each breast, and place roasted pepper strips on top of the cheese. Starting at the filling end, carefully roll the breasts up tightly. Use a toothpick to hold chicken breast together.

3. In small bowl, whisk together egg white and water. Put bread crumbs on a plate. Dip each chicken roll in egg white mixture, then in bread crumbs. Heat oil in nonstick skillet sprayed with vegetable spray. Cook over high heat for 3 minutes, turning often, or until browned on all sides. Transfer to prepared baking sheet and bake for 10 to 15 minutes. Remove toothpicks before serving.

Choices Per Serving

1	Carbohydrate
4	Meat & Alternatives

Nutritional Analysis Per Serving			
Calories	258	Fat, total	7 g
Carbohydrate	17 g	Fat, saturated	2 g
Fiber	0 g	Sodium	714 mg
Protein	30 g	Cholesterol	65 mg

Tips

Try other nuts, such as cashews or pecans.

Try veal or turkey scallopini instead of chicken.

Serve with couscous and Green Beans and Diced Tomatoes (page 243) for an eye-catching meal.

Make Ahead

Bread chicken breasts and prepare sauce earlier in the day. Cook just before serving.

Almond Chicken Breasts with Creamy Tarragon Mustard Sauce

1 lb	skinless, boneless chicken breasts	500 g
3 tbsp	all-purpose flour	45 mL
1	egg white	1
3 tbsp	water	45 mL
1/3 cup	finely chopped almonds	75 mL
1/2 cup	seasoned bread crumbs	125 mL
2 tsp	vegetable oil	10 mL

SAUCE

1/4 cup	light mayonnaise	50 mL
1/4 cup	light sour cream	50 mL
1 tsp	Dijon mustard	5 mL
1 tsp	dried tarragon	5 mL

1. Between sheets of waxed paper, pound breasts to 1/4-inch (5 mm) thickness. Dust with flour. In shallow bowl, whisk together egg white and water. Combine almonds and bread crumbs and place on a plate.

2. In nonstick skillet sprayed with vegetable spray, heat oil over medium-high heat. Dip breasts in egg wash, then in crumb mixture. Cook for 3 minutes on one side; turn and cook for 2 minutes longer or until just done at center.

3. Meanwhile, in small saucepan whisk together mayonnaise, sour cream, mustard and tarragon; heat over low heat just until warm. Serve over chicken.

Choices Per Serving

1 Carbohydrate

3½ Meat & Alternatives

Nutritional Analysis Per Serving			
Calories	340	Fat, total	17 g
Carbohydrate	19 g	Fat, saturated	3 g
Fiber	2 g	Sodium	536 mg
Protein	27 g	Cholesterol	61 mg

Preheat oven to
425°F (220°C)

Baking sheet sprayed
with vegetable spray

Tips

Turkey, veal or
pork scallopini can
replace chicken.

A stronger cheese, such
as Swiss, can replace
mozzarella.

A great dish to reheat
the next day.

The chicken together
with the cheese in the
recipe provides 5 Meat
& Alternatives choices.
If your meal plan calls for
less, use smaller chicken
breasts in the recipe.

Using plain bread crumbs
instead of seasoned bread
crumbs will reduce the
sodium to 463 mg/serving.

Make Ahead

Prepare earlier in the
day, refrigerate and bake
at 350°F (180°C) until
warm (approximately
10 minutes).

Chicken and Eggplant Parmesan

4	crosswise slices of eggplant, skin on, approximately ½ inch (1 cm) thick	4
1	whole egg	1
1	egg white	1
1 tbsp	water or milk	15 mL
⅔ cup	seasoned bread crumbs	150 mL
3 tbsp	chopped fresh parsley (or 2 tsp/10 mL dried)	45 mL
1 tbsp	grated Parmesan cheese	15 mL
1 lb	skinless, boneless chicken breasts (about 4)	500 g
2 tsp	vegetable oil	10 mL
1 tsp	minced garlic	5 mL
½ cup	tomato pasta sauce	125 mL
½ cup	grated mozzarella cheese	125 mL

1. In small bowl, whisk together whole egg, egg white and water. On plate stir together bread crumbs, parsley and Parmesan. Dip eggplant slices in egg wash, then coat with bread-crumb mixture. Place on prepared pan and bake for 20 minutes, or until tender, turning once.

2. Meanwhile, pound chicken breasts between sheets of waxed paper to ¼-inch (5 mm) thickness. Dip chicken in remaining egg wash, then coat with remaining bread-crumb mixture. Heat oil and garlic in nonstick skillet sprayed with vegetable spray and cook for 4 minutes, or until golden brown, turning once.

Choices Per Serving

1   Carbohydrate

5   Meat & Alternatives

Nutritional Analysis Per Serving

Calories	325	Fat, total	11 g
Carbohydrate	19 g	Fat, saturated	5 g
Fiber	0 g	Sodium	924 mg
Protein	35 g	Cholesterol	127 mg

3. Spread 1 tbsp (15 mL) of tomato sauce on each eggplant slice. Place one chicken breast on top of each eggplant slice. Spread another 1 tbsp (15 mL) of tomato sauce on top of each chicken piece. Sprinkle with cheese and bake for 5 minutes or until cheese melts.

• • • • • • • • • • • • • • • •

Preheat broiler

• • • • • • • • • • • • • • • •

Tips

Try this dish with macaroni or penne instead of spaghetti.

Substitute fresh tuna or swordfish for the chicken.

Substituting low-fat Cheddar cheese (20% M.F.) for regular Cheddar will reduce the fat content of this recipe by 3 g and the saturated fat by 2 g/serving.

For a change, substitute 4 oz (125 g) cooked seafood for the chicken.

Chicken Tetrazzini

8 oz	spaghetti	250 g
4 tsp	margarine	20 mL
1½ tsp	crushed garlic	7 mL
1 cup	chopped onion	250 mL
1 cup	chopped sweet red pepper	250 mL
1 cup	sliced mushrooms	250 mL
3 tbsp	all-purpose flour	45 mL
1½ cups	chicken stock	375 mL
1 cup	2% milk	250 mL
3 tbsp	white wine	45 mL
1½ tsp	Dijon mustard	7 mL
4 oz	cooked boneless skinless chicken pieces	125 g
½ cup	shredded Cheddar cheese	125 mL
1 tbsp	grated Parmesan cheese	15 mL
	Chopped fresh parsley	

1. In saucepan of boiling water, cook spaghetti according to package directions or until firm to the bite; drain.

2. Meanwhile, in nonstick saucepan, melt margarine; sauté garlic, onion, red pepper and mushrooms until softened, approximately 5 minutes. Add flour and cook, stirring, for 1 minute.

3. Add stock, milk, wine and mustard; cook, stirring, for 3 minutes or until thickened. Add chicken.

4. Add sauce to spaghetti and toss to mix well; place in baking dish. Sprinkle Cheddar and Parmesan cheeses over top; bake until top is golden, approximately 5 minutes. Garnish with parsley.

Choices Per Serving

2½ Carbohydrates

2   Meat & Alternatives

½   Fat

Nutritional Analysis Per Serving

Calories	355	Fat, total	12 g
Carbohydrate	40 g	Fat, saturated	6 g
Fiber	2 g	Sodium	603 mg
Protein	18 g	Cholesterol	34 mg

Tip

Using regular chicken stock and adding the optional salt boosts sodium to 700 mg/serving.

White-Hot Chicken Chili

2 tbsp	vegetable oil	25 mL
1	onion, chopped	1
1	stalk celery, chopped	1
1¼ lb	boneless skinless chicken breasts, cubed	625 g
2	cloves garlic, minced	2
2	jalapeno peppers, chopped	2
1 tbsp	chili powder	15 mL
1 tsp	ground cumin	5 mL
1 tsp	dried oregano	5 mL
Pinch	salt, optional	Pinch
Pinch	cayenne pepper	Pinch
2 cups	low-sodium chicken stock	500 mL
1	can (19 oz/540 mL) white kidney beans, drained and rinsed	1
¼ cup	chopped fresh coriander or parsley	50 mL

1. In large saucepan, heat half of the oil over medium heat; cook onion and celery for 5 minutes. Push to one side. Heat remaining oil on other side of pan over high heat; brown chicken on all sides, about 5 minutes.

2. Stir in garlic, jalapeno peppers, chili powder, cumin, oregano, optional salt and cayenne; cook, stirring, for 1 minute. Stir in stock; bring to boil. Cover and reduce heat; simmer for 15 minutes. Uncover and simmer for 10 minutes. Stir in beans; cook for 5 minutes, stirring occasionally.

3. Taste and adjust seasoning if necessary. Serve sprinkled with coriander.

Choices Per Serving

½ Carbohydrate

4 Meat & Alternatives

Nutritional Analysis Per Serving			
Calories	247	Fat, total	7 g
Carbohydrate	17 g	Fat, saturated	1 g
Fiber	6 g	Sodium	574 mg
Protein	28 g	Cholesterol	55 mg

Tips

Great combination of ratatouille and chili in one dish.

Great as a family meal. Serve with French bread.

Ground pork, veal or chicken can replace turkey.

Make Ahead

Prepare up to a day ahead and reheat gently, adding extra chicken stock if too thick.

Turkey Ratatouille Chili

2 tsp	vegetable oil	10 mL
2 tsp	minced garlic	10 mL
1 cup	chopped onions	250 mL
1²⁄₃ cups	chopped zucchini	400 mL
1²⁄₃ cups	chopped peeled eggplant	400 mL
1½ cups	chopped mushrooms	375 mL
12 oz	ground turkey	375 g
2 tbsp	tomato paste	25 mL
1	can (19 oz/540 mL) tomatoes, puréed	1
2 cups	chicken stock	500 mL
1⅓ cups	peeled chopped potatoes	325 mL
1 cup	canned red kidney beans, drained	250 mL
1 tbsp	chili powder	15 mL
1½ tsp	dried basil	7 mL
1	bay leaf	1

1. In large nonstick saucepan sprayed with vegetable spray, heat oil over medium heat. Add garlic, onions, zucchini and eggplant; cook for 5 minutes or until softened. Add mushrooms and cook 2 minutes longer. Remove vegetables from skillet and set aside. Add turkey to skillet and cook for 3 minutes, stirring to break it up, or until no longer pink. Drain fat and add cooked vegetables to skillet.

2. Add tomato paste, tomatoes, stock, potatoes, beans, chili powder, basil and bay leaf; bring to a boil. Cover, reduce heat to low and simmer for 40 minutes, stirring occasionally.

Choices Per Serving

2 Carbohydrates

2½ Meat & Alternatives

Nutritional Analysis Per Serving

Calories	250	Fat, total	4 g
Carbohydrate	36 g	Fat, saturated	1 g
Fiber	7 g	Sodium	615 mg
Protein	20 g	Cholesterol	37 mg

Meat

There are many Meat & Alternatives choices that can balance a meal. Meat is one tasty choice that forms the basis of many main entrées. Today's meat is much leaner than it used to be. Meat is also a great source of iron and nutrients. In fact, the iron in meat called "heme" iron is absorbed more readily by the body than iron found in other sources. Always choose lean cuts of meat, trimmed of fat, as they will contain less total fat and saturated fat.

Preheat oven to
375°F (190°C)

Shallow 12- by 8-inch
(2.5 L) baking dish

Tips

Unless you're using
expensive tomato paste
from a tube, what do you
do with leftover canned
tomato paste? You can
freeze leftover tomato
paste in ice-cube trays,
but I prefer to drop
tablespoonfuls (you'll get
10 from a 5½ oz/156 mL
can) onto a baking sheet
lined with plastic wrap
and freeze. When firm,
transfer to a plastic
storage bag or container
and place in freezer.
What's nice about
this method is that
you need only add the
already-measured
amount to your recipe.

This dish is a good
source of vitamin C
and an excellent source
of zinc, niacin and
vitamin B$_{12}$.

Shepherd's Pie

1 lb	lean ground beef or ground veal	500 g
8 oz	mushrooms, sliced or chopped	250 g
1	medium onion, finely chopped	1
2	cloves garlic, minced	2
½ tsp	dried thyme	2 mL
½ tsp	dried marjoram	2 mL
3 tbsp	all-purpose flour	50 mL
1½ cups	beef stock	375 mL
2 tbsp	tomato paste	25 mL
2 tsp	Worcestershire sauce	10 mL
	Salt and pepper	
1	can (12 oz/341 mL) corn niblets, drained	1
2 lbs	potatoes (about 6 medium), peeled and cubed	1 kg
¾ cup	milk or buttermilk	175 mL
2 tbsp	dry bread crumbs	25 mL
2 tbsp	Parmesan cheese	25 mL
¼ tsp	paprika	1 mL

1. In a large nonstick skillet, cook beef over medium-high heat, breaking up with back of a spoon, for 5 minutes or until no longer pink.

2. Add mushrooms, onion, garlic, thyme and marjoram; cook, stirring often, for 5 minutes or until softened. Sprinkle with flour; stir in stock, tomato paste and Worcestershire sauce. Bring to a boil; reduce heat and simmer, covered, for 8 minutes. Season with salt, if necessary, and pepper to taste.

3. Spread meat mixture in baking dish; layer with corn.

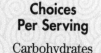

Choices Per Serving	
3	Carbohydrates
2½	Meat & Alternatives
1	Fat

Nutritional Analysis Per Serving			
Calories	385	Fat, total	13 g
Carbohydrate	46 g	Fat, saturated	5 g
Fiber	4 g	Sodium	496 mg
Protein	23 g	Cholesterol	45 mg

4. Meanwhile, in a large saucepan of boiling salted water, cook potatoes until tender. Drain and mash using a potato masher or electric mixer; beat in milk until smooth. Season with salt and pepper to taste. Place small spoonfuls of potato over corn and spread evenly. (The recipe can be prepared up to this point earlier in the day or the day before, then covered and refrigerated.)

5. In a small bowl, combine bread crumbs, Parmesan and paprika; sprinkle over top of shepherd's pie.

6. Bake in preheated oven for 25 to 30 minutes (40 minutes, if refrigerated) or until filling is bubbly.

Slow cooker

Make Ahead

This dish can be partially prepared the night before it is cooked. Make mashed potatoes, cover and refrigerate. Complete Steps 1 and 2, chilling cooked meat and onion mixture separately. Refrigerate overnight. The next morning, continue cooking as directed in Step 3.

Shepherd's Pie with Creamy Corn Filling

1 tbsp	vegetable oil	15 mL
1 lb	lean ground beef	500 g
2	onions, finely chopped	2
4	cloves garlic, minced	4
2 tsp	paprika	10 mL
1 tsp	salt, optional	5 mL
½ tsp	cracked black peppercorns	2 mL
2 tbsp	all-purpose flour	25 mL
1 cup	condensed beef broth (undiluted)	250 mL
2 tbsp	tomato paste	25 mL
1	can (19 oz/540 mL) cream-style corn	1
4 cups	mashed potatoes, seasoned with 1 tbsp (15 mL) butter, ½ tsp (2 mL) salt, optional and ¼ tsp (1 mL) black pepper	1 L
¼ cup	shredded Cheddar cheese	50 mL

1. In a skillet, heat oil over medium-high heat. Add beef and cook, breaking up with the back of a spoon, until meat is no longer pink. Using a slotted spoon, transfer to slow cooker stoneware. Drain off liquid.

2. Reduce heat to medium. Add onions to pan and cook until softened. Add garlic, paprika, optional salt and pepper and cook, stirring, for 1 minute. Sprinkle flour over mixture, stir and cook for 1 minute. Add beef broth and tomato paste, stir to combine and cook, stirring, until thickened.

3. Transfer mixture to slow cooker stoneware. Spread corn evenly over mixture and top with mashed potatoes. Sprinkle cheese on top, cover and cook on Low for 4 to 6 hours or on High for 3 to 4 hours, until hot and bubbly.

Choices Per Serving

3 Carbohydrates
2½ Meat & Alternatives
½ Fat

Nutritional Analysis Per Serving			
Calories	422	Fat, total	16 g
Carbohydrate	51 g	Fat, saturated	7 g
Fiber	4 g	Sodium	601 mg
Protein	23 g	Cholesterol	53 mg

Best-Ever Meat Loaf

Tips

Using oatmeal as
a binder gives a
coarser texture to the
meat loaf (bread crumbs
produce a finer one).
Use whichever binder
you prefer.

Double the recipe and
wrap the extra cooked
meat loaf in plastic
wrap, then in foil, for
the freezer. Defrost
overnight in the fridge.
To reheat, cut into slices
and place in saucepan.
Moisten with about
½ cup (125 mL) beef
stock; set over medium
heat until piping hot. Or
place meat loaf and stock
in casserole dish and
microwave at Medium
until heated through.

1 tbsp	vegetable oil	15 mL
1	medium onion, chopped	1
2	cloves garlic, minced	2
1 tsp	dried basil	5 mL
1 tsp	dried marjoram	5 mL
¾ tsp	salt	4 mL
¼ tsp	pepper	1 mL
1	egg	1
¼ cup	chili sauce or ketchup	50 mL
1 tbsp	Worcestershire sauce	15 mL
2 tbsp	chopped fresh parsley	25 mL
1½ lbs	lean ground beef	750 g
¾ cup	rolled oats	175 mL
	or	
½ cup	dry bread crumbs	125 mL

1. In a large nonstick skillet, heat oil over medium heat. Add onion, garlic, basil, marjoram, salt and pepper; cook, stirring, for 3 minutes or until softened. (Or place in microwave-safe bowl; microwave, covered, at High for 3 minutes.) Let cool slightly.

2. In a large bowl, beat the egg; stir in onion mixture, chili sauce, Worcestershire sauce and parsley. Crumble beef over mixture and sprinkle with rolled oats. Using a wooden spoon or with your hands, gently mix until evenly combined.

3. Pack meat mixture lightly into loaf pan. Bake in preheated oven for 1 hour or until meat thermometer registers 170°F (75°C). Let stand for 5 minutes; drain fat in pan, turn out onto a plate and cut into thick slices.

Choices Per Serving	
1	Carbohydrate
3	Meat & Alternatives
1	Fat

Nutritional Analysis Per Serving			
Calories	345	Fat, total	21 g
Carbohydrate	13 g	Fat, saturated	7 g
Fiber	2 g	Sodium	498 mg
Protein	25 g	Cholesterol	100 mg

Tips

Mashed sweet potatoes contrast nicely with lightly curried ground beef in this comforting supper dish. If you are freezing it, do not add almonds; sprinkle them over top just before serving.

To reduce fat by 6 g/serving or about 1 Fat choice/serving, eliminate the almonds.

Further reduce the fat by eliminating the 1 tbsp (15 mL) vegetable oil. Sauté the onion and ginger in a non-stick skillet with a little water instead.

Nutrient packed, this recipe is an excellent source of vitamins A, E, niacin and B_{12}, as well as iron and zinc.

Baked Curried Beef and Sweet Potatoes

4	small sweet potatoes	4
1 tbsp	margarine or butter	15 mL
	Salt and pepper	
2 tbsp	chopped fresh parsley	25 mL
1 tbsp	vegetable oil	15 mL
1	onion, chopped	1
1 tbsp	minced fresh ginger	15 mL
1 lb	lean ground beef	500 g
2 tbsp	curry powder	25 mL
1 tsp	ground cumin	5 mL
1 tsp	ground coriander	5 mL
2 cups	beef stock	500 mL
2 tbsp	tomato paste	25 mL
⅓ cup	raisins	75 mL
⅓ cup	slivered almonds	75 mL

1. Pierce sweet potatoes several times with fork. Bake in 400°F (200°C) oven for about 1 hour or until tender. (Or peel and cut in large chunks; boil in water for 20 minutes or microwave on High for 7 to 15 minutes.) Peel and mash with butter, and salt and pepper to taste. Stir in parsley. Transfer to 4-cup (1 L) casserole. (Potatoes can be covered and refrigerated for up to 1 day or frozen for up to 2 months. Thaw in refrigerator and bring to room temperature for 30 minutes before proceeding.)

2. Meanwhile, in large skillet, heat oil over medium heat; cook onion and ginger for 5 minutes. Add beef, breaking up with spoon; cook until no longer pink, about 7 minutes. Drain off fat.

Choices Per Serving

3	Carbohydrates
3½	Meat & Alternatives
2½	Fats

Nutritional Analysis Per Serving

Calories	583	Fat, total	31 g
Carbohydrate	50 g	Fat, saturated	8 g
Fiber	7 g	Sodium	507 mg
Protein	29 g	Cholesterol	64 mg

3. Stir in curry powder, cumin and coriander. Add stock and tomato paste; bring to boil. Reduce heat and simmer for 20 to 25 minutes or until most of the liquid has evaporated. Stir in raisins and almonds. Taste and adjust seasoning. Transfer to 4-cup (1 L) casserole. (Beef mixture can be covered and refrigerated for up to 2 days, or frozen for up to 2 months; thaw in refrigerator and bring to room temperature for 30 minutes before proceeding.)

4. Reheat both casseroles, covered, in 350°F (180°C) oven for about 30 minutes or until bubbly. To serve, spoon sweet potatoes onto heated platter; make a well in center and spoon in curried beef.

Slow cooker

Make Ahead

This dish can be partially prepared the night before it is cooked. Complete Step 2, heating 1 tbsp (15 mL) oil in pan before softening onions, carrots and celery. Cover and refrigerate mixture overnight. The next morning, brown steak (Step 1), or skip this step and place steak directly in stoneware. Continue cooking as directed. Alternatively, cook steak overnight and refrigerate. When ready to serve, bring to a boil in a large skillet and simmer for 10 minutes, until meat is heated through and sauce is hot and bubbling.

Saucy Swiss Steak

1 tbsp	vegetable oil	15 mL
2 lbs	round steak or "simmering" steak	1 kg
2	medium onions, finely chopped	2
¼ cup	thinly sliced carrots	50 mL
1	small carrot, thinly sliced, about ¼ cup (50 mL)	1
I	small stalk celery, thinly sliced, about ¼ cup (50 mL)	1
½ tsp	salt	2 mL
¼ tsp	black pepper	1 mL
2 tbsp	all-purpose flour	25 mL
1	can (28 oz/796 mL) plum tomatoes, drained and chopped, ½ cup (125 mL) juice reserved	1
1 tbsp	Worcestershire sauce	15 mL
1	bay leaf	1

1. In a skillet, heat oil over medium-high heat. Add steak, in pieces, if necessary, and brown on both sides. Transfer to slow cooker stoneware.

2. Reduce heat to medium-low. Add onion, carrots, celery, salt and pepper to pan. Cover and cook until vegetables are softened, about 8 minutes. Sprinkle flour over vegetables and cook for 1 minute, stirring. Add tomatoes, reserved juice and Worcestershire sauce. Bring to a boil, stirring until slightly thickened. Add bay leaf.

3. Pour tomato mixture over steak and cook on Low for 8 to 10 hours or on High for 4 to 5 hours, until meat is tender. Discard bay leaf.

Choices Per Serving

1 Carbohydrate

5 Meat & Alternatives

Nutritional Analysis Per Serving

Calories	196	Fat, total	4 g
Carbohydrate	11 g	Fat, saturated	1 g
Fiber	2 g	Sodium	330 mg
Protein	28 g	Cholesterol	49 mg

Tip

Change the kind of vegetables used for a variation.

Make Ahead

If possible, marinate overnight to enhance the flavor of the steak. Turn occasionally. Leftover marinade can be used as part of the liquid to cook plain rice, which is then served with the kabobs.

Steak Kabobs with Honey Garlic Marinade

2 tbsp	soya sauce	25 mL
2 tbsp	sherry or rice vinegar	25 mL
4 tsp	honey	20 mL
2 tsp	crushed garlic	10 mL
1½ tsp	sesame oil	7 mL
4 tsp	vegetable oil	20 mL
1 tbsp	water	15 mL
¾ lb	lean steak, cut into cubes	375 g
16	pieces (1-inch/2.5cm) sweet green pepper	16
16	pieces (1-inch/2.5cm) onion	16
16	small mushrooms	16
16	snow peas	16

1. In bowl, combine soya sauce, sherry, honey, garlic, sesame and vegetable oils and water. Add steak and marinate for 30 minutes, or longer in refrigerator.

2. Remove beef from marinade. Place marinade in small saucepan and cook for 3 to 5 minutes or until thick and syrupy.

3. Thread beef, green pepper, onion, mushrooms and snow peas alternately onto 8 metal skewers. Place on greased grill and barbecue for 10 to 15 minutes, turning often and brushing with marinade, or until cooked as desired. Serve with any remaining marinade.

Choices Per Serving

1   Carbohydrate

3½   Meat & Alternatives

Nutritional Analysis Per Serving			
Calories	252	Fat, total	9 g
Carbohydrate	22 g	Fat, saturated	1 g
Fiber	3 g	Sodium	541 mg
Protein	24 g	Cholesterol	37 mg

Preheat oven to
425°F (220°C)

13- by 9-inch (3 L)
baking dish sprayed
with vegetable spray

Tip

This recipe is an
excellent source
of vitamins A and C,
niacin, calcium,
phosphorus and zinc.

Spicy Beef Polenta Layered Casserole

8 oz	lean ground beef	250 g
3/4 cup	diced onions	175 mL
2 tsp	minced garlic	10 mL
3/4 cup	diced green bell peppers	175 mL
3/4 cup	diced carrots	175 mL
2 tsp	minced jalapeno peppers (optional) or 1/2 tsp (2 mL) dried chili flakes	10 mL
1	can (19 oz/540 mL) tomatoes, crushed	1
3/4 cup	canned or frozen corn kernels	175 mL
1/3 cup	sliced black olives	75 mL
1	bay leaf	1
1 tbsp	chili powder	15 mL
1 1/2 tsp	Italian seasoning	7 mL
6 cups	chicken stock or beef stock	1.5 L
1 1/2 cup	cornmeal	375 mL
1 cup	shredded low-fat mozzarella cheese	250 mL
2 tbsp	grated low-fat Parmesan cheese	25 mL

1. In a nonstick saucepan sprayed with vegetable spray, cook beef over medium-high heat, stirring, for 3 minutes or until no longer pink. Add onions and garlic; cook for 3 minutes or until softened. Add green peppers, carrots and jalapeno peppers; cook for 2 minutes. Add tomatoes, corn, black olives, bay leaf, chili powder and Italian seasoning; bring to a boil. Reduce heat to low; cook, covered, for 20 minutes or until thickened and vegetables are tender.

Choices Per Serving

2   Carbohydrates

2 1/2   Meat & Alternatives

Nutritional Analysis Per Serving

Calories	306	Fat, total	11 g
Carbohydrate	33 g	Fat, saturated	6 g
Fiber	4 g	Sodium	515 mg
Protein	20 g	Cholesterol	38 mg

2. In a nonstick saucepan over medium-high heat, bring stock to a boil. Reduce heat to low; gradually whisk in cornmeal. Cook, stirring, for 5 minutes. Spread half of meat sauce over bottom of prepared baking dish; top with half of polenta. Repeat layers; sprinkle with mozzarella cheese and Parmesan cheese. Cover pan with foil. Bake in preheated oven for 15 minutes or until heated through; let stand for 5 minutes before serving.

Tips

Serve with rice noodles, instead of traditional pasta. Complete the meal with a no-sugar-added fruit-flavored yogurt.

Look for a large iceberg lettuce to get the best quality leaves.

Use other vegetables such as celery and oyster mushrooms as substitutes.

Make Ahead

Prepare entire beef mixture earlier in the day. Reheat gently before placing in lettuce leaves.

Oriental Beef Bundles in Lettuce

12 oz	lean ground beef	375 g
SAUCE		
2 tbsp	hoisin sauce	25 mL
1 tbsp	rice wine vinegar	15 mL
2 tsp	minced garlic	10 mL
1½ tsp	minced gingerroot	7 mL
1 tsp	sesame oil	5 mL
1 tsp	vegetable oil	5 mL
⅓ cup	finely chopped carrots	75 mL
¾ cup	finely chopped red or green peppers	175 mL
¾ cup	finely chopped mushrooms	175 mL
½ cup	chopped water chestnuts	125 mL
2	green onions, chopped	2
2 tbsp	hoisin sauce	25 mL
1 tbsp	water	15 mL
8	large iceberg lettuce leaves	8

1. *Sauce:* In small bowl, whisk together hoisin, vinegar, garlic, gingerroot and sesame oil; set aside.

2. In nonstick skillet sprayed with vegetable spray, cook beef over medium heat for 5 minutes, or until browned; remove from skillet. Drain any excess liquid.

3. In same nonstick skillet, heat oil over medium heat. Add carrots and cook for 3 minutes. Add red peppers and mushrooms and cook for 3 minutes or until softened. Return beef to pan along with water chestnuts and green onions. Add sauce and cook for 2 minutes.

4. Combine hoisin sauce and water in small bowl. Place a little over leaves. Divide beef mixture among lettuce leaves. Serve open or rolled up.

Choices Per Serving

1 Carbohydrate

2½ Meat & Alternatives

1 Fat

Nutritional Analysis Per Serving

Calories	301	Fat, total	17 g
Carbohydrate	16 g	Fat, saturated	6 g
Fiber	2 g	Sodium	302 mg
Protein	20 g	Cholesterol	53 mg

Start barbecue or
preheat oven to
450°F (230°C)

Tips

Ground chicken or veal
can replace beef.

Serve these burgers on
kaiser rolls or pita buns.

Make Ahead

Prepare beef mixture up
to a day ahead and form
into burgers. Freeze up
to 6 weeks.

Hoisin Garlic Burgers

1 lb	lean ground beef	500 g
¼ cup	bread crumbs	50 mL
¼ cup	chopped green onions (about 2 medium)	50 mL
3 tbsp	chopped coriander or parsley	45 mL
2 tbsp	hoisin sauce	25 mL
2 tsp	minced garlic	10 mL
1 tsp	minced gingerroot	5 mL
1	egg	1
2 tbsp	water	25 mL
2 tbsp	hoisin sauce	25 mL
1 tsp	sesame oil	5 mL

1. In bowl combine beef, bread crumbs, green onions, coriander, hoisin sauce, garlic, gingerroot and egg; mix well. Make 4 to 5 burgers.

2. In small bowl whisk together water, hoisin sauce and sesame oil. Brush half of the sauce over top of burgers.

3. Place on greased grill and barbecue, or place on rack on baking sheet and bake for 10 to 15 minutes (or until no longer pink inside). Turn patties once and brush with remaining sauce.

Choices Per Serving

½ Carbohydrate

3 Meat & Alternatives

½ Fat

Nutritional Analysis Per Serving

Calories	292	Fat, total	18 g
Carbohydrate	10 g	Fat, saturated	7 g
Fiber	1 g	Sodium	305 mg
Protein	21 g	Cholesterol	100 mg

Tip

Enjoy this quick skillet supper with a green salad and low-fat dressing. Finish with sliced fruit topped with a fat-free no-sugar-added yogurt.

Tex-Mex Pork Chops with Black Bean–Corn Salsa

4	pork chops	4
1	clove garlic, minced	1
2 tsp	chili powder	10 mL
1 tsp	ground cumin	5 mL
1 tsp	dried oregano	5 mL
¼ tsp	hot pepper flakes	1 mL
	Salt and pepper	
1 tbsp	vegetable oil	15 mL
1	can (19 oz/540 mL) black beans, drained and rinsed	1
1 cup	corn kernels (frozen or canned)	250 mL
1 cup	bottled salsa (preferably chunky)	250 mL
⅓ cup	chopped fresh coriander	75 mL

1. Trim any fat from chops. Combine garlic, chili powder, cumin, oregano, hot pepper flakes and ¼ tsp (1 mL) each of the salt and pepper; rub all over chops.

2. In large heavy skillet, heat oil over medium-high heat; cook chops for 5 minutes on each side; reducing heat if starting to stick. Remove to plate.

3. Remove any fat and burnt bits from pan. Return chops and any juices. Add beans, corn and salsa. (Recipe can be prepared to this point, covered and refrigerated for up to 8 hours. Bring to room temperature for 30 minutes before proceeding.)

4. Bring to boil, reduce heat and simmer for about 8 minutes or until sauce is hot. Taste and adjust seasoning if necessary. Serve sprinkled with coriander.

Choices Per Serving

2   Carbohydrates

4   Meat & Alternatives

Nutritional Analysis Per Serving			
Calories	400	Fat, total	10 g
Carbohydrate	45 g	Fat, saturated	2 g
Fiber	12 g	Sodium	218 mg
Protein	35 g	Cholesterol	51 mg

Tips

Use beef steak or boneless chicken breast instead of pork.

Serve over pasta or rice.

This recipe is high in carbohydrate when compared to most other meat entrées. Using a granulated sugar substitute in place of the brown sugar may alter the taste slightly, but will reduce the total carbohydrate content to 20 g/serving and the Carbohydrate choices to 1.

Using low-sodium chicken stock and low-sodium soya sauce in this recipe will reduce the sodium to 500 mg/serving.

. . . .

Make Ahead

Prepare sauce up to a day before.

Pork Stir-fry with Sweet-and-Sour Sauce, Snow Peas and Red Peppers

SAUCE

1 cup	chicken stock	250 mL
1/3 cup	brown sugar	75 mL
1/3 cup	ketchup	75 mL
2 tbsp	rice wine vinegar	25 mL
1 tbsp	soya sauce	15 mL
2 tsp	sesame oil	10 mL
4 tsp	cornstarch	20 mL
2 tsp	minced garlic	10 mL
1 1/2 tsp	minced gingerroot	7 mL
12 oz	pork loin, cut into thin strips	375 g
1 tsp	vegetable oil	5 mL
1 1/2 cups	snow peas or sugar snap peas	375 mL
1 1/4 cups	red pepper strips	300 mL
3/4 cup	green pepper strips	175 mL
1/2 cup	chopped green onions (about 4 medium)	125 mL

1. In small bowl combine stock, brown sugar, ketchup, vinegar, soya sauce, sesame oil, cornstarch, garlic and ginger; set aside.

2. In nonstick wok or skillet sprayed with vegetable spray, cook the pork strips over high heat for 2 minutes, stirring constantly, or until just done at center; remove from wok.

3. Add oil to wok. Cook snow peas, red and green peppers for 3 minutes, stirring constantly, or until tender-crisp. Stir sauce again and add to wok along with pork. Cook for 45 seconds or until thickened. Garnish with green onions.

Nutritional Analysis Per Serving

Calories	291	Fat, total	7 g
Carbohydrate	37 g	Fat, saturated	2 g
Fiber	3 g	Sodium	862 mg
Protein	22 g	Cholesterol	55 mg

Choices Per Serving

2 1/2	Carbohydrates
3	Meat & Alternatives

• • • • • • • • • • • • • • •

Preheat oven to
350°F (180°C)

Roasting pan with rack

• • • • • • • • • • • • • • •

Tips

It may appear that you
have too much stuffing
when you first tie the
pork. But once all the
strings are in place, it's
easy to enclose the meat
completely around
the fruit mixture.

This delicious roast is
likely to be more Meat &
Alternatives choices
than most meal plans
allow for. Either choose
a smaller serving size or
balance it by eating
less from the Meat &
Alternatives group at
another meal.

Company Pork Roast with Fruit Stuffing

STUFFING

1 tbsp	margarine or butter	15 mL
⅓ cup	chopped green onions	75 mL
1 tsp	ground cumin	5 mL
½ tsp	curry powder	2 mL
1 cup	chopped mixed dried fruits, such as apricots, prunes, apples, cranberries	250 mL
½ cup	soft bread crumbs	125 mL
1 tsp	grated orange rind	5 mL
1	egg, beaten	1
	Salt and pepper	
3 lbs	boneless pork loin roast	1.5 kg
2 tsp	vegetable oil	10 mL
1	large clove garlic, minced	1
1 tsp	rubbed sage	5 mL
½ tsp	dried thyme	2 mL
1 tbsp	all-purpose flour	15 mL
½ cup	white wine or chicken stock	125 mL
¾ cup	chicken stock	175 mL

1. *Stuffing:* In a small skillet, melt butter over medium heat. Add green onions, cumin and curry powder; cook, stirring, for 2 minutes or until softened.

2. In a bowl combine onion mixture, dried fruits, bread crumbs, orange rind and egg; season with salt and pepper.

3. Remove strings from pork roast; unfold roast and trim excess fat. Place pork roast, boned side up, on work surface. Cover with plastic wrap and pound using a meat mallet to flatten slightly. Season with salt and pepper; spread stuffing down center of meat. Roll the pork around the stuffing and tie securely at 6 intervals with butcher's string.

Nutritional Analysis Per Serving			
Calories	258	Fat, total	8 g
Carbohydrate	12 g	Fat, saturated	3 g
Fiber	1 g	Sodium	173 mg
Protein	32 g	Cholesterol	119 mg

**Choices
Per Serving**

1   Carbohydrate

4½   Meat & Alternatives

4. Place roast on rack in roasting pan. In a small bowl, combine oil, garlic, sage and thyme; spread over pork roast and season with salt and pepper.

5. Roast in preheated oven for $1\frac{1}{2}$ to $1\frac{3}{4}$ hours or until meat thermometer registers 160°F (70°C).

6. Remove roast to cutting board; tent with foil and let stand for 10 minutes before carving.

7. Pour off fat in pan. Place over medium heat; sprinkle with flour. Cook, stirring, for 1 minute or until lightly colored. Add wine or stock; cook until partially reduced. Add stock and bring to a boil, scraping any brown bits from bottom of pan. Season with salt and pepper to taste. Strain sauce through a fine sieve into a warm sauceboat. Cut pork into thick slices and serve accompanied with gravy.

* * * * * * * * * * * * *

Deep baking dish,
measuring about 12 by
16 inches (30 by 40 cm)

* * * * * * * * * * * * *

Tips

Baked beans take many
forms around the world,
and cassoulet is the
version favored in the
well-fed northern
regions of France.
There, any number of
fatty meats (goose and/or
pork fat, for example)
are mixed with beans
and baked under an
equally fatty crust. Here
we "Mediterraneanize"
the original recipe, using
additional vegetables
and a lot less fat. Still,
this is a hefty and lengthy
dish that requires cool
weather, a suitable
occasion (to justify
the effort), and a
well-ventilated room.

This recipe is an
excellent source of
vitamin A, the B vitamins,
iron, magnesium,
phosphorus and zinc.

Cassoulet with Pork and Zucchini

1 tbsp	olive oil	15 mL
¼ tsp	salt, optional	1 mL
¼ tsp	freshly ground black pepper	1 mL
1 lb	pork tenderloin, cut into 1-inch (2.5 cm) cubes	500 g
1 tbsp	finely chopped garlic	15 mL
1 tbsp	olive oil	15 mL
½ tsp	salt, optional	2 mL
½ tsp	freshly ground black pepper	2 mL
1 cup	finely diced onions	250 mL
2	medium leeks, trimmed, washed and finely chopped (about 3 cups/750 mL)	2
2	stalks celery with leaves, finely chopped	2
Half	green pepper, finely diced	Half
1	large carrot, scraped and finely diced (about 4 oz/125 g)	1
8 oz	mushrooms, trimmed and quartered	250 g
1 lb	tomatoes, peeled and finely chopped (about 2 cups/500 mL) or canned tomatoes	500 g
1 tbsp	tomato paste, diluted in 1 cup (250 mL) water	15 mL
1 tsp	red wine vinegar	5 mL
1 tsp	dried basil	5 mL
1 tsp	dried oregano	5 mL
2 cups	cooked white kidney beans or 1 can (19 oz/540 mL), rinsed and drained	500 mL
2 cups	cooked red Romano beans or 1 can (19 oz/540 mL), rinsed and drained	500 mL

Choices Per Serving

3½   Carbohydrates

3   Meat & Alternatives

Nutritional Analysis Per Serving			
Calories	476	Fat, total	12 g
Carbohydrate	57 g	Fat, saturated	2 g
Fiber	5 g	Sodium	383 mg
Protein	31 g	Cholesterol	87 mg

1	medium zucchini cut into ¼-inch (5 mm) rounds (about 8 oz/250 g)	1
2 cups	low-sodium chicken stock	500 mL

TOPPING

2 cups	breadcrumbs	500 mL
1 tbsp	finely chopped garlic	15 mL
½ tsp	ground allspice	2 mL
2	eggs, beaten	2
2 tbsp	olive oil	25 mL
1 cup	dry white vermouth or white wine	250 mL
	Few sprigs fresh parsley, chopped	

1. In a large nonstick frying pan, heat 1 tbsp (15 mL) olive oil, optional ¼ tsp (1 mL) salt and pepper over high heat for 30 seconds. Add pork and stir-fry for 2 minutes, turning meat often so that all the pieces are thoroughly browned. Add garlic and stir-fry 1 more minute. Transfer contents of the frying pan to a large saucepan.

2. Return the frying pan to high heat. Add 1 tbsp (15 mL) olive oil, optional ½ tsp (2 mL) salt and pepper; heat for 30 seconds. Add onions, leeks, celery, green pepper, carrot and mushrooms; cook, stirring, for 4 minutes or until the vegetables are softened and a little oily. Transfer vegetables to saucepan with meat.

3. Stir in tomatoes, diluted tomato paste, vinegar, dried basil and oregano. Bring to a boil, cover tightly, reduce heat to medium-low and cook for 25 to 30 minutes or until the meat is cooked through. Remove from heat.

4. Preheat oven to 375°F (190°C). Add white kidney beans, red Romano beans, zucchini and chicken stock to the stew. Gently fold to mix everything thoroughly. Transfer this mixture to baking dish. Spread mixture over bottom of dish, making a layer about 1½ inches (4 cm) deep.

5. *Topping:* In a bowl stir together the breadcrumbs, garlic and allspice until combined. In a small bowl, combine the eggs, olive oil and vermouth. Add this liquid to the breadcrumbs and stir to mix until combined (it'll be wet and lumpy).

recipe continues on page 222

6. As evenly as possible, spread this topping over the stew. Bake uncovered for 30 minutes. Remove from oven and press the topping (which will have browned a little) just into the stew, but leaving it still on top. Put back in the oven and bake another 30 minutes until the topping is nicely crusted and the stew is bubbling underneath.

7. Remove from oven and let rest 10 minutes. Portion onto plates, keeping breadcrumbs on top; garnish with chopped parsley and serve immediately.

Tips

Apples have always been paired with pork but pears deserve equal treatment. Here they make an especially delicious companion to this versatile meat.

Serve with rice and a steamed green vegetable such as snow peas, along with red pepper or broccoli.

You can replace the honey with a sugar substitute to save 5 g carbohydrate/serving.

Pork with Pears, Honey and Thyme

1 tbsp	vegetable oil	15 mL
1 lb	thin boneless pork loin chops (about 8)	500 g
2	pears, peeled, cored and thinly sliced	2
3	green onions, chopped	3
1 tbsp	honey	15 mL
½ tsp	dried thyme	2 mL
½ cup	chicken stock	125 mL
1 tbsp	cider vinegar	15 mL
1 tsp	cornstarch	5 mL
¼ tsp	salt	1 mL
¼ tsp	pepper	1 mL

1. In a large nonstick skillet, heat oil over medium-high heat; brown pork for 2 minutes on each side. Remove to a plate and keep warm. Add pears, green onions, honey and thyme to skillet; cook, stirring, for 2 to 3 minutes or until pears are softened.

2. Meanwhile, in a bowl, combine stock, vinegar, cornstarch, salt and pepper. Pour into skillet; cook, stirring, until slightly thickened. Return pork and any accumulated juices to skillet and cook, turning occasionally, for 1 to 2 minutes or until heated through.

Choices Per Serving

1	Carbohydrate
3½	Meat & Alternatives

Nutritional Analysis Per Serving			
Calories	265	Fat, total	10 g
Carbohydrate	18 g	Fat, saturated	2 g
Fiber	3 g	Sodium	279 mg
Protein	26 g	Cholesterol	62 mg

Slow cooker

Tip

Ghee is a type of clarified butter highly valued in Indian cooking as it can be heated to a very high temperature. It is available in grocery stores specializing in Indian ingredients and will keep, refrigerated, for as long as a year.

Make Ahead

This dish must be assembled the night before it is cooked as it needs to be marinated overnight. Follow preparation directions and refrigerate overnight. The next day, transfer to stoneware and cook as directed.

Pork Vindaloo

1 tbsp	cumin seeds	15 mL
2 tsp	coriander seeds	10 mL
1 tbsp	clarified butter or ghee (see tip)	15 mL
1	onion, finely chopped	1
8	cloves garlic, minced	8
1 tbsp	minced gingerroot	15 mL
1	piece cinnamon stick, about 2 inches (5 cm)	1
6	whole cloves	6
½ tsp	salt	2 mL
2 tsp	mustard seeds	10 mL
¼ tsp	cayenne pepper	1 mL
2 lbs	stewing pork, cut into 1-inch (2.5 cm) cubes	1 kg
4	bay leaves	4
½ cup	red wine vinegar	125 mL

1. In a skillet, over medium heat, cook cumin and coriander seeds, stirring constantly, until they release their aroma and just begin to turn golden. Remove pan from heat and transfer seeds to a mortar or a cutting board. Using a pestle or a rolling pin, crush seeds coarsely. Set aside.

2. In a skillet, heat butter or ghee over medium heat. Add onion, garlic and gingerroot and cook for 1 minute. Add cumin and coriander seeds, cinnamon, cloves, salt, mustard seeds and cayenne and cook for 1 more minute. Remove from heat. Let cool.

3. Place pork in a mixing bowl. Add bay leaves and contents of pan. Add vinegar and stir to combine. Cover and marinate overnight in refrigerator. The next day, transfer to slow cooker stoneware, cover and cook on Low for 8 to 10 hours or on High for 4 to 5 hours, until pork is tender. Discard bay leaves, cinnamon stick and whole cloves.

Nutritional Analysis Per Serving

Calories	181	Fat, total	6 g
Carbohydrate	4 g	Fat, saturated	2 g
Fiber	1 g	Sodium	225 mg
Protein	26 g	Cholesterol	82 mg

Choices Per Serving

3½ Meat & Alternatives

Chicken Kabobs with Ginger Lemon Marinade page 192

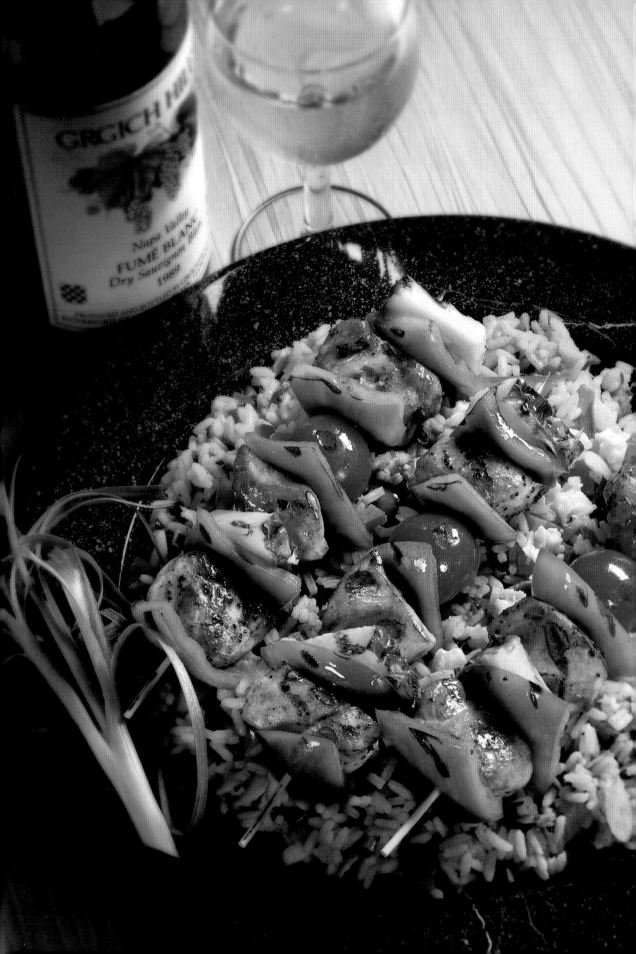

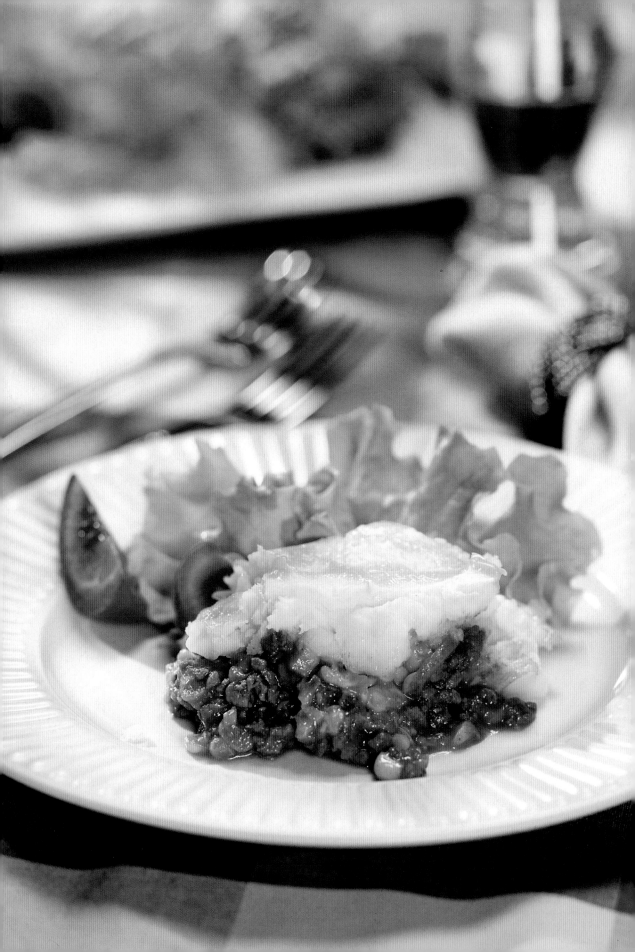

Tips

Lamb can be butterflied and filled, then gently folded over and tied with a string.

Complete this meal with a simple dessert of fresh fruit topped with ½ cup (125 mL) of fat-free no-sugar-added vanilla pudding. If your meal plan allows additional Carbohydrates choices, add a couple of plain cookies.

Make Ahead

Prepare pesto up to 2 days before and keep refrigerated. Can also be frozen for up to 4 weeks.

Choices Per Serving

2   Carbohydrates

3½   Meat & Alternatives

Leg of Lamb with Pesto and Wild Rice

STUFFING

1 tsp	vegetable oil	5 mL
2 tsp	minced garlic	10 mL
1 cup	chopped onions	250 mL
1 cup	chopped red or green peppers	250 mL
¾ cup	wild rice	175 mL
¾ cup	white rice	175 mL
3 cups	beef or chicken stock	750 mL
⅓ cup	pesto (see recipe, page 118)	75 mL
3 lb	boneless leg of lamb with a pocket	1.5 kg
1 tsp	vegetable oil	5 mL
1 tsp	minced garlic	5 mL
⅔ cup	beef stock	150 mL
½ cup	red or white wine	125 mL

1. In saucepan, heat oil over medium heat. Add garlic and onions and cook for 3 minutes or until softened. Add red peppers and cook for 2 minutes longer. Add rices and cook, stirring, for 3 minutes. Add stock; bring to a boil, cover, reduce heat to medium-low and simmer covered for 20 to 25 minutes or until rice is tender and liquid absorbed. Stir in pesto. Set aside to cool.

2. Stuff leg of lamb with some of the cooled rice mixture; put leftover stuffing in a casserole dish and cover. Rub lamb with oil and garlic and place on rack in roasting pan. Truss lamb with string. Pour stock and wine under lamb. Bake covered for 20 minutes, basting with pan juices every 10 minutes. Uncover lamb and bake another 20 to 25 minutes, basting every 10 minutes. Add extra stock if liquids evaporate. Put casserole dish with leftover stuffing in the oven for the last 20 minutes. Serve meat with juices.

Nutritional Analysis Per Serving			
Calories	335	Fat, total	10 g
Carbohydrate	30 g	Fat, saturated	3 g
Fiber	2 g	Sodium	704 mg
Protein	28 g	Cholesterol	72 mg

Shepherd's Pie with Creamy Corn Filling page 206

Curried Lamb Casserole with Sweet Potatoes

¾ lb	lamb, cut into ¾-inch (2 cm) cubes	375 g
	All-purpose flour for dusting	
1 tbsp	vegetable oil	15 mL
2 tsp	crushed garlic	10 mL
1 cup	chopped onion	250 mL
1 cup	finely chopped carrots	250 mL
½ cup	finely chopped sweet green peppers	125 mL
1 cup	cubed peeled sweet potatoes	250 mL
1½ cups	sliced mushrooms	375 mL
2½ cups	beef stock	625 mL
⅓ cup	red wine	75 mL
3 tbsp	tomato paste	45 mL
2 tsp	curry powder	10 mL

1. Dust lamb with flour.

2. In large nonstick Dutch oven, heat oil, sauté lamb for 2 minutes or just until seared all over. Remove lamb and set aside.

3. To skillet, add garlic, onion, carrots, green pepper and sweet potatoes; cook, stirring often, for 8 to 10 minutes or until tender. Add mushrooms and cook until softened, approximately 3 minutes.

4. Add stock, wine, tomato paste and curry powder. Return lamb to pan; cover and simmer for 1½ hours, stirring occasionally.

Nutritional Analysis Per Serving

Calories	310	Fat, total	9 g
Carbohydrate	32 g	Fat, saturated	2 g
Fiber	5 g	Sodium	783 mg
Protein	23 g	Cholesterol	61 mg

Veal Paprikash

Tips

Fettuccine or other long noodles make a delicious companion to this creamy veal in mushroom sauce.

The most flavorful paprika comes from Hungary, where it ranges in strength from mild (sweet) to hot.

This recipe is an excellent source of iron, zinc, phosphorus and B vitamins.

2 tbsp	vegetable oil	25 mL
1 lb	grain-fed veal scallops or boneless beef sirloin, cut into thin strips	500 g
4 cups	quartered mushrooms (about 12 oz/375 g)	1 L
1	large onion, halved lengthwise and thinly sliced	1
2	cloves garlic, minced	2
4 tsp	sweet Hungarian paprika	20 mL
½ tsp	dried marjoram	2 mL
½ tsp	salt	2 mL
¼ tsp	pepper	1 mL
1 tbsp	all-purpose flour	15 mL
¾ cup	chicken stock	175 mL
½ cup	sour cream	125 mL
	Salt and pepper	

1. In a large nonstick skillet, heat half the oil over high heat; stir-fry veal in 2 batches, each for 3 minutes or until browned but still pink inside. Transfer to a plate along with pan juices; keep warm.

2. Reduce heat to medium. Add remaining oil. Add mushrooms, onion, garlic, paprika, marjoram, salt and pepper; cook, stirring often, for 7 minutes or until lightly colored.

3. Sprinkle mushroom mixture with flour; pour in stock. Cook, stirring, for 2 minutes or until thickened. Stir in sour cream. Return veal and accumulated juices to pan; cook 1 minute more or until heated through. Adjust seasoning with salt and pepper to taste; serve immediately.

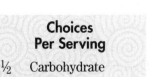

Choices Per Serving

½ Carbohydrate

4 Meat & Alternatives

Nutritional Analysis Per Serving

Calories	266	Fat, total	11 g
Carbohydrate	12 g	Fat, saturated	1 g
Fiber	2 g	Sodium	462 mg
Protein	30 g	Cholesterol	107 mg

Preheat oven to
400°F (200°C)

Tips

If the veal seems tough,
marinate it in milk
2 hours before using.
Be sure not to overcook
the veal, which will
make it tough.

You can substitute
boneless chicken breasts
for the veal.

Make Ahead

Assemble and refrigerate
veal rolls early in the
day. Make sauce ahead
of time but add sour
cream after reheating.

Veal Stuffed with Cheese in Mushroom Sauce

1 lb	veal cutlets	500 g
1 tsp	vegetable oil	5 mL
½ cup	finely diced mushrooms	125 mL
¼ cup	finely diced onions	50 mL
1 tsp	crushed garlic	5 mL
⅓ cup	shredded mozzarella cheese	75 mL
¼ cup	beef stock	50 mL
	Chopped fresh parsley	

SAUCE

1 tbsp	margarine	15 mL
1½ cups	sliced mushrooms	375 mL
2 tbsp	all-purpose flour	25 mL
1 cup	beef stock	250 mL
1 tbsp	sherry (optional)	15 mL
2 tbsp	light sour cream	25 mL

1. Pound veal until flat and divide into 4 serving pieces.

2. In small nonstick skillet, heat oil; sauté mushrooms, onions and garlic until softened, approximately 3 minutes. Remove from heat.

3. Divide vegetable mixture among cutlets. Sprinkle cheese over top. Roll up and secure with toothpick. Place in baking dish and add stock. Cover and bake for 8 to 10 minutes or just until veal is tender. Remove rolls to serving platter. Keep warm.

4. *Sauce:* In small nonstick skillet, melt margarine; sauté mushrooms until softened and liquid is released. Add flour and cook, stirring, for 1 minute. Add stock, and sherry (if using); cook until thickened, approximately 2 minutes, stirring constantly. If too thick, add more stock. Remove from heat and stir in sour cream; pour over veal. Garnish with parsley.

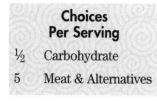

Choices Per Serving

½ Carbohydrate

5 Meat & Alternatives

Nutritional Analysis Per Serving			
Calories	266	Fat, total	11 g
Carbohydrate	7 g	Fat, saturated	4 g
Fiber	1 g	Sodium	559 mg
Protein	33 g	Cholesterol	11 mg

Baking sheet sprayed
with nonstick
vegetable spray

Tips

Chicken can be
substituted for the veal.

Adjust the chili powder
to your taste.

Serve on a bed of rice
or pasta with steamed
broccoli or green beans
on the side. Complete the
meal with Frozen Vanilla
Yogurt (page 363).

Make Ahead

Prepare and refrigerate
meatballs up to a
day before serving,
then reheat on
low temperature.

Spicy Veal Meatballs with Tomato Sauce

12 oz	ground veal	375 g
¼ cup	finely chopped onion	50 mL
2 tsp	crushed garlic	10 mL
¼ cup	finely chopped sweet red pepper	50 mL
1	egg	1
1½ tsp	grated Parmesan cheese	7 mL
⅓ cup	dry bread crumbs	75 mL
2 tbsp	chili sauce or ketchup	25 mL
2 tbsp	chopped fresh basil (or 1 tsp/5 mL dried)	25 mL
1 tsp	chili powder	5 mL
1¾ cups	tomato sauce, heated	425 mL

1. In large bowl, mix together veal, onion, garlic,
red pepper, egg, cheese, bread crumbs, chili sauce,
basil and chili powder until well combined. Roll into
1-inch (2.5 cm) balls and place on baking sheet.

2. Bake for approximately 10 minutes or until no longer
pink inside. Place in serving dish and pour tomato sauce
over top.

Choices Per Serving

1	Carbohydrate
2	Meat & Alternatives

Nutritional Analysis Per Serving			
Calories	172	Fat, total	6 g
Carbohydrate	14 g	Fat, saturated	2 g
Fiber	2 g	Sodium	589 mg
Protein	16 g	Cholesterol	88 mg

Veal with Pineapple Lime Sauce and Pecans

1 lb	veal scallopini	500 g
2 tsp	oil	10 mL
3 tbsp	flour	45 mL

SAUCE

1/4 cup	chopped green onions (about 2 medium)	50 mL
2 tbsp	chopped pecans	25 mL
1/4 cup	pineapple juice concentrate	50 mL
1/4 cup	water	50 mL
1 tbsp	honey	15 mL
1 tbsp	fresh lime juice	15 mL
1 tsp	grated lime zest	5 mL

1. Between sheets of waxed paper pound veal to 1/4-inch (5 mm) thickness. In large nonstick skillet sprayed with vegetable spray, heat oil over medium-high heat. Dredge veal in flour and cook for 2 1/2 minutes per side or until just done at center. Place on a serving dish and cover.

2. Add green onions and pecans to skillet. Cook for 2 minutes. Add pineapple juice concentrate, water, honey, lime juice and lime zest. Bring to a boil for 1 minute, or until slightly syrupy and thickened. Serve sauce over veal.

Choices Per Serving

| 1 | Carbohydrate |
| 2 1/2 | Meat & Alternatives |

Nutritional Analysis Per Serving			
Calories	210	Fat, total	7 g
Carbohydrate	19 g	Fat, saturated	1 g
Fiber	1 g	Sodium	68 mg
Protein	18 g	Cholesterol	67 mg

Vegetarian Main Dishes

Many people are trying to incorporate more meatless recipes into their everyday meals. Combinations of legumes, beans, nuts and seeds and whole grains provide complete protein with less saturated fat than main courses containing animal sources of protein.

These delicious vegetarian main dishes may inspire you to venture further into the world of alternative protein choices. *Canada's Food Guide* recommends "incorporating dried beans, peas and lentils more often." This is a great place to start.

Preheat oven to
350°F (180°C)

13- by 9-inch (3 L)
baking dish

Tips

This shepherd's pie
rivals the beef
version — creamy,
thick and rich tasting.
Beans provide the
meat-like texture.

For a different twist,
try sweet potatoes.

Try other cheeses such
as mozzarella or Swiss.

Make Ahead

Prepare up to 1 day in
advance. Reheat gently.

Freeze for up to 3 weeks.

Vegetarian Shepherd's Pie with Peppered Potato Topping

2 tsp	vegetable oil	10 mL
2 tsp	minced garlic	10 mL
1 cup	chopped onions	250 mL
¾ cup	finely chopped carrots	175 mL
1½ cups	prepared tomato pasta sauce	375 mL
1 cup	canned red kidney beans, rinsed and drained	250 mL
1 cup	canned chickpeas, rinsed and drained	250 mL
½ cup	vegetable stock (see recipe, page 53) or water	125 mL
1½ tsp	dried basil	7 mL
2	bay leaves	2
4 cups	diced potatoes	1 L
½ cup	2% milk	125 mL
⅓ cup	light sour cream	75 mL
¼ tsp	freshly ground black pepper	1 mL
¾ cup	shredded Cheddar cheese	175 mL
3 tbsp	grated Parmesan cheese	45 mL

1. In a saucepan heat oil over medium-high heat. Add garlic, onions and carrots; cook 4 minutes or until onion is softened. Stir in tomato sauce, kidney beans, chickpeas, stock, basil and bay leaves; reduce heat to medium-low, cover and cook 15 minutes or until vegetables are tender. Remove bay leaves. Transfer sauce to a food processor; pulse on and off just until chunky. Spread over bottom of baking dish.

Choices Per Serving

2½ Carbohydrates

½ Meat & Alternative

1 Fat

Nutritional Analysis Per Serving

Calories	322	Fat, total	11 g
Carbohydrate	42 g	Fat, saturated	6 g
Fiber	6 g	Sodium	466 mg
Protein	15 g	Cholesterol	27 mg

2. Place potatoes in a saucepan; add cold water to cover. Bring to a boil, reduce heat and simmer 10 to 12 minutes or until tender. Drain; mash with milk, sour cream and pepper. Spoon on top of sauce in baking dish. Sprinkle with cheeses.

3. Bake, uncovered, 20 minutes or until hot.

Spicy Rice, Bean and Lentil Casserole

2 tsp	vegetable oil	10 mL
2 tsp	minced garlic	10 mL
1 cup	chopped onions	250 mL
¾ cup	chopped green peppers	175 mL
3¾ cups	basic vegetable stock (see recipe, page 55)	950 mL
¾ cup	brown rice	175 mL
½ cup	green lentils	125 mL
1 tsp	dried basil	5 mL
1 tsp	chili powder	5 mL
1	can (19 oz/540 mL) red kidney beans, rinsed and drained	1
1 cup	canned or frozen corn kernels, drained	250 mL
1 cup	medium salsa	250 mL

1. In a nonstick saucepan, heat oil over medium-high heat. Add garlic, onions and green peppers; cook 3 minutes. Stir in stock, brown rice, lentils, basil and chili powder; bring to a boil, cover, reduce heat to medium-low and cook 30 to 40 minutes, stirring occasionally, until rice and lentils are tender and liquid is absorbed.

2. Stir in beans, corn and salsa; cover and cook 5 minutes or until heated through.

Choices Per Serving

3½ Carbohydrates
1½ Meat & Alternatives

Nutritional Analysis Per Serving

Calories	341	Fat, total	3 g
Carbohydrate	65 g	Fat, saturated	0 g
Fiber	11 g	Sodium	362 mg
Protein	17 g	Cholesterol	0 mg

Tips

If using whole dried mushrooms, slice after soaking.

Use any combination of wild mushrooms. If not available, use common mushrooms.

Vegetables supply the majority of the carbohydrate in this recipe.

- - - - - - - - - - - - -

Make Ahead

Prepare up to 1 day in advance. Reheat gently, adding more stock if too thick.

Three-Mushroom Tomato Potato Stew

1 cup	sliced dried mushrooms	250 mL
2 tsp	vegetable oil	10 mL
1½ cups	chopped onions	375 mL
2 tsp	minced garlic	10 mL
1 cup	chopped carrots	250 mL
4 cups	thinly sliced oyster mushrooms	1 L
3 cups	thinly sliced button mushrooms	750 mL
2 cups	basic vegetable stock (see recipe, page 55)	500 mL
1	can (19 oz/540 mL) tomatoes	1
¾ cup	chopped peeled sweet potatoes	175 mL
¾ cup	chopped peeled potatoes	175 mL
2 tbsp	tomato paste	25 mL
2	bay leaves	2
1 tsp	dried basil	5 mL
1 tsp	dried thyme	5 mL
¼ tsp	coarsely ground black pepper	1 mL

1. In a small bowl, add 2 cups (500 mL) boiling water to cover dried mushrooms. Soak 15 minutes. Drain, reserving soaking liquid; measure out 1 cup (250 mL).

2. In a large nonstick saucepan sprayed with vegetable spray, heat oil over medium-high heat. Add onions, garlic and carrots; cook, stirring occasionally, 5 minutes or until softened and browned. Stir in fresh mushrooms; cook 8 minutes longer, stirring occasionally, or until all liquid is absorbed.

3. Stir in dried mushrooms, reserved 1 cup (250 mL) mushroom liquid, stock, tomatoes, sweet potatoes, potatoes, tomato paste, bay leaves, basil, thyme and pepper. Bring to a boil, reduce heat to medium-low, cover, and cook 20 minutes or until potatoes are tender.

Choices Per Serving

3	Carbohydrates
½	Fat

Nutritional Analysis Per Serving			
Calories	252	Fat, total	4 g
Carbohydrate	53 g	Fat, saturated	0 g
Fiber	9 g	Sodium	440 mg
Protein	8 g	Cholesterol	0 mg

Tips

Serve in a pita or tortilla
with lettuce, tomatoes
and onions.

Another simple topping
can be made with 3 parts
2% yogurt and 1 part
Dijon mustard.

Substitute black beans
with another bean of
your choice.

Make Ahead

Prepare mixture and
sauce up to 1 day in
advance. Reheat gently.

Bean Burgers with Dill Sauce

BURGERS

2 cups	canned black beans, rinsed and drained	500 mL
½ cup	dry seasoned bread crumbs	125 mL
⅓ cup	chopped fresh dill	75 mL
⅓ cup	chopped red onions	75 mL
¼ cup	finely chopped carrots	50 mL
2 tbsp	cornmeal	25 mL
1	egg	1
1½ tsp	minced garlic	7 mL
¼ tsp	salt	1 mL

SAUCE

3 tbsp	light sour cream	45 mL
2 tbsp	light mayonnaise	25 mL
2 tsp	freshly squeezed lemon juice	10 mL
¼ to ½ tsp	minced garlic	1 to 2 mL
1 tbsp	chopped fresh dill (or ½ tsp/2 mL dried)	15 mL

1. In a food processor, combine black beans, bread crumbs, dill, onions, carrots, cornmeal, egg, garlic and salt. Pulse on and off until well combined. With wet hands, scoop up ¼ cup (50 mL) of mixture and form into a patty. Put on prepared baking sheet. Repeat procedure for remaining patties.

2. Bake 15 minutes, turning at the halfway point.

3. *Meanwhile, make the sauce:* In a small bowl, stir together sour cream, mayonnaise, lemon juice, garlic and dill.

4. Serve burgers hot with sauce on side.

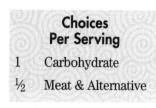

Choices Per Serving

1 Carbohydrate
½ Meat & Alternative

Nutritional Analysis Per Serving

Calories	122	Fat, total	3 g
Carbohydrate	19 g	Fat, saturated	1 g
Fiber	5 g	Sodium	491 mg
Protein	6 g	Cholesterol	27 mg

Tips

Replace coriander with dill or parsley.

Peanut butter can replace tahini.

These burgers are an excellent meatless main dish. The tahini is the source of most of the fat in this recipe. Like other nuts and seeds, the fat is primarily from monounsaturated sources.

Make Ahead

Prepare burgers early in the day and refrigerate until ready to cook. Prepare sauce to up a day ahead.

Falafel Burgers with Creamy Sesame Sauce

2 cups	drained canned chick peas	500 mL
1/4 cup	chopped green onions	50 mL
1/4 cup	chopped fresh coriander	50 mL
1/4 cup	finely chopped carrots	50 mL
1/4 cup	bread crumbs	50 mL
3 tbsp	lemon juice	45 mL
3 tbsp	water	45 mL
2 tbsp	tahini (puréed sesame seeds)	25 mL
2 tsp	minced garlic	10 mL
1/4 tsp	ground black pepper	1 mL
2 tsp	vegetable oil	10 mL

SAUCE

1/4 cup	light sour cream	50 mL
2 tbsp	tahini	25 mL
2 tbsp	chopped fresh coriander	25 mL
2 tbsp	water	25 mL
2 tsp	lemon juice	10 mL
1/2 tsp	minced garlic	2 mL

1. Put chick peas, green onions, coriander, carrots, bread crumbs, lemon juice, water, tahini, garlic and black pepper in food processor; pulse on and off until finely chopped. With wet hands, form each 1/4 cup (50 mL) into a patty.

2. In small bowl, whisk together sour cream, tahini, coriander, water, lemon juice and garlic.

3. In nonstick skillet sprayed with vegetable spray, heat 1 tsp (5 mL) of oil over medium heat. Add 4 patties and cook for 3 1/2 minutes or until golden; turn and cook 3 1/2 minutes longer or until golden and hot inside. Remove from pan. Heat remaining 1 tsp (5 mL) oil and cook remaining patties. Serve with sesame sauce.

Choices Per Serving

2	Carbohydrates
1	Meat & Alternative
2	Fats

Nutritional Analysis Per Serving

Calories	305	Fat, total	14 g
Carbohydrate	36 g	Fat, saturated	3 g
Fiber	6 g	Sodium	87 mg
Protein	12 g	Cholesterol	6 mg

Tips

Use a 10-oz (300 g)
package of frozen spinach
instead of fresh spinach.
All ricotta or all cottage
cheese can be used,
but ricotta gives a
creamy texture.

Serve this quiche with
fresh whole grain bread.
Half a cup (125 mL)
of no-sugar-added
raspberry yogurt served
over 1 cup (250 mL) of
fresh raspberries or
a sliced peach make
the meal complete.

Make Ahead

Prepare mixture early in
the day. Bake just before
serving. Great reheated
gently the next day.

Crustless Dill Spinach Quiche with Mushrooms and Cheese

10 oz	fresh spinach	300 g
2 tsp	vegetable oil	10 mL
1 tsp	minced garlic	5 mL
¾ cup	chopped onions	175 mL
¾ cup	chopped mushrooms	175 mL
⅔ cup	5% ricotta cheese	150 mL
⅔ cup	2% cottage cheese	150 mL
⅓ cup	grated Cheddar cheese	75 mL
2 tbsp	grated Parmesan cheese	25 mL
1	whole egg	1
1	egg white	1
3 tbsp	chopped fresh dill (or 2 tsp/10 mL dried)	45 mL
¼ tsp	ground black pepper	1 mL

1. Wash spinach and shake off excess water. In the water clinging to the leaves, cook the spinach over high heat just until it wilts. Squeeze out excess moisture, chop and set aside.

2. In large nonstick skillet, heat oil over medium heat; add garlic, onions and mushrooms and cook for 5 minutes or until softened. Remove from heat and add chopped spinach, ricotta, cottage, Cheddar and Parmesan cheeses, whole egg, egg white, dill and pepper; mix well. Pour into prepared pan and bake for 35 to 40 minutes or until knife inserted in center comes out clean.

Choices Per Serving

½ Carbohydrate

2 Meat & Alternatives

Nutritional Analysis Per Serving			
Calories	177	Fat, total	10 g
Carbohydrate	7 g	Fat, saturated	5 g
Fiber	2 g	Sodium	302 mg
Protein	14 g	Cholesterol	62 mg

Vegetables and Other Sides

Vegetables come in all shapes, sizes and flavors. Studies tell us that Canadians are consuming fewer than the recommended number of vegetable servings each day. Most are great sources of nutrients, and many contain phyto-chemicals, which have been linked to potential protective effects against cancer, heart disease, osteoporosis and diabetes.

Many of the side dishes here are based on Grains & Starches choices, which provide both soluble and insoluble fiber and other nutrients. Keep in mind that, most often, ½ cup (125 mL) cooked grains equals one serving of Grains & Starches.

continued on next page

Tips

Try making this dish with green beans. Trim and cut into 1½-inch (4 cm) lengths and cook in boiling water for about 5 minutes or until tender-crisp.

Asparagus makes this recipe an excellent source of folic acid.

Asparagus with Parmesan and Toasted Almonds

1½ lbs	asparagus	750 g
1/4 cup	sliced blanched almonds	50 mL
2 tbsp	margarine or butter	25 mL
2	cloves garlic, finely chopped	2
1/4 cup	freshly grated Parmesan cheese	50 mL
	Salt and freshly ground black pepper	

1. Snap off asparagus ends; cut spears on the diagonal into 2-inch (5 cm) lengths. In a large nonstick skillet, bring ½ cup (125 mL) water to a boil; cook asparagus for 2 minutes (start timing when water returns to a boil) or until just tender-crisp. Run under cold water to chill; drain and reserve.

2. Dry the skillet and place over medium heat. Add almonds and toast, stirring often, for 2 to 3 minutes or until golden. Remove and reserve.

3. Increase heat to medium-high. Add butter to skillet; cook asparagus and garlic, stirring, for 4 minutes or until asparagus is just tender.

4. Sprinkle with Parmesan; season with salt and pepper. Transfer to serving bowl; top with almonds.

Choices Per Serving

| ½ | Meat & Alternative |
| 1 | Fat |

Nutritional Analysis Per Serving			
Calories	107	Fat, total	8 g
Carbohydrate	7 g	Fat, saturated	4 g
Fiber	2 g	Sodium	113 mg
Protein	5 g	Cholesterol	14 mg

• • • • • • • • • • • • • • •

Tips

Adjust the lemon to taste.

If asparagus is not available, try broccoli.

This recipe is a good source of folate and vitamin C. A delicious accompaniment to a meal.

• • • • • • • • • • • • • • •

Make Ahead

Make this early in day if it is to be served cold, to allow the asparagus a chance to marinate.

Asparagus with Lemon and Garlic

½ lb	asparagus, trimmed	250 g
2 tsp	vegetable oil	10 mL
1 tsp	crushed garlic	5 mL
¼ cup	diced sweet red pepper	50 mL
1	green onion, sliced	1
2 tbsp	white wine	25 mL
4 tsp	lemon juice	20 mL
2 tbsp	chicken stock	25 mL
	Pepper	

1. Steam or boil asparagus just until tender-crisp. Do not overcook. Drain and set aside.

2. In large nonstick skillet, heat oil; sauté garlic and red pepper until softened.

3. Reduce heat and add green onion, wine, lemon juice, chicken stock, pepper to taste and asparagus. Cook for 1 minute. Place asparagus mixture in serving dish.

Choices
Per Serving

½   Fat

Nutritional Analysis Per Serving			
Calories	39	Fat, total	2 g
Carbohydrate	3 g	Fat, saturated	0 g
Fiber	1 g	Sodium	46 mg
Protein	1 g	Cholesterol	0 mg

Add a sprinkle of fresh herbs such as parsley or basil to oil mixture.

An excellent source of vitamin C.

Green Beans and Diced Tomatoes

8 oz	green beans, trimmed	250 g
1½ tsp	vegetable oil	7 mL
1 tsp	crushed garlic	5 mL
¾ cup	chopped onion	175 mL
⅓ cup	chopped sweet red or yellow pepper	75 mL
1½ cups	diced tomatoes	375 mL
½ tsp	dried basil (or 1 tbsp/15 mL fresh)	2 mL
½ tsp	dried oregano	2 mL
2 tbsp	chicken stock	25 mL
2 tsp	lemon juice	10 mL
2 tsp	grated Parmesan cheese (optional)	10 mL

1. Steam or microwave green beans just until tender. Set aside.

2. In nonstick skillet, heat oil; sauté garlic, onion and red pepper just until tender.

3. Add green beans, tomatoes, basil, oregano, stock and lemon juice; cook for 2 minutes, stirring constantly. Serve sprinkled with Parmesan (if using).

Choices Per Serving

½ Carbohydrate

½ Fats

Nutritional Analysis Per Serving

Calories	77	Fat, total	3 g
Carbohydrate	13 g	Fat, saturated	0 g
Fiber	3 g	Sodium	74 mg
Protein	3 g	Cholesterol	1 mg

Tips

To make fresh bread
crumbs, process 2 thick
slices crusty bread in a
food processor until fine.

This recipe is an
excellent source of
vitamin C, magnesium
and folic acid.

Baked White Beans with Garlic Crumb Crust

3 tbsp	olive oil	45 mL
2 cups	chopped Spanish onion	500 mL
3	cloves garlic, finely chopped	3
2 tbsp	balsamic vinegar	25 mL
5	tomatoes, seeded and diced	5
1 tbsp	chopped fresh thyme or 1 tsp (5 mL) dried thyme leaves	15 mL
1	large bay leaf	1
	Salt and freshly ground black pepper	
2	zucchini, halved lengthwise, thickly sliced	2
1	red bell pepper, diced	1
1	yellow bell pepper, diced	1
2	cans (each 19 oz/ 540 mL) white kidney beans, drained and rinsed	2

GARLIC CRUMB CRUST

1½ cups	soft fresh bread crumbs (see tip)	375 mL
¼ cup	chopped fresh parsley	50 mL
2	cloves garlic, minced	2
2 tbsp	olive oil	25 mL

1. In a Dutch oven or large saucepan, heat oil over medium heat. Cook onions and garlic, stirring often, for 5 minutes or until softened. Add balsamic vinegar and cook until evaporated. Add tomatoes, thyme and bay leaf; season with salt and pepper. Bring to boil. Reduce heat, cover and simmer for 20 minutes.

2. Add zucchini and peppers; cook for 5 to 7 minutes or until vegetables are tender-crisp. Gently stir in beans.

Choices Per Serving

1½ Carbohydrates

2 Fats

Nutritional Analysis Per Serving			
Calories	261	Fat, total	10 g
Carbohydrate	37 g	Fat, saturated	1 g
Fiber	11 g	Sodium	475 mg
Protein	10 g	Cholesterol	0 mg

3. Spoon mixture into prepared baking dish. (Can be prepared up to this point, covered and refrigerated for up to one day.)

4. *Garlic Crumb Crust:* In a bowl, combine bread crumbs, parsley and garlic. Drizzle with olive oil and toss to coat. Sprinkle crumb topping over beans; bake for 35 to 45 minutes or until bubbly and top is golden.

Tips

The simple addition of cashews and red onions to this dish transforms ordinary green beans into a formidable companion to any gourmet main course.

Both the cashews and the oil contribute fat to this delicious dish. As with most plant sources of fat, the majority of fat supplied is monounsaturated. Nutrient recommendations suggest that most of our fat (80%) come from these sources.

Green Beans with Cashews

1 lb	green beans, trimmed	500 g
2 tbsp	olive oil	25 mL
½ cup	slivered red onions	125 mL
⅓ cup	raw cashews	75 mL
¼ tsp	salt	1 mL
¼ tsp	black pepper	1 mL
	Few sprigs fresh parsley, chopped	

1. Blanch green beans in a pot of boiling water for 5 minutes. Drain and immediately refresh in a bowl of ice-cold water. Drain and set aside.

2. In a large frying pan heat olive oil over medium-high heat for 30 seconds. Add onions, cashews, salt and pepper and stir-fry for 2 to 3 minutes, until the onions are softened. Add cooked green beans, raise heat to high, and stir-fry actively for 2 to 3 minutes, until the beans feel hot to the touch. (Take care that you don't burn any cashews in the process.) Transfer to a serving plate and garnish with chopped parsley. Serve immediately.

**Choices
Per Serving**

1   Carbohydrate

2½   Fats

Nutritional Analysis Per Serving

Calories	172	Fat, total	12 g
Carbohydrate	14 g	Fat, saturated	2 g
Fiber	3 g	Sodium	215 mg
Protein	4 g	Cholesterol	0 mg

● ● ● ● ● ● ● ● ● ● ● ● ● ● ●

Tips

While North American
tastes are generally
restricted to broccoli
florets, Asian cooking
also uses broccoli stalks
extensively. So don't
throw them away — trim
the woody bottoms and
peel the stalks using
a paring knife; then cut
the tender, mild interior
into slices or strips.

Broccoli and peppers are
a winning combination,
providing excellent
sources of vitamins A
and C and folic acid.

Orange Broccoli with Red Pepper

1/3 cup	orange juice	75 mL
1/2 tsp	cornstarch	2 mL
1 tbsp	olive oil	15 mL
4 cups	small broccoli florets and stalks, cut into 1 1/2- by 1/2-inch (4 by 1 cm) lengths	1 L
1	sweet red pepper, cut into 2- by 1/2-inch (5 by 1 cm) strips	1
1	clove garlic, minced	1
1 tsp	grated orange rind	5 mL
1/4 tsp	salt	1 mL
1/4 tsp	pepper	1 mL

1. In a glass measuring cup, stir together orange juice and cornstarch until smooth; reserve.

2. Heat oil in a large nonstick skillet over high heat. Add broccoli, red pepper and garlic; cook, stirring, for 2 minutes.

3. Add orange juice mixture; cover and cook 1 to 2 minutes or until vegetables are tender-crisp. Sprinkle with orange rind; season with salt and pepper. Serve immediately.

Choices Per Serving

1/2   Carbohydrate

1/2   Fat

Nutritional Analysis Per Serving

Calories	78	Fat, total	4 g
Carbohydrate	10 g	Fat, saturated	1 g
Fiber	3 g	Sodium	161 mg
Protein	3 g	Cholesterol	0 mg

Tips

Brussels sprouts can have a slightly bitter taste, especially if overcooked. The addition of sweet potatoes and pecans balances the flavor.

Toast pecans in 400°F (200°C) oven or in skillet on top of stove for 2 minutes or until brown.

With relatively little change in taste, the brown sugar or honey can be replaced with granulated sugar substitute to save about 5 g of carbohydrate/serving.

Brussels Sprouts with Pecans and Sweet Potatoes

1½ cups	cubed peeled sweet potatoes	375 mL
¾ lb	brussels sprouts, cut in half	375 g
1 tbsp	margarine	15 mL
½ cup	chopped onion	125 mL
1 tsp	crushed garlic	5 mL
¼ cup	chicken stock	50 mL
4 tsp	brown sugar or honey	20 mL
¼ tsp	cinnamon	1 mL
2 tbsp	pecan pieces, toasted	25 mL

1. In saucepan of boiling water, cook sweet potatoes until just tender; drain and reserve. Repeat with brussels sprouts. Set aside.

2. In nonstick skillet, melt margarine; sauté onion and garlic just until tender. Add sweet potatoes, brussels sprouts, stock, sugar, cinnamon and pecans; cook for 3 minutes or until vegetables are tender.

Choices Per Serving

1½ Carbohydrates
1   Fat

Nutritional Analysis Per Serving

Calories	186	Fat, total	6 g
Carbohydrate	32 g	Fat, saturated	1 g
Fiber	6 g	Sodium	152 mg
Protein	6 g	Cholesterol	0 mg

Tips

For a modern spin of an Oktoberfest dinner, spoon cabbage in center of serving plates and top with grilled sausages or smoked pork chops.

Honey provides 5 g of carbohydrate. A sugar substitute can replace this and reduce the Carbohydrate choice to ½.

Sweet-and-Spicy Cabbage

1	large pear or apple	1
2 tbsp	vegetable oil	25 mL
½	red onion, cut into thin wedge strips	½
½ tsp	hot pepper flakes or to taste	2 mL
½	small Savoy cabbage, finely shredded	½
2 tbsp	rice vinegar	25 mL
1 tbsp	liquid honey	15 mL
	Salt	

1. Cut pear into quarters and core (not necessary to peel). Thinly slice, then cut slices in half.

2. In a large nonstick skillet, heat oil over high heat until almost smoking. Add pear, onion and hot pepper flakes; stir-fry for 1 minute. Add cabbage and stir-fry for 1 minute more or until wilted.

3. Stir in rice vinegar and honey; cook, stirring, for 30 seconds. Season with salt to taste; serve immediately.

Choices Per Serving

1	Carbohydrate
1½	Fats

Nutritional Analysis Per Serving

Calories	125	Fat, total	7 g
Carbohydrate	17 g	Fat, saturated	1 g
Fiber	3 g	Sodium	16 mg
Protein	2 g	Cholesterol	0 mg

● ● ● ● ● ● ● ● ● ● ● ● ● ● ● ●

Tips

If doubling the recipe, glaze vegetables in a large nonstick skillet to evaporate the stock quickly.

Try this tasty treatment with a combination of blanched carrots, rutabaga and parsnip strips, too.

This recipe contains almost 3 days' supply of vitamin A.

Lemon-Glazed Baby Carrots

1 lb	peeled baby carrots	500 g
¼ cup	chicken stock or vegetable stock (see recipe, page 53)	50 mL
1 tbsp	margarine or butter	15 mL
1 tbsp	brown sugar	15 mL
1 tbsp	lemon juice	15 mL
½ tsp	grated lemon rind	2 mL
¼ tsp	salt	1 mL
	Pepper to taste	
1 tbsp	finely chopped fresh parsley or chives	15 mL

1. In a medium saucepan, cook carrots in boiling salted water for 5 to 7 minutes (start timing when water returns to a boil) or until just tender-crisp; drain and return to saucepan.

2. Add stock, butter, brown sugar, lemon juice and rind, salt and pepper. Cook, stirring often, 3 to 5 minutes or until liquid has evaporated and carrots are nicely glazed.

3. Sprinkle with parsley or chives and serve.

Choices Per Serving

1	Carbohydrate
½	Fat

Nutritional Analysis Per Serving

Calories	91	Fat, total	3 g
Carbohydrate	15 g	Fat, saturated	2 g
Fiber	3 g	Sodium	261 mg
Protein	2 g	Cholesterol	8 mg

Tips

A colorful, emphatically dressed combination of lush red pepper and the oft-neglected cauliflower, this salad travels well on picnics in the summer, just as it helps to liven up a cozy dinner in winter.

This is an excellent source of vitamins A and C.

Cauliflower and Red Pepper

1	head cauliflower, florets only	1
2	red bell peppers, roasted, skinned and cut into thick strips	2
¼ tsp	salt	1 mL
¼ tsp	black pepper	1 mL
2 tbsp	lemon juice	25 mL
1 tbsp	Dijon mustard	15 mL
1 tsp	vegetable oil	5 mL
1 tsp	black mustard seeds	5 mL
½ tsp	turmeric	2 mL
½ tsp	whole coriander seeds	2 mL
2	cloves garlic	2
2 tbsp	olive oil	25 mL

1. Blanch cauliflower florets in a large saucepan of boiling water for 5 to 6 minutes, until just cooked. Drain, refresh in iced water, drain again and transfer to a bowl. Add red peppers to cauliflower. Sprinkle with salt and pepper and toss.

2. In a small bowl whisk together the lemon juice and Dijon mustard until blended. Set aside.

3. In a small frying pan heat vegetable oil over medium heat for 1 minute. Add mustard seeds, turmeric and coriander seeds, and stir-fry for 2 to 3 minutes, or until the seeds begin to pop. With a rubber spatula, scrape cooked spices from the pan into the lemon-mustard mixture. Squeeze garlic through a garlic press and add to the mixture. Add olive oil and whisk until the dressing has emulsified.

4. Add dressing to the cauliflower–red pepper mixture. Toss gently but thoroughly to dress all the pieces evenly. Transfer to a serving bowl, propping up the red pepper ribbons to properly accent the yellow-tinted cauliflower. This salad benefits greatly from a 1- or 2-hour wait, after which it should be served at room temperature.

Choices Per Serving

½	Carbohydrate
1	Fat

Nutritional Analysis Per Serving

Calories	83	Fat, total	6 g
Carbohydrate	7 g	Fat, saturated	1 g
Fiber	2 g	Sodium	142 mg
Protein	2 g	Cholesterol	0 mg

Preheat oven to
350°F (180°C)

2-quart (2 L) casserole
dish sprayed with
vegetable spray

Tips

Be sure to use
evaporated milk — it's
what gives this dish
its creaminess.

Leeks can have a lot of
hidden dirt — to clean
thoroughly, slice in half
lengthwise and wash
under cold running water,
getting between the
layers where dirt hides.

Use fresh parsley, basil or
coriander instead of dill.

Reheat leftovers gently.

Make Ahead

Cook vegetables early
in day. Bake dish just
before serving.

Corn, Leek and Red Pepper Casserole

1 tsp	vegetable oil	5 mL
1 tsp	minced garlic	5 mL
1 cup	sliced leeks	250 mL
1 cup	chopped red peppers	250 mL
2 cups	corn kernels	500 mL
2½ tbsp	all-purpose flour	35 mL
2	whole eggs	2
2	egg whites	2
1⅓ cups	2% evaporated milk	325 mL
¼ cup	chopped fresh dill (or 2 tsp/10 mL dried)	50 mL
¼ cup	bread crumbs	50 mL
½ tsp	margarine or butter	2 mL

1. In nonstick skillet sprayed with vegetable spray, heat oil over medium heat. Add garlic, leeks and red peppers and cook for 7 minutes, or until tender, stirring occasionally; set aside.

2. Put 1 cup (250 mL) of corn in food processor with flour; purée. Add whole eggs, egg whites, evaporated milk and dill; process until smooth.

3. In large bowl, combine sautéed vegetables, corn purée and remaining 1 cup (250 mL) corn. Pour into prepared dish. Combine bread crumbs and margarine until crumbly. Sprinkle over top casserole and bake for 30 minutes or until set at center.

Choices Per Serving

1½ Carbohydrates

1 Fat

Nutritional Analysis Per Serving			
Calories	169	Fat, total	5 g
Carbohydrate	26 g	Fat, saturated	1 g
Fiber	2 g	Sodium	110 mg
Protein	8 g	Cholesterol	76 mg

Preheat oven to
425°F (220°C)

Baking sheet sprayed
with vegetable spray

Tips

These mushrooms can
serve as a wonderful
appetizer or side dish
with a main meal.

Use fresh parsley or
spinach to replace basil,
or use a combination.

Toast pine nuts in a
nonstick skillet for
2 minutes until browned.

Make Ahead

Prepare filling up to a day
ahead. Fill mushrooms
early in the day. Bake just
before serving.

Cheesy Pesto Stuffed Mushrooms

14 oz	large stuffing mushrooms (approximately 16)	350 g
3/4 cup	packed basil leaves	175 mL
1 1/2 tbsp	olive oil	20 mL
1 1/2 tbsp	toasted pine nuts	20 mL
1 tbsp	grated Parmesan cheese	15 mL
1/2 tsp	minced garlic	2 mL
2 tbsp	chicken stock or water	25 mL
1/4 cup	5% ricotta cheese	50 mL

1. Wipe mushrooms clean and gently remove stems; reserve for another purpose. Put caps on baking sheet.

2. Put basil, olive oil, pine nuts, Parmesan and garlic in food processor; process until finely chopped, scraping down sides of bowl once. Add stock through the feed tube and process until smooth. Add ricotta and process until mixed.

3. Divide mixture evenly among mushroom caps. Bake for 10 to 15 minutes or until hot.

Choices Per Serving	
1/2	Meat & Alternative
1/2	Fat

Nutritional Analysis Per Serving

Calories	68	Fat, total	5 g
Carbohydrate	4 g	Fat, saturated	1 g
Fiber	1 g	Sodium	62 mg
Protein	3 g	Cholesterol	4 mg

Slow cooker

Tip

This is a great dish to serve with roasted poultry or meat. If your guests like spice, pass hot pepper sauce at the table.

New Orleans Braised Onions

2 to 3	large Spanish onions	2 to 3
6 to 9	whole cloves	6 to 9
½ tsp	salt	2 mL
½ tsp	cracked black peppercorns	2 mL
Pinch	ground thyme	Pinch
	Grated zest and juice of 1 orange	
½ cup	condensed beef broth, undiluted	125 mL
	Finely chopped fresh parsley, optional	
	Hot pepper sauce, optional	

1. Stud onions with cloves. Place in slow cooker stoneware and sprinkle with salt, peppercorns, thyme and orange zest. Pour orange juice and beef broth over onions, cover and cook on Low for 8 hours or on High for 4 hours, until onions are tender.

2. Keep onions warm. In a saucepan over medium heat, reduce cooking liquid by half.

3. When ready to serve, cut onions into quarters. Place on a deep platter and cover with sauce. Sprinkle with parsley, if desired, and pass the hot pepper sauce, if desired.

Choices Per Serving

1   Extra

Nutritional Analysis Per Serving

Calories	20	Fat, total	0 g
Carbohydrate	4 g	Fat, saturated	0 g
Fiber	1 g	Sodium	188 mg
Protein	1 g	Cholesterol	0 mg

Oriental Beef Bundles in Lettuce *page 214*
Overleaf: Curried Lamb Casserole with Sweet Potatoes *page 226*

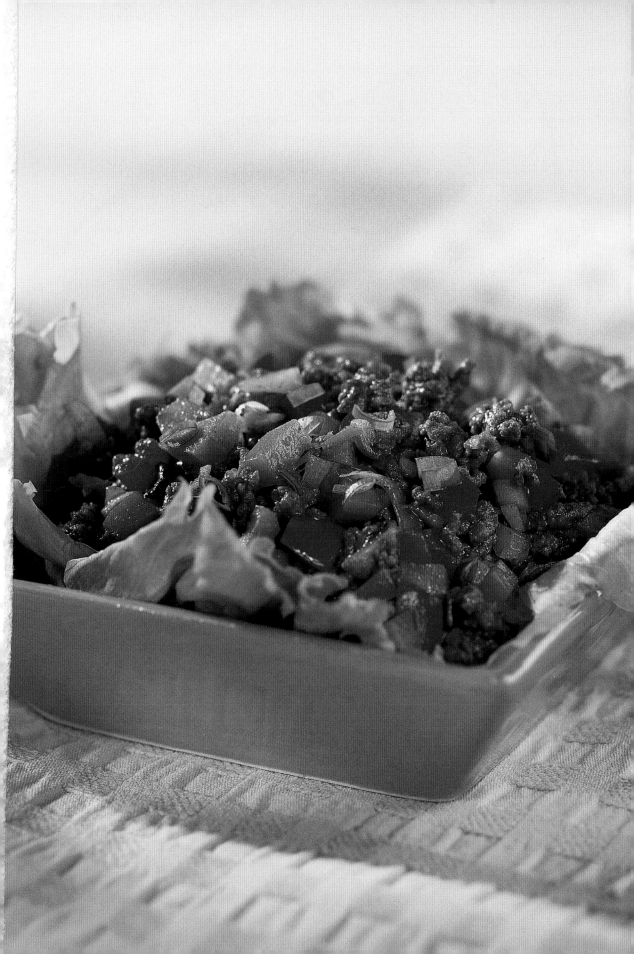

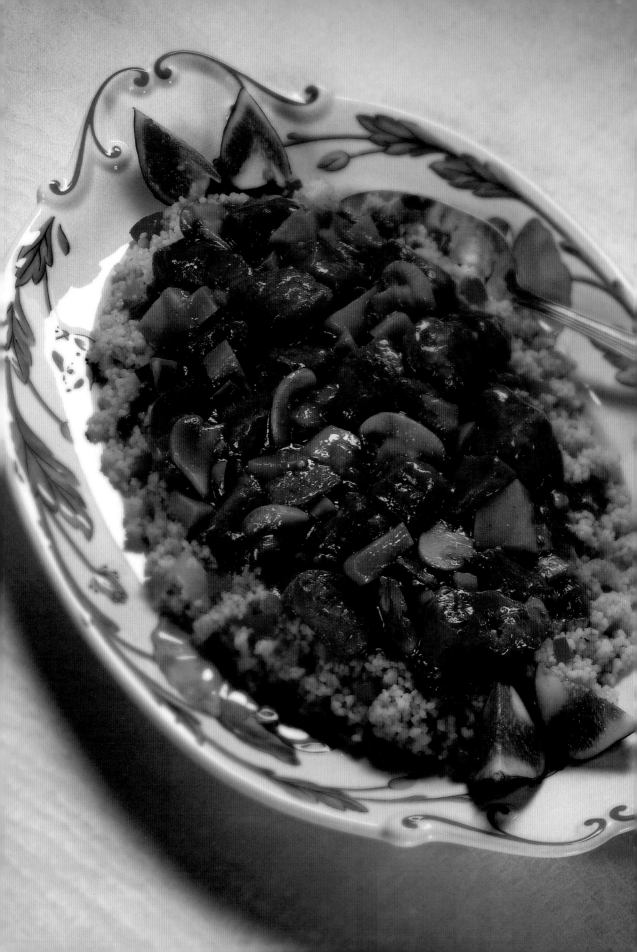

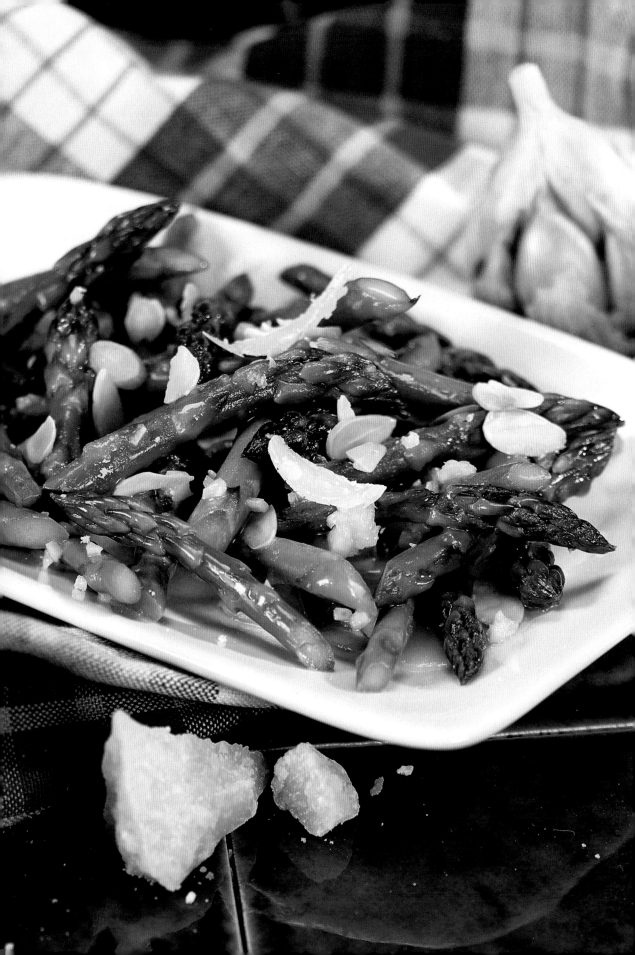

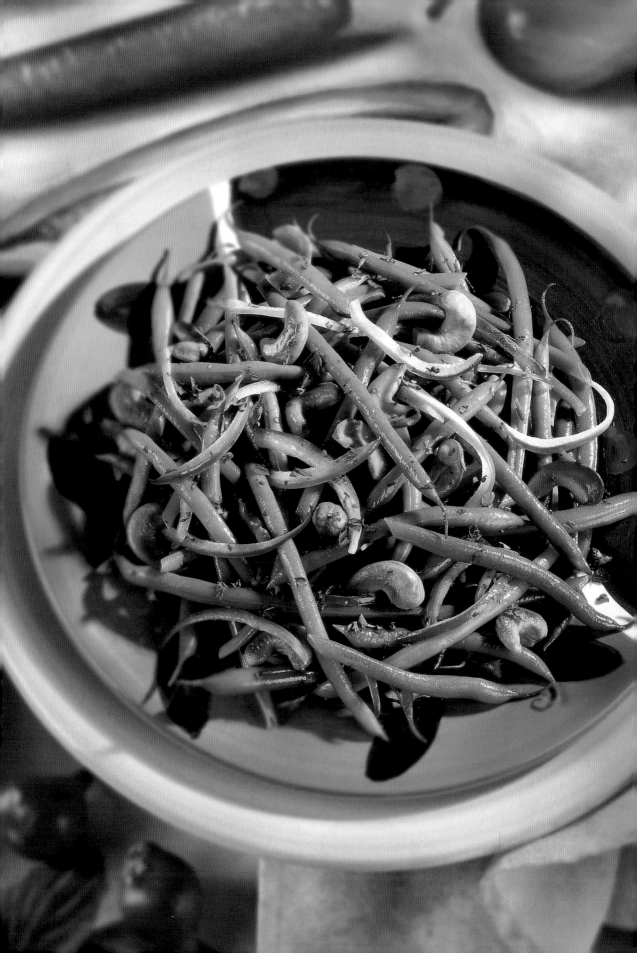

Use any other combination of vegetables. Keep colors contrasting.

A delicious combination of vegetables serving as an excellent source of vitamins A and C. Serve with traditional meals to brighten up any ordinary supper.

Remember to cook on a high heat and not to overcook.

Teriyaki Sesame Vegetables

1½ tsp	vegetable oil	7 mL
1 tsp	crushed garlic	5 mL
Half	large sweet red or yellow pepper, sliced thinly	Half
Half	large sweet green pepper, sliced thinly	Half
1½ cups	snow peas	375 mL
1	large carrot, sliced thinly	1
½ tsp	sesame seeds	2 mL

SAUCE

1 tsp	crushed garlic	5 mL
1 tbsp	soya sauce	15 mL
1 tbsp	rice wine vinegar or white wine vinegar	15 mL
½ tsp	minced gingerroot	2 mL
½ tsp	sesame oil	2 mL
1 tbsp	water	15 mL
1 tbsp	brown sugar	15 mL
1½ tsp	vegetable oil	7 mL

1. *Sauce:* In small saucepan, combine garlic, soya sauce, vinegar, ginger, sesame oil, water, sugar and vegetable oil; cook for 3 to 5 minutes or until thickened and syrupy.

2. In large nonstick skillet, heat oil; sauté garlic, red and green peppers, snow peas and carrot, stirring constantly, for 2 minutes.

3. Add sauce; sauté for 2 minutes or just until vegetables are tender-crisp. Place in serving dish and sprinkle with sesame seeds.

Choices Per Serving

½ Carbohydrate

1½ Fats

Nutritional Analysis Per Serving			
Calories	128	Fat, total	8 g
Carbohydrate	13 g	Fat, saturated	1 g
Fiber	2 g	Sodium	256 mg
Protein	3 g	Cholesterol	0 mg

Tips

The potatoes can also
be diced.

Substitute another
cheese of your choice,
such as Swiss or
mozzarella.

The milk and cheese
in this casserole make
it an excellent source
of calcium. Using
low-fat cheese can
reduce the fat content
in this recipe to
7 g/serving or eliminate
1 Fats choice.

Make Ahead

This casserole can be
prepared and refrigerated
up to 24 hours ahead of
time and baked just prior
to eating.

Potato Cheese Casserole

4	medium potatoes, peeled and thinly sliced	4
1½ tsp	margarine	7 mL
1 cup	chopped onions	250 mL
1 tsp	crushed garlic	5 mL
2 tbsp	all-purpose flour	25 mL
1¾ cups	2% warm milk	425 mL
3 tbsp	chopped fresh dill (or 1 tsp/5 mL dried dillweed)	45 mL
	Salt and pepper	
½ cup	shredded Cheddar cheese	125 mL

1. In saucepan of boiling water, cook potatoes just until fork-tender, approximately 10 minutes; drain. Arrange in baking dish just large enough to lay in single layer of overlapping slices.

2. In medium nonstick saucepan, melt margarine; sauté onions and garlic for 5 minutes or until softened. Add flour and cook, stirring, for 1 minute. Slowly stir in milk, simmer until thickened, stirring constantly, 3 to 4 minutes. Add dill; season with salt and pepper to taste.

3. Pour sauce over potatoes; sprinkle with cheese. Cover and bake for approximately 1 hour or until potatoes are tender.

**Choices
Per Serving**

1½   Carbohydrates

1   Meat & Alternative

1½   Fats

Nutritional Analysis Per Serving			
Calories	252	Fat, total	11 g
Carbohydrate	27 g	Fat, saturated	7 g
Fiber	2 g	Sodium	263 mg
Protein	12 g	Cholesterol	32 mg

Tips

Smoked salmon freezes
well for up to 4 weeks.
Use as needed.

Red onions or sweet
Vidalia onions can
replace green onions.

If in a hurry, microwave
potatoes. Each potato
cooks in approximately
8 minutes at high power.

Make Ahead

Prepare filling up to a day
ahead and fill potatoes.
Bake just before serving.

Baked Potatoes Stuffed with Smoked Salmon and Broccoli

4	medium baking potatoes	4
1 cup	chopped broccoli florets	250 mL
2/3 cup	light sour cream	150 mL
1/4 cup	2% milk	50 mL
1/4 cup	grated Parmesan cheese	50 mL
2 tbsp	chopped fresh dill (or 2 tsp/10 mL dried)	25 mL
1/4 cup	chopped green onions (about 2 medium)	50 mL
3 oz	smoked salmon, chopped	75 g

1. Bake the potatoes for 1 hour or until easily pierced with a fork; let cool slightly. Meanwhile, in a saucepan of boiling water or in microwave, cook the broccoli for 1 minute or until tender-crisp. Drain and set aside.

2. Cut potatoes in half lengthwise, and carefully scoop out flesh, leaving skins intact. Mash potato with sour cream and milk; stir in 2 tbsp (25 mL) of the Parmesan, the dill, green onions, smoked salmon and broccoli. Spoon mixture back into potato skin shells; sprinkle with remaining 2 tbsp (25 mL) Parmesan. Bake for 10 to 15 minutes, or until heated through.

Choices Per Serving

1	Carbohydrate
1/2	Meat & Alternative
1/2	Fat

Nutritional Analysis Per Serving

Calories	118	Fat, total	4 g
Carbohydrate	15 g	Fat, saturated	2 g
Fiber	2 g	Sodium	154 mg
Protein	6 g	Cholesterol	14 mg

....

....

Tip

Leave the skins on potatoes, scrub thoroughly and dry on paper towels. Cut in half any that are larger than 1 inch (2.5 cm) in diameter.

....

Make Ahead

This dish can be partially prepared the night before it is cooked. Complete Steps 1 and 2 and refrigerate overnight. The next day, continue cooking as directed in Step 3.

New Potato Curry

2 tbsp	vegetable oil or clarified butter	25 mL
1 lb	small new potatoes, about 10 new potatoes (see tip)	500 g
2	onions, finely chopped	2
1	clove garlic, minced	1
1 tsp	curry powder, preferably Madras	5 mL
½ tsp	salt	2 mL
½ tsp	cracked black peppercorns	2 mL
½ cup	water or vegetable or chicken stock	125 mL
2 tbsp	lemon juice	25 mL
¼ cup	finely chopped cilantro	50 mL

1. In a skillet, heat butter or oil over medium-high heat. Add potatoes and cook just until they begin to brown. Transfer to slow cooker stoneware.

2. Reduce heat to medium. Add onions and cook, stirring, until softened. Add garlic, curry powder, salt and pepper. Stir and cook for 1 minute. Add water or stock, bring to a boil and pour over potatoes.

3. Cover and cook on Low for 8 to 10 hours or on High for 4 to 5 hours, until potatoes are tender. Stir in lemon juice and garnish with cilantro.

Choices Per Serving

1 Carbohydrate

1 Fat

Nutritional Analysis Per Serving			
Calories	111	Fat, total	4 g
Carbohydrate	17 g	Fat, saturated	3 g
Fiber	2 g	Sodium	288 mg
Protein	3 g	Cholesterol	10 mg

Preheat oven to
350°F (180°C)

Baking dish sprayed with
nonstick vegetable spray

Tips

The darker the skin of
the sweet potato, the
moister it is.

This recipe should be
reserved for special
occasions as it is
relatively high in
carbohydrate for an
everyday meal. The
honey or maple syrup
can be replaced with
granulated sugar
substitute to save about
14 g of carbohydrate/
serving and reduce the
Carbohydrate choice
to 1½.

Chopped dates or
apricots can replace
the raisins.

Make Ahead

Prepare casserole
without apples up to the
day before. Add apples,
toss and bake just
prior to serving.

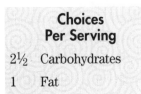

Choices Per Serving	
2½	Carbohydrates
1	Fat

Sweet Potato, Apple and Raisin Casserole

1 lb	sweet potatoes, peeled and cubed	500 g
¾ tsp	ground ginger	4 mL
¼ cup	honey or maple syrup	50 mL
¾ tsp	ground cinnamon	4 mL
2 tbsp	margarine, melted	25 mL
¼ cup	raisins	50 mL
2 tbsp	chopped walnuts	25 mL
¾ cup	cubed peeled sweet apples	175 mL

1. Steam or microwave sweet potatoes just until slightly underdone. Drain and place in baking dish.

2. In small bowl, combine ginger, honey, cinnamon, margarine, raisins, walnuts and apples; mix well. Pour over sweet potatoes and bake, uncovered, for 20 minutes or until tender.

Nutritional Analysis Per Serving			
Calories	216	Fat, total	6 g
Carbohydrate	42 g	Fat, saturated	1 g
Fiber	3 g	Sodium	60 mg
Protein	2 g	Cholesterol	0 mg

Tips

Gnocchi is the Italian version of dumplings, usually made from potatoes or flour. This sweet potato version is served the traditional way with a sauce. It makes a wonderful side dish.

The sweet potatoes help to make this recipe an excellent source of vitamins A and E.

Sweet Potato Gnocchi with Parmesan Sauce

1½ lbs	sweet potatoes, scrubbed	750 g
⅓ cup	5% ricotta cheese	75 mL
1	large egg	1
¼ tsp	ground cinnamon	1 mL
⅛ tsp	freshly ground black pepper	0.5 mL
Pinch	salt	Pinch
1½ cups	all-purpose flour	375 mL

PARMESAN SAUCE

2 tsp	margarine or butter	10 mL
1½ tbsp	all-purpose flour	20 mL
1 cup	low-fat milk	250 mL
⅔ cup	vegetable stock (see recipe, page 53) or chicken stock	150 mL
3 tbsp	grated low-fat Parmesan cheese	45 mL

1. In a saucepan over medium-high heat, cover sweet potatoes with cold water; bring to a boil. Cook for 30 minutes or until tender when pierced with a fork; drain. When cool enough to handle, peel potatoes; mash. Add ricotta cheese, egg, cinnamon, pepper and salt; mash until well combined. Mix in flour.

2. On a lightly floured wooden board, roll about one-quarter of dough into a rope as thick as your thumb. With a sharp knife, cut into ¾-inch (2 cm) pieces. Repeat with remaining dough. Keep gnocchi pieces separate to avoid sticking.

3. In a large pot of boiling water, cook gnocchi (in batches of about 20) for 3 minutes or until they rise to the top; cook for another 30 seconds. Remove with a slotted spoon to a warm serving dish.

Choices Per Serving

2	Carbohydrates
½	Fat

Nutritional Analysis Per Serving

Calories	214	Fat, total	4 g
Carbohydrate	39 g	Fat, saturated	1 g
Fiber	3 g	Sodium	115 mg
Protein	7 g	Cholesterol	33 mg

4. *Sauce:* In a small nonstick saucepan, heat margarine over low heat. Add flour; cook, stirring, for 1 minute. Add milk and stock; bring to a boil, whisking constantly. Reduce heat to low; cook for 5 minutes. Remove from heat. Add Parmesan cheese.

5. In a serving bowl combine gnocchi and sauce; toss well. Serve immediately.

Garden Paella

Tip

This recipe is an excellent source of vitamin C and folic acid.

2 tbsp	olive oil	25 mL
1	sweet red pepper, cut in strips	1
1	onion, finely chopped	1
2	cloves garlic, minced	2
2	tomatoes, peeled and chopped	2
1½ cups	Arborio or other short-grain rice	375 mL
3 cups	chicken or vegetable stock (see recipe, page 53)	750 mL
¾ tsp	salt, optional	4 mL
¼ tsp	saffron threads, crushed	1 mL
1 lb	asparagus	500 g
½ cup	sliced unblanched almonds	125 mL
2	hard-cooked eggs, cut in wedges	2
	Pepper	

1. In large deep skillet, heat oil over medium-high heat; cook red pepper, onion and garlic for 5 minutes, stirring occasionally. Add tomatoes; cook for about 3 minutes, stirring constantly, until thickened and most of the liquid has evaporated. Remove from heat.

2. Stir in rice to coat. Stir in stock, optional salt and saffron. Return skillet to heat; bring to boil. Reduce heat to low; simmer, covered, for 15 minutes or until rice is almost tender.

3. Cut each asparagus spear into thirds crosswise; arrange over rice. Cook, covered, for 5 to 8 minutes or until rice and asparagus are tender and liquid is absorbed. With fork, stir in almonds. Serve garnished with eggs and sprinkled with pepper to taste.

Choices Per Serving

2½ Carbohydrates
½ Meat & Alternative
1½ Fats

Nutritional Analysis Per Serving

Calories	280	Fat, total	10 g
Carbohydrate	38 g	Fat, saturated	2 g
Fiber	2 g	Sodium	297 mg
Protein	10 g	Cholesterol	54 mg

Sautéed Rice with Almonds, Curry and Ginger

1 tbsp	vegetable oil	15 mL
1 tsp	crushed garlic	5 mL
1½ cups	thinly sliced bok choy or nappa cabbage	375 mL
1 cup	snow peas	250 mL
½ cup	chopped sweet red pepper	125 mL
⅓ cup	chopped carrot	75 mL
1 tsp	ground ginger	5 mL
1 tsp	curry powder	5 mL
¾ cup	chicken stock	175 mL
4 tsp	soya sauce	20 mL
1	egg	1
2 cups	cooked rice	500 mL
2 tbsp	toasted chopped almonds	25 mL
2 tbsp	chopped green onion	25 mL

1. In large nonstick skillet, heat oil; sauté garlic, cabbage, snow peas, red pepper and carrot for 3 minutes or just until tender, stirring constantly. Add ginger, curry powder, stock and soya sauce; cook for 1 minute.

2. Add egg and rice; cook for 1 minute or until egg is well incorporated. Place in serving dish and sprinkle with almonds and green onions.

Nutritional Analysis Per Serving			
Calories	249	Fat, total	7 g
Carbohydrate	39 g	Fat, saturated	1 g
Fiber	2 g	Sodium	630 mg
Protein	8 g	Cholesterol	54 mg

Moors and Christians

Tips

Although there are several different versions of how this classic Cuban dish got its name, all lead back to the eighth century, when Spain was invaded by its enemy, the Moors.

This dish is also delicious cold and makes a nice addition to a buffet as a rice salad.

An excellent source of vitamin C.

1	roasted red bell pepper, finely chopped	1
1 tbsp	vegetable oil	15 mL
2	medium onions, finely chopped	2
4	large cloves garlic, minced	4
2 tsp	dried oregano leaves	10 mL
2 tsp	cumin seeds	10 mL
1	medium tomato, peeled, seeded and chopped	1
1	can (19 oz/540 mL) black beans, rinsed and drained, or 1 cup (250 mL) dried black beans, cooked and drained	1
½ cup	condensed chicken broth (undiluted)	125 mL
2 cups	long-grain rice	500 mL
1	green bell pepper, finely chopped	1
2 tbsp	lemon or lime juice	25 mL
¼ cup	finely chopped cilantro	50 mL
4	green onions, white part only, finely chopped	4

1. In a skillet, heat oil over medium heat. Add onion and cook until soft. Add garlic, oregano and cumin seeds and cook for 1 minute. Stirring, add roasted red pepper, tomato, beans and chicken broth and bring to a boil. Transfer to slow cooker stoneware.

2. Cover and cook on Low for 8 to 10 hours or on High for 4 to 5 hours.

3. When bean mixture is cooked, make rice. In a heavy pot with a tight-fitting lid, combine rice with 4 cups (1 L) water. Cover, bring to a rapid boil, then turn off the heat, leaving the pot on the warm element. Do not lift the lid or move the pot until rice is ready, which will take about 20 minutes.

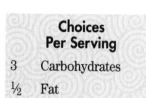

Choices Per Serving

3   Carbohydrates
½   Fat

Nutritional Analysis Per Serving			
Calories	247	Fat, total	3 g
Carbohydrate	49 g	Fat, saturated	0 g
Fiber	3 g	Sodium	101 mg
Protein	7 g	Cholesterol	0 mg

4. Meanwhile, add green pepper to contents of slow cooker and stir well. Cover and cook on High for 20 to 30 minutes, until pepper is tender.

5. Stir cooked rice into slow cooker. Add lemon or lime juice, cilantro and green onions and stir to combine thoroughly. Serve hot as a main course or cold as a salad.

Tips

This is delicious warm or cold.

Toast almonds in small skillet on top of stove or in 400°F (200°C) oven for 2 minutes.

For a special dinner menu, use 1 cup (250 mL) wild rice and omit the white rice.

Make Ahead

If serving cold, prepare early in day and stir just prior to serving.

Wild Rice, Snow Peas and Almond Casserole

2 tsp	margarine	10 mL
½ cup	chopped onion	125 mL
1 tsp	crushed garlic	5 mL
½ cup	wild rice	125 mL
½ cup	white rice	125 mL
3¼ cups	chicken stock	800 mL
¾ cup	chopped snow peas	175 mL
¼ cup	diced sweet red pepper	50 mL
¼ cup	toasted sliced almonds	50 mL
1 tbsp	grated Parmesan cheese	15 mL

1. In large nonstick saucepan, melt margarine; sauté onion and garlic until softened. Add wild and white rice; stir for 2 minutes.

2. Add stock; reduce heat, cover and simmer just until rice is tender and liquid is absorbed, 30 to 40 minutes.

3. Add snow peas, red pepper and almonds; cook for 2 minutes. Place in serving bowl and sprinkle with cheese.

Choices Per Serving

2½	Carbohydrates
1	Meat & Alternative
½	Fat

Nutritional Analysis Per Serving

Calories	281	Fat, total	8 g
Carbohydrate	42 g	Fat, saturated	1 g
Fiber	2 g	Sodium	654 mg
Protein	12 g	Cholesterol	1 mg

5. When absorbed, continue adding 1 cup (250 mL) stock at a time, stirring almost constantly, for 15 minutes. Add mushroom mixture; cook, stirring often, adding more stock when absorbed, until rice is just tender but slightly firm in the center. Mixture should be creamy; add more stock or water, if necessary. (Total cooking time will be 20 to 25 minutes.)

6. Add Parmesan cheese; adjust seasoning with salt and pepper to taste. Spoon into warm shallow serving bowls or onto plates. Sprinkle with parsley; serve immediately.

Tip

Other nuts, such as skinned hazelnuts or unblanched almonds, can be substituted for the walnuts.

Mushroom Barley Pilaf

1 tbsp	margarine or butter	15 mL
2 cups	sliced mushrooms	500 mL
1	small onion, chopped	1
½ tsp	dried thyme or marjoram leaves	2 mL
1 cup	pearl barley, rinsed	250 mL
2½ cups	chicken or vegetable stock (see recipe, page 53) (approx.)	625 mL
⅓ cup	finely chopped walnuts or pecans	75 mL
¼ cup	freshly grated Parmesan cheese	50 mL
2 tbsp	chopped fresh parsley	25 mL
	Salt and freshly ground black pepper	

1. In a medium saucepan, heat butter over medium heat. Add mushrooms, onion and thyme; cook, stirring, for 5 minutes or until softened.

2. Stir in barley and stock; bring to a boil. Reduce heat, cover and simmer, stirring occasionally and adding more stock if necessary, for 30 minutes or until barley is tender.

3. Stir in walnuts, Parmesan and parsley; season with salt and pepper to taste.

Choices Per Serving	
2	Carbohydrates
½	Meat & Alternative
1	Fat

Nutritional Analysis Per Serving

Calories	222	Fat, total	8 g
Carbohydrate	30 g	Fat, saturated	3 g
Fiber	3 g	Sodium	405 mg
Protein	9 g	Cholesterol	8 mg

Tip

This recipe makes an excellent lunch base. Round out the meal by adding any missing choices for your meal plan, such as additional Meat & Alternatives, some whole-grain bread and a Milk & Alternatives serving.

Barley with Tomato, Red Onion, Goat Cheese and Basil

3 cups	vegetable stock (see recipe, page 53) or chicken stock	750 mL
¾ cup	pearl barley	175 mL
3 cups	chopped ripe plum tomatoes	750 mL
1 cup	chopped red onions	250 mL
¾ cup	chopped fresh basil (or 1 tsp/5 mL dried)	175 mL
2 oz	goat cheese, crumbled	50 g

DRESSING

1 tbsp	olive oil	15 mL
1 tbsp	fresh lemon juice	15 mL
1 tbsp	balsamic vinegar	15 mL
1 tsp	minced garlic	5 mL

1. In a saucepan over medium-high heat, bring stock to a boil. Add barley; reduce heat to medium-low. Cook, covered, for 45 minutes or until tender and liquid is absorbed. Transfer to a large serving bowl. Add tomatoes, red onions, basil and goat cheese; toss well.

2. *Dressing:* In a bowl combine olive oil, lemon juice, balsamic vinegar and garlic. Pour over barley mixture; toss to coat well. Serve warm or at room temperature.

Choices Per Serving

2½	Carbohydrates
½	Meat & Alternative
1	Fat

Nutritional Analysis Per Serving			
Calories	267	Fat, total	8 g
Carbohydrate	44 g	Fat, saturated	3 g
Fiber	6 g	Sodium	102 mg
Protein	9 g	Cholesterol	7 mg

Tips

Although barley is rarely used this way, this dish proves how wonderful it is with tomatoes and feta cheese.

Try goat cheese, instead of feta, for a change.

Using low-sodium chicken stock in this recipe will reduce the sodium to 559 mg/serving.

Make Ahead

Make early in day and refrigerate; reheat on low to serve. Also delicious at room temperature.

Barley with Sautéed Vegetables and Feta Cheese

1 tbsp	vegetable oil	15 mL
2 tsp	crushed garlic	10 mL
¾ cup	chopped sweet green pepper	175 mL
¾ cup	chopped mushrooms	175 mL
¾ cup	pot barley	175 mL
1½ cups	crushed canned tomatoes	375 mL
3 cups	chicken stock	750 mL
1½ tsp	dried basil (or 2 tbsp/25 mL chopped fresh)	7 mL
½ tsp	dried oregano	2 mL
3 oz	feta cheese, crumbled	75 g

1. In large nonstick saucepan, heat oil; sauté garlic, green pepper and mushrooms until softened, approximately 5 minutes. Add barley and sauté for 2 minutes, stirring constantly.

2. Add tomatoes, stock, basil and oregano; cover and simmer for approximately 30 minutes or until barley is tender. Pour into serving dish and sprinkle with cheese.

Choices Per Serving

1½	Carbohydrates
½	Meat & Alternative
1	Fat

Nutritional Analysis Per Serving

Calories	187	Fat, total	6 g
Carbohydrate	28 g	Fat, saturated	3 g
Fiber	3 g	Sodium	1017 mg
Protein	6 g	Cholesterol	13 mg

Preheat oven to
425°F (220°C)

Baking sheet sprayed
with vegetable spray

Tips

Couscous has been a
staple of North African
cuisine for centuries. It
is made with coarsely
ground semolina — a
hard wheat flour used for
pasta. Couscous is loaded
with fiber, vitamins and
minerals. For extra flavor,
try cooking it with stock
or tomato sauce. It's a
wonderful replacement
for pasta, rice or
other grains.

These cakes make terrific
vegetarian burgers! Just
place in a pita lined with
lettuce, tomatoes and
onions. Drizzle with
sauce and serve.

Greek Couscous Cakes

1½ cups	vegetable stock (see recipe, page 53) or chicken stock	375 mL
1 cup	couscous	250 mL
½ cup	minced red bell peppers	125 mL
⅓ cup	minced green onions	75 mL
⅓ cup	minced red onions	75 mL
¼ cup	minced black olives	50 mL
1 tsp	minced garlic	5 mL
1 tsp	dried oregano	5 mL
1½ oz	light feta cheese, crumbled	40 g
2	large egg whites	2
1	large egg	1
2 tbsp	fresh lemon juice	25 mL

SAUCE

½ cup	low-fat sour cream	125 mL
2 tsp	chopped fresh dill (or ⅛ tsp/0.5 mL dried)	10 mL
1 tsp	fresh lemon juice	5 mL
¼ tsp	minced garlic	1 mL

1. In a saucepan over high heat, bring stock to a boil. Add couscous; remove from heat. Let stand, covered, for 5 minutes or until liquid is absorbed and grain is tender. Fluff with a fork; set aside to cool.

2. In a bowl combine cooled couscous, red peppers, green onions, red onions, black olives, garlic, oregano, feta cheese, egg whites, whole egg and lemon juice. Form each ⅓ cup (75 mL) mixture into a flat patty, squeezing together in your hands. Place patties on prepared baking sheet. Bake in preheated oven, turning at halfway point, for 20 minutes or until golden.

3. *Sauce:* In a bowl combine sour cream, dill, lemon juice and garlic. Serve warm patties with sauce.

Choices Per Serving

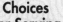

2	Carbohydrates
1	Meat & Alternative

Nutritional Analysis Per Serving			
Calories	192	Fat, total	4 g
Carbohydrate	30 g	Fat, saturated	1 g
Fiber	2 g	Sodium	98 mg
Protein	9 g	Cholesterol	39 mg

Vegetable Couscous

2 tbsp	vegetable oil	25 mL
1	onion, cut in 2-inch (5 cm) chunks	1
1 tbsp	minced fresh ginger	15 mL
½ tsp	paprika	2 mL
½ tsp	pepper	2 mL
½ tsp	turmeric	2 mL
½ tsp	ground cumin	2 mL
Pinch	cayenne	Pinch
1	clove garlic, minced	1
3	carrots, cut in 2-inch (5 cm) chunks	3
3	parsnips, cut in 2-inch (5 cm) chunks	3
2	small white turnips, peeled and cut in wedges	2
2	tomatoes, peeled and quartered	2
1	can (19 oz/540 mL) chick-peas, drained and rinsed	1
2½ cups	chicken or vegetable stock (see recipe, page 53)	625 mL
2 cups	sliced green beans	500 mL
½ cup	seedless raisins	125 mL
	Salt	
1 cup	couscous	250 mL

1. In large wide heavy saucepan, heat oil over medium heat; cook onion for 2 minutes. Add ginger, paprika, pepper, turmeric, cumin and cayenne; cook for 3 minutes, stirring often.

2. Add garlic, carrots, parsnips, turnips, tomatoes, chick-peas and stock; bring to boil. Reduce heat to low; simmer, covered, for 15 minutes or until vegetables are almost tender.

Choices Per Serving

3½ Carbohydrates

1 Meat & Alternative

Nutritional Analysis Per Serving			
Calories	344	Fat, total	6 g
Carbohydrate	62 g	Fat, saturated	1 g
Fiber	8 g	Sodium	292 mg
Protein	13 g	Cholesterol	0 mg

3. Add beans and raisins; cook, uncovered, for 10 minutes or until beans are tender-crisp and liquid has thickened slightly. Season with salt to taste. (Stew can be prepared to this point, cooled, covered and refrigerated for up to 1 day. In this case, just cook 5 minutes after adding beans. Reheat gently.)

4. Meanwhile, in medium saucepan, boil $1\frac{1}{2}$ cups (375 mL) water; add couscous and $\frac{1}{2}$ tsp (2 mL) salt. Remove from heat. Let stand, covered, for 5 minutes or until couscous is tender and water is absorbed; fluff with fork. Spoon onto large heated platter; make well in center. Spoon in vegetable mixture.

Tips

This dish is fine served at room temperature.

Couscous is a delicious alternative to traditional Grains & Starches choices. This pellet made from semolina flour is typically found in the specialty section of most supermarkets.

Make Ahead

Prepare up to the day before, then gently reheat over low heat.

Couscous with Raisins, Dates and Curry

1¼ cups	chicken stock	300 mL
¾ cup	couscous	175 mL
1 tbsp	margarine	15 mL
¾ cup	finely chopped onions	175 mL
1 tsp	crushed garlic	5 mL
1 cup	finely chopped sweet red pepper	250 mL
¼ cup	raisins	50 mL
1 tsp	curry powder	5 mL
5	dried dates or apricots, chopped	5

1. In small saucepan, bring chicken stock to boil. Stir in couscous and remove from heat. Cover and let stand until liquid is absorbed, 5 to 8 minutes. Place in serving bowl.

2. Meanwhile, in nonstick saucepan, melt margarine; sauté onions, garlic and red pepper until softened, approximately 5 minutes. Add raisins, curry powder and dates; mix until combined. Add to couscous and mix well.

Choices Per Serving

3   Carbohydrates

½   Fat

Nutritional Analysis Per Serving

Calories	237	Fat, total	2 g
Carbohydrate	49 g	Fat, saturated	0 g
Fiber	4 g	Sodium	480 mg
Protein	6 g	Cholesterol	0 mg

Tips

Originally from Russia, kasha is the name given to buckwheat seeds that have been hulled and, most often, either finely or coarsely ground. (Despite its name, buckwheat isn't a type of wheat; in fact, it is not a cereal at all.) Toasting the kernels enhances their nutty flavor and keeps them from sticking together.

This recipe is an excellent source of vitamins A and C, niacin and folic acid, as well as iron, magnesium and phosphorus.

Kasha with Beans and Salsa Dressing

DRESSING

½ cup	chopped fresh coriander	125 mL
⅓ cup	medium salsa	75 mL
¼ cup	low-fat sour cream	50 mL
3 tbsp	light mayonnaise	45 mL
2 tbsp	water	25 mL
1 tsp	minced garlic	5 mL

SALAD

1½ cups	vegetable stock (see recipe, page 53) or chicken stock	375 mL
¾ cup	whole grain kasha	175 mL
½ cup	canned red kidney beans, rinsed and drained	125 mL
½ cup	canned chickpeas, rinsed and drained	125 mL
½ cup	chopped red onions	125 mL

1. *Dressing:* In a bowl combine coriander, salsa, sour cream, mayonnaise, water and garlic. Set aside.

2. *Salad:* In a saucepan over high heat, bring stock to boil. Meanwhile, in a nonstick saucepan set over medium-high heat, toast kasha for 1 minute. Add hot stock; return to a boil, stirring. Reduce heat to medium-low; cook, covered, for 10 minutes or until kasha is tender and liquid is absorbed. Set aside to cool.

3. In a serving bowl, combine cooled kasha, red kidney beans, chickpeas and red onions. Pour dressing over; toss to coat well. Serve at room temperature or heat in microwave to serve warm.

Choices Per Serving

2½ Carbohydrates
½ Meat & Alternative
½ Fat

Nutritional Analysis Per Serving

Calories	238	Fat, total	5 g
Carbohydrate	42 g	Fat, saturated	0 g
Fiber	3 g	Sodium	210 mg
Protein	9 g	Cholesterol	0 mg

Preheat oven to
425°F (220°C)

8-inch (2 L) square
baking dish sprayed
with vegetable spray

Large baking sheet
lined with foil

Tips

Chèvre is a white,
tart-flavored cheese
made from goat's milk.
At least, it's supposed to
be — some cheese sold
as chèvre contains cow's
milk, so read the label
carefully! Depending on
the producer, goat cheese
can be drier or creamier
in texture. Either way,
at only 15% M.F., it is a
lower-fat cheese. And
because it's so flavorful,
a little goes a long way.

Using low-sodium
vegetable or chicken
stock in this recipe will
reduce the sodium to
427 mg/serving.

Polenta with Chèvre and Roasted Vegetables

POLENTA

3 cups	vegetable or chicken stock	750 mL
1 cup	cornmeal	250 mL
1	medium red bell pepper, cut into quarters	1
1	medium yellow pepper, cut into quarters	1
1	medium red onion, sliced	1
2	small zucchini (about 8 oz/250 g), cut in half lengthwise	2
1 tbsp	olive oil	15 mL
1	small head garlic, top ½ inch (1 cm) cut off	1
1 tbsp	balsamic vinegar	15 mL
2 oz	goat cheese (chèvre)	50 g

1. In a deep saucepan over medium-high heat, bring stock to a boil. Reduce heat to low; gradually whisk in cornmeal. Cook, stirring, for 5 minutes. Pour into baking dish, smoothing top; chill.

2. In a bowl combine red pepper, yellow pepper, onion, zucchini and olive oil; transfer to prepared baking sheet. Wrap garlic loosely in foil; add to baking sheet. Roast vegetables in preheated oven, turning occasionally, for 45 minutes or until tender. Squeeze garlic out of skins; chop remaining vegetables. Transfer all to a bowl. Sprinkle with balsamic vinegar; toss to coat well.

3. Turn polenta onto cutting board; cut into 4 squares. In a large nonstick frying pan sprayed with vegetable spray, cook polenta over medium-high heat for 2 minutes or until golden. Turn; cook for 1 minute. Spoon polenta onto serving plates. Top with vegetable mixture; sprinkle with goat cheese. Serve.

**Choices
Per Serving**

2½	Carbohydrates
½	Meat & Alternative
1	Fat

Nutritional Analysis Per Serving

Calories	258	Fat, total	8 g
Carbohydrate	39 g	Fat, saturated	3 g
Fiber	4 g	Sodium	1172 mg
Protein	9 g	Cholesterol	7 mg

Sandwiches and Wraps

Tasty, satisfying and great choices, the selections in this chapter provide you with almost a complete meal in one neat package. Whether you're looking for vegetarian, chicken, fish or pork, these sandwiches and wrap choices contribute Grains & Starches, Meat & Alternatives, Fats and vegetables and provide plenty of nutrients and ways to spice up mealtime. All you need to round out the meal is a serving of milk and a fruit choice.

Using a selection of whole-grain breads and wraps increases the variety of taste and the nutrients consumed. With breads such as pumpernickel and with spices such as coriander, curry or dill, the ho-hum can become extraordinary!

Dilled Salmon and Egg Salad on Pumpernickel

Tips

To prevent cucumber from turning soggy, assemble sandwiches the same day they are served.

To reduce the sodium content of this recipe, eliminate the salt and, if available, use fresh poached salmon instead of canned.

These nutritious sandwiches are an excellent source of vitamins B_{12} and D, niacin and phosphorus.

Make Ahead

Filling can be prepared through step 1 and refrigerated, covered, for up to two days.

3	hard-cooked eggs, finely chopped	3
1	can (7½ oz/213 g) sockeye salmon, drained and flaked	1
¼ cup	light mayonnaise	50 mL
1	large green onion, finely chopped	1
2 tbsp	chopped fresh dill or parsley	25 mL
1 tsp	grated lemon zest	5 mL
¼ tsp	salt	1 mL
¼ tsp	freshly ground black pepper	1 mL
8	slices pumpernickel bread	8
½	seedless cucumber, thinly sliced	½

1. In a bowl, combine eggs, salmon, mayonnaise, green onion, dill, lemon zest, salt and pepper.

2. Divide salad among pumpernickel slices, spreading evenly. Layer with cucumber slices. Serve open-faced or sandwich together. Cut in half.

Choices Per Serving

2	Carbohydrates
2	Meat & Alternatives
1	Fat

Nutritional Analysis Per Serving			
Calories	354	Fat, total	15 g
Carbohydrate	35 g	Fat, saturated	2 g
Fiber	4 g	Sodium	956 mg
Protein	20 g	Cholesterol	175 mg

Preheat oven to
425°F (220°C)

Baking sheet sprayed
with vegetable spray

Tips

Seafood or any firm
white fish can substitute
for the salmon.

Substitute chopped
broccoli for snow peas.

Handle cooked
salmon gently, since
it flakes easily.

Make Ahead

Prepare sauce up to
one day in advance.
Keep refrigerated.

Salmon Fajitas in Hoisin Sauce

SAUCE

2 tbsp	hoisin sauce	25 mL
1 tbsp	honey	15 mL
2 tsp	low-sodium soya sauce	10 mL
2 tsp	lemon juice	10 mL
2 tsp	sesame oil	10 mL
1½ tsp	minced garlic	7 mL
1 tsp	minced ginger root	5 mL
½ tsp	cornstarch	2 mL
8 oz	salmon, thinly sliced	250 g
1 tsp	vegetable oil	5 mL
1¼ cups	halved snow peas	300 mL
1¼ cups	thinly sliced red or green peppers	300 mL
⅓ cup	chopped green onions (about 3 medium)	75 mL
3 tbsp	chopped fresh coriander or parsley	45 mL
6	small tortillas	6

1. *Sauce:* In small bowl whisk together hoisin sauce, honey, soya sauce, lemon juice, sesame oil, garlic, ginger and cornstarch; set aside.

2. In nonstick skillet sprayed with vegetable spray, cook salmon over high heat for 2 minutes, or until just barely done at center; set aside.

3. Heat oil in nonstick skillet over medium heat. Add snow peas and red peppers; cook for 4 minutes or until tender. Stir sauce again and add to vegetables, along with green onions and coriander. Cook for 1 minute, or until slightly thickened. Remove from heat and gently stir in salmon.

4. Divide salmon filling among tortillas; roll up and put on prepared baking sheet. Bake for 5 minutes or until heated through.

Nutritional Analysis Per Serving

Calories	481	Fat, total	15 g
Carbohydrate	62 g	Fat, saturated	2 g
Fiber	5 g	Sodium	613 mg
Protein	25 g	Cholesterol	42 mg

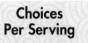

**Choices
Per Serving**

4 Carbohydrates

3 Meat & Alternatives

● ● ● ● ● ● ● ● ● ● ● ● ● ● ●

Tips

If peanut allergies are
a concern, there
are a number of good
substitutes for the peanut
butter used in the sauce.
Try soya nut butter,
which is made from
dry-roasted soya beans.
It's "soya good," you
won't know the
difference! Other
great-tasting nut butters
include those made from
almonds, pecans — even
macadamias! Try making
your own nut butters by
puréeing roasted dried
nuts with some oil until
the mixture forms a
smooth consistency.

Don't think of these
tortilla bites just as party
appetizers — they make
a great dinner for the
entire family. Don't
bother slicing them; just
"wrap and roll" and enjoy.
Make early in the day,
cover and serve at room
temperature or heat
in the oven at 400°F
(200°C) for 10 minutes.

This is an excellent
source of vitamin C.

Tortilla Bites Stuffed with Chicken, Pasta and Peanut Sauce

4 oz	boneless skinless chicken breast	125 g
2 oz	wide rice noodles	50 g
1¼ cups	julienned red bell peppers	300 mL
1¼ cups	julienned snow peas	300 mL
½ cup	chopped green onions	125 mL
⅓ cup	chopped fresh coriander	75 mL

PEANUT SAUCE

3 tbsp	peanut butter	45 mL
3 tbsp	water	45 mL
1½ tbsp	rice wine vinegar	20 mL
1½ tbsp	honey	20 mL
1 tbsp	sesame oil	15 mL
1 tbsp	light soya sauce	15 mL
1½ tsp	minced garlic	7 mL
1½ tsp	minced gingerroot	7 mL
¾ tsp	hot Asian chili sauce (optional)	4 mL

6	8-inch (20 cm) flour tortillas	6

1. In a nonstick frying pan sprayed with vegetable spray
or on a preheated grill, cook chicken over medium-high
heat, turning once, for 12 minutes or until cooked
through; cut into thin slices.

2. In a pot of boiling water, cook noodles for 5 minutes
or until soft; drain. Rinse under cold running water;
chop noodles.

3. In a nonstick frying pan sprayed with vegetable spray,
cook red peppers and snow peas over medium-high heat
for 3 minutes or until tender-crisp. Remove from heat;
add chicken, noodles, green onions and coriander.

Choices Per Serving	
2½	Carbohydrates
1	Meat & Alternative
1	Fat

Nutritional Analysis Per Serving			
Calories	287	Fat, total	9 g
Carbohydrate	40 g	Fat, saturated	2 g
Fiber	3 g	Sodium	259 mg
Protein	11 g	Cholesterol	11 mg

4. *Peanut Sauce:* In a bowl combine peanut butter, water, vinegar, honey, sesame oil, soya sauce, garlic, ginger and chili sauce; whisk well. Add $\frac{1}{4}$ cup (50 mL) sauce to vegetable-noodle mixture.

5. Spread about $\frac{3}{4}$ cup (175 mL) vegetable-noodle mixture evenly over each tortilla; roll up. Cut each tortilla diagonally into 4 pieces. Wrap in plastic and chill or serve warm with remaining peanut sauce for dipping.

Curried Chicken Salad Sandwiches

Tips

Simmer 2 boneless chicken breasts (½ lb/250 g) in lightly salted water or chicken stock for 10 minutes; remove from heat. Let cool in stock for 15 minutes.

These tasty sandwiches are high in carbohydrate due to the sugar in mango chutney. Reducing the chutney to 1 tbsp (15 mL) can save about 7 g of carbohydrate/serving, lowering the Carbohydrates choice to 3.

8 tbsp	light mayonnaise	125 mL
2 tbsp	bottled mango chutney	25 mL
1 tsp	mild curry paste or powder	5 mL
1½ cups	finely diced cooked chicken	375 mL
½ cup	finely diced unpeeled apple	125 mL
⅓ cup	finely diced radishes	75 mL
2 tbsp	finely chopped green onions	25 mL
	Salt	
4	slices thick-cut whole-grain bread	4
	Red leaf or Boston lettuce	

1. In a bowl, blend 6 tablespoons (90 mL) mayonnaise with chutney and curry paste. Stir in chicken, apple, radishes and green onions; season with salt to taste.

2. Spread bread slices with remaining mayonnaise. Spread two bread slices generously with chicken mixture; top with lettuce and remaining bread. Cut in half.

Choices Per Serving

3½   Carbohydrates

4   Meat & Alternatives

Nutritional Analysis Per Serving			
Calories	520	Fat, total	20 g
Carbohydrate	58 g	Fat, saturated	2 g
Fiber	6 g	Sodium	771 mg
Protein	31 g	Cholesterol	72 mg

New Orleans Braised Onions *page 256*
Overleaf: New Potato Curry *page 262*

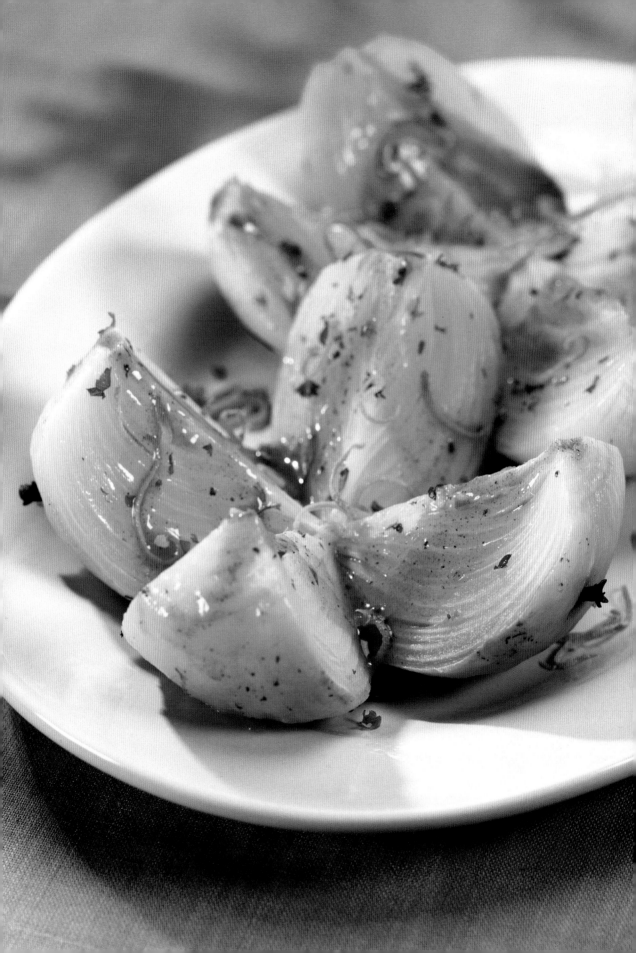

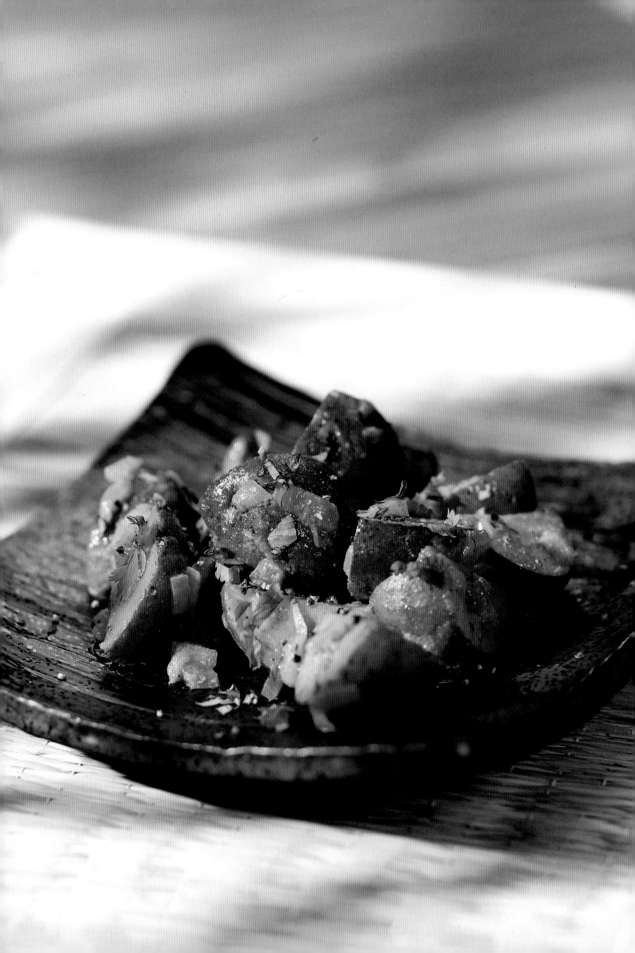

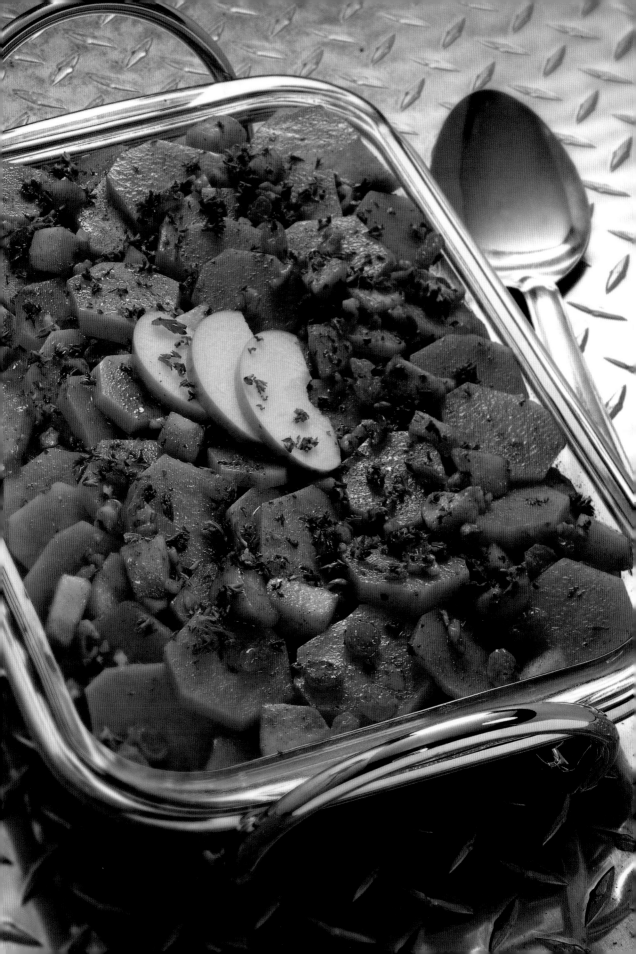

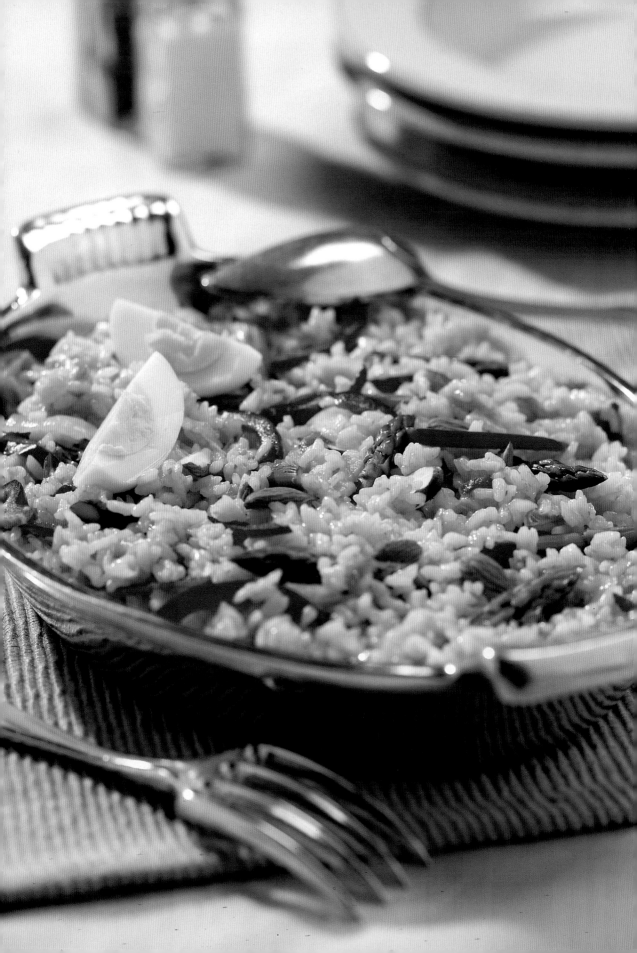

Tip

Pork makes this recipe an excellent source of thiamin; peppers make it an excellent source of vitamin C.

Pork Fajitas with Salsa, Onions and Rice Noodles

3 oz	wide rice noodles	75 g
8 oz	pork or beef tenderloin	250 g
2 tsp	vegetable oil	10 mL
1 cup	thinly sliced red onions	250 mL
2 tsp	minced garlic	10 mL
1 cup	thinly sliced green bell peppers	250 mL
1 cup	thinly sliced red bell peppers	250 mL
1	large green onion, sliced	1
3/4 cup	medium salsa	175 mL
1/3 cup	chopped fresh coriander	75 mL
8	8-inch (20 cm) flour tortillas	8
3/4 cup	shredded low-fat Cheddar cheese	175 mL
1/3 cup	low-fat sour cream	75 mL

1. In a pot of boiling water, cook rice noodles for 5 minutes or until tender; drain. Rinse under cold running water; drain. Set aside.

2. In a nonstick frying pan sprayed with vegetable spray or on a preheated grill, cook pork tenderloin over medium-high heat, turning once, for 15 minutes or until just cooked through. Slice thinly.

3. In a nonstick frying pan sprayed with vegetable spray, heat oil over medium-high heat; add red onions and garlic. Cook for 2 minutes or until softened. Add green peppers and red peppers; cook, stirring frequently, for 2 minutes or until tender-crisp. Add green onion, rice noodles and pork; remove from heat. Add salsa and coriander; combine well.

4. Sprinkle tortillas with Cheddar cheese. Place about 1/2 cup (125 mL) filling in center of each tortilla. Add sour cream; fold bottom end up over filling. Tuck sides in; roll up tightly. Serve immediately.

Choices Per Serving

2½ Carbohydrates

2 Meat & Alternatives

Nutritional Analysis Per Serving			
Calories	306	Fat, total	9 g
Carbohydrate	37 g	Fat, saturated	3 g
Fiber	3 g	Sodium	376 mg
Protein	18 g	Cholesterol	30 mg

Garden Paella *page 266*
Overleaf: Sweet Potato, Apple and Raisin Casserole *page 263*

●●●●●●●●●●●●●●●●

Preheat oven to
425°F (220°C)

Baking sheet sprayed
with vegetable spray

●●●●●●●●●●●●●●●●

Tips

Use pork chops or pork
cutlets or substitute
boneless chicken or beef
steak. Mozzarella cheese
can replace Cheddar.

If you use low-fat cheese
the total fat will be 14 g,
with only 6 g of saturated
fat, and the Fat choice
will be reduced to $\frac{1}{2}$.

●●●●●●●●●●●●●●●●

Make Ahead

Prepare pork mixture
earlier in the day. Reheat
gently and fill tortillas.

Pork Fajitas with Sweet Peppers, Coriander and Cheese

8 oz	pork tenderloin, cut into thin strips	250 g
2 tsp	vegetable oil	10 mL
1½ tsp	minced garlic	7 mL
1½ cups	thinly sliced onions	375 mL
1½ cups	red pepper strips	375 mL
¼ cup	fresh chopped coriander or parsley	50 mL
3 tbsp	chopped green onions (about 2 medium)	45 mL
4	large flour tortillas	4
½ cup	grated Cheddar cheese	125 mL
⅓ cup	bottled salsa	75 mL
¼ cup	light sour cream	50 mL

1. In nonstick skillet sprayed with vegetable spray, cook the pork strips over high heat for 2 minutes, or until just done at center. Remove from skillet. Add oil. Cook garlic and onions for 4 minutes until browned. Add red pepper strips and cook over medium heat for 5 minutes, or until softened.

2. Remove from heat and stir in coriander, green onions and pork. Divide among tortillas. Top with Cheddar, salsa and sour cream. Roll up, place on baking sheet and bake for 5 minutes or until heated through.

Choices Per Serving	
2	Carbohydrates
3	Meat & Alternatives
1	Fat

Nutritional Analysis Per Serving

Calories	405	Fat, total	19 g
Carbohydrate	33 g	Fat, saturated	9 g
Fiber	4 g	Sodium	434 mg
Protein	27 g	Cholesterol	72 mg

Quinoa (pronounced KEEN-wah) may be unfamiliar to many North Americans, but it's not exactly new. In fact, it was a staple of the ancient Incas, who described it as the "mother grain." And it seems that they were right! Quinoa contains more protein than any other grain. I like to use it in soups, as part of a main or side dish, in salads and as a substitute for rice.

While it's incredibly nutritious, quinoa can have a slightly bitter taste. But you can eliminate the bitterness by rinsing the quinoa thoroughly, drying it and then toasting it lightly in a nonstick skillet.

A sugar substitute can replace the honey and reduce the carbohydrate by 5 g/serving, lowering the Carbohydrates choice to 2.

Quinoa Wraps with Hoisin Vegetables

1 cup	quinoa, rinsed	250 mL
2 cups	vegetable stock (see recipe, page 53) or chicken stock	500 mL
1 tsp	minced garlic	5 mL
1 tsp	minced gingerroot	5 mL
½ cup	diced red bell peppers	125 mL
½ cup	diced snow peas	125 mL
½ cup	diced water chestnuts	125 mL
¼ cup	chopped green onions	50 mL
¼ cup	hoisin sauce	50 mL
¼ cup	light mayonnaise	50 mL
2 tbsp	honey	25 mL
¼ cup	chopped fresh coriander or parsley	50 mL
8	6-inch (15 cm) flour tortillas	8

1. In a small nonstick skillet, toast quinoa over medium-high heat for 2 minutes.

2. In a saucepan over medium-high heat, bring stock to a boil. Add quinoa; reduce heat to medium-low. Cook, covered, for 15 minutes or until grain is tender and liquid is absorbed. Set aside.

3. In a nonstick frying pan sprayed with vegetable spray, cook garlic, ginger, red peppers, snow peas and water chestnuts over medium-high heat for 3 minutes or until softened. Add green onions; cook for 1 minute. Remove from heat; add to quinoa.

4. In a bowl combine hoisin sauce, mayonnaise, honey and coriander; spread over tortillas. Place about ⅓ cup (75 mL) quinoa mixture in center of each tortilla. Fold right side over filling; roll up from the bottom. Serve.

Nutritional Analysis Per Serving			
Calories	241	Fat, total	5 g
Carbohydrate	43 g	Fat, saturated	1 g
Fiber	3 g	Sodium	307 mg
Protein	6 g	Cholesterol	0 mg

Tips

Flavored tortillas — such as pesto, sun-dried tomato, herb or whole wheat — are now appearing in many supermarkets. The different colors make these wraps an attractive dish for entertaining.

Try substituting other herbs — such as coriander, basil or parsley — for the dill.

If tahini is unavailable, use peanut butter.

Make Ahead

Prepare hummus up to 3 days in advance. Sauté vegetables early in day and reheat before serving.

1 cup	canned chickpeas, rinsed and drained	250 mL
¼ cup	tahini	50 mL
¼ cup	water	50 mL
2 tbsp	freshly squeezed lemon juice	25 mL
4 tsp	olive oil	20 mL
1 tbsp	chopped fresh parsley	15 mL
¾ tsp	minced garlic	4 mL
2 tsp	vegetable oil	10 mL
1 cup	diced onions	250 mL
1¼ cups	diced red bell peppers	300 mL
1¼ cups	chopped snow peas	300 mL
¼ cup	chopped fresh dill (or 2 tsp/10 mL dried)	50 mL
4	10-inch (25 cm) flour tortillas, preferably different flavors, if available	4

1. *Make the hummus:* In a food processor, combine chickpeas, tahini, water, lemon juice, oil, parsley and garlic; process until creamy and smooth. Transfer to a bowl and set aside.

2. In a large nonstick saucepan, heat oil over medium-high heat. Add onions and sauté 4 minutes or until soft and browned. Add red peppers and sauté 4 minutes until soft. Add snow peas and sauté 2 minutes or until tender-crisp. Stir in dill and remove from heat.

3. Divide hummus equally among tortillas, spreading to within ½ inch (1 cm) of edge. Divide vegetable mixture between tortillas. Form each tortilla into a packet by folding bottom edge over filling, then sides, then top, to enclose filling completely.

Choices Per Serving

2½   Carbohydrates

1   Meat & Alternative

2½   Fats

Nutritional Analysis Per Serving

Calories	382	Fat, total	18 g
Carbohydrate	47 g	Fat, saturated	2 g
Fiber	7 g	Sodium	269 mg
Protein	12 g	Cholesterol	0 mg

Just for Kids

Life's fondest memories often involve family mealtimes, where favorite recipes become comfort foods. In this chapter, you'll find variations on many old favorites that are chock full of nutrients and are simple to prepare. Some of the recipes here are sure to become family favorites for after the big game or the bike ride. When you serve these dishes, you'll likely hear words such as "crunchy," "spicy" and "yummy" issuing from your kids' mouths.

Most kids are eager to help with food preparation; their reward is the satisfaction of having contributed to the family mealtime — not to mention the delicious food! Round out the meals with some vegetables and a heaping serving of calcium, such as a lower-fat yogurt or a milk-based dessert, and you will have scored a crowd pleaser.

Preheat oven to
425°F (220°C)

Baking sheet sprayed
with vegetable spray

Tips

Children devour these
tasty egg rolls. Double
the recipe if necessary.

Ground chicken or veal
can replace beef.

Cheddar cheese can
replace mozzarella for a
more intense flavor.

Roll the wrappers
any way that's easy.
Wetting the edges of
the wrappers with water
may help secure roll.

Make Ahead

Prepare these up to
a day ahead and keep
refrigerated. Bake an
extra 5 minutes. These
can also be prepared and
frozen for up to a month.

Italian Pizza Egg Rolls

1 tsp	vegetable oil	5 mL
1 tsp	minced garlic	5 mL
¼ cup	finely chopped carrots	50 mL
¼ cup	finely chopped onions	50 mL
¼ cup	finely chopped green peppers	50 mL
3 oz	lean ground beef	75 g
½ cup	tomato pasta sauce	125 mL
½ cup	grated mozzarella cheese (1½ oz/40 g)	125 mL
1 tbsp	grated Parmesan cheese	15 mL
9	egg roll wrappers (5½ inches/13 cm square)	9

1. In nonstick skillet sprayed with vegetable spray, heat oil over medium heat. Add garlic, carrots and onions; cook for 8 minutes, or until softened and browned. Add peppers and cook 2 minutes longer. Add beef and cook for 2 minutes, stirring to break it up, or until it is no longer pink. Remove from heat and stir in tomato sauce, mozzarella and Parmesan cheeses.

2. Keeping rest of wrappers covered with a cloth to prevent drying out, put one wrapper on work surface with a corner pointing towards you. Put 2 tbsp (25 mL) of the filling in the center. Fold the lower corner up over the filling, fold the 2 side corners in over the filling, and roll the bundle away from you. Put on prepared pan and repeat until all wrappers are filled. Bake for 14 minutes, until browned, turning the pizza rolls at the halfway mark.

Choices
Per Serving

1½   Carbohydrates

1   Meat & Alternative

Nutritional Analysis Per Serving

Calories	184	Fat, total	6 g
Carbohydrate	23 g	Fat, saturated	3 g
Fiber	1 g	Sodium	332 mg
Protein	10 g	Cholesterol	17 mg

Turkey Macaroni Chili

Tips

Great mild-tasting chili that children love. Can be served as a soup or alongside rice or pasta.

Ground turkey can be replaced with ground chicken, beef or veal.

Red kidney beans can be replaced with white beans or chick peas.

Make Ahead

Can be prepared up to 2 days ahead and reheated. Can be frozen for up to 3 weeks.

Great for leftovers.

1½ tsp	vegetable oil	7 mL
1 tsp	minced garlic	5 mL
½ cup	finely chopped carrots	125 mL
1 cup	chopped onions	250 mL
8 oz	ground turkey	250 g
1	can (19 oz/540 mL) tomatoes, crushed	1
2 cups	chicken stock	500 mL
1½ cups	peeled, diced potatoes	375 mL
¾ cup	canned red kidney beans, drained	175 mL
¾ cup	corn kernels	175 mL
2 tbsp	tomato paste	25 mL
1½ tsp	chili powder	7 mL
1½ tsp	dried oregano	7 mL
1½ tsp	dried basil	7 mL
⅓ cup	elbow macaroni	75 mL

1. In large nonstick saucepan, heat oil over medium heat; add garlic, carrots and onions and cook for 8 minutes or until softened, stirring occasionally. Add turkey and cook, stirring to break it up, for 2 minutes or until no longer pink. Add tomatoes, stock, potatoes, beans, corn, tomato paste, chili, oregano and basil; bring to a boil, reduce heat to low, cover and simmer for 20 minutes.

2. Bring to a boil and add macaroni; cook for 12 minutes or until pasta is tender but firm.

Choices
Per Serving

1½ Carbohydrates

1 Meat & Alternative

Nutritional Analysis Per Serving			
Calories	182	Fat, total	4 g
Carbohydrate	28 g	Fat, saturated	1 g
Fiber	4 g	Sodium	557 mg
Protein	10 g	Cholesterol	22 mg

Tips

Ground chicken, turkey or veal can replace the beef.

Chick peas can be replaced with kidney beans.

Make Ahead

Prepare up to a day ahead, adding more stock if too thick. Great for leftovers.

Spicy Meatball and Pasta Stew

MEATBALLS

8 oz	lean ground beef	250 g
1	egg	1
2 tbsp	ketchup or chili sauce	25 mL
2 tbsp	seasoned bread crumbs	25 mL
1 tsp	minced garlic	5 mL
½ tsp	chili powder	2 mL

STEW

2 tsp	vegetable oil	10 mL
1 tsp	minced garlic	5 mL
1¼ cups	chopped onions	300 mL
¾ cup	chopped carrots	175 mL
3½ cups	low-sodium beef stock	875 mL
1	can (19 oz/540 mL) tomatoes, crushed	1
¾ cup	canned chick peas, drained	175 mL
1 tbsp	tomato paste	15 mL
2 tsp	granulated sugar	10 mL
2 tsp	chili powder	10 mL
1 tsp	dried oregano	5 mL
1¼ tsp	dried basil	6 mL
⅔ cup	small shell pasta	150 mL

1. *Meatballs:* In large bowl, combine ground beef, egg, ketchup, bread crumbs, garlic and chili powder; mix well. Form each ½ tbsp (7 mL) into a meatball and place on a baking sheet; cover and set aside.

Choices Per Serving

1½ Carbohydrates

1   Meat & Alternative

½   Fat

Nutritional Analysis Per Serving			
Calories	203	Fat, total	7 g
Carbohydrate	26 g	Fat, saturated	2 g
Fiber	3 g	Sodium	564 mg
Protein	11 g	Cholesterol	43 mg

2. *Stew:* In large nonstick saucepan, heat oil over medium heat. Add garlic, onions and carrots and cook for 5 minutes or until onions are softened. Stir in stock, tomatoes, chick peas, tomato paste, sugar, chili powder, oregano and basil; bring to a boil, reduce heat to medium-low, cover and let cook for 20 minutes. Bring to a boil again and stir in pasta and meatballs; let simmer for 10 minutes or until pasta is tender but firm, and meatballs are cooked.

Preheat oven to
350°F (180°C)

10- to 11-inch
(25 to 28 cm) pizza
or springform baking
pan sprayed with
vegetable spray

Make Ahead

Prepare pasta crust
and sauce early in day.
Do not pour sauce over
top until ready to bake.

Pizza Pasta with Beef-Tomato Sauce and Cheese

6 oz	macaroni	150 g
1	egg	1
1/3 cup	2% milk	75 mL
3 tbsp	grated Parmesan cheese	45 mL
1 tsp	vegetable oil	5 mL
2 tsp	crushed garlic	10 mL
3/4 cup	finely chopped onions	175 mL
1/2 cup	finely chopped sweet green peppers	125 mL
1/3 cup	finely chopped carrots	75 mL
8 oz	ground beef or chicken	250 g
1	can (19 oz/540 mL) tomatoes, crushed	1
2 tbsp	tomato paste	25 mL
1 1/2 tsp	dried basil	7 mL
1 tsp	dried oregano	5 mL
1 cup	low-fat mozzarella cheese, shredded	250 mL

1. Cook pasta in boiling water according to package instructions or until firm to the bite. Drain and place in serving bowl. Add egg, milk and cheese. Mix well. Place in baking pan as a crust and bake for 20 minutes.

2. Meanwhile, in medium nonstick saucepan sprayed with vegetable spray, heat oil; sauté garlic, onions, green peppers and carrots until tender, approximately 5 minutes. Add beef and sauté until no longer pink, approximately 4 minutes. Add tomatoes, paste, basil and oregano. Cover and simmer on low heat for 15 minutes, stirring occasionally.

3. Pour sauce into pasta crust. Sprinkle with cheese; bake for 10 minutes or until cheese melts.

Choices Per Serving

1½ Carbohydrates

2½ Meat & Alternatives

Nutritional Analysis Per Serving			
Calories	303	Fat, total	13 g
Carbohydrate	27 g	Fat, saturated	6 g
Fiber	2 g	Sodium	435 mg
Protein	20 g	Cholesterol	67 mg

Preheat oven to
400°F (200°C)

Baking sheet, with
greased rack

Tips

You can also make
extra batches of the
crumb mixture and
store in the freezer.

Instead of boneless
chicken breasts,
prepare skinless chicken
drumsticks in the same
way but bake in a
375°F (190°C) oven
for 35 to 40 minutes
or until tender.

Adding salt brings the
sodium to 674 mg/serving.

Yummy Parmesan Chicken Fingers

½ cup	finely crushed soda cracker crumbs (about 16 crackers)	125 mL
⅓ cup	freshly grated Parmesan cheese	75 mL
½ tsp	dried basil leaves	2 mL
½ tsp	dried marjoram leaves	2 mL
½ tsp	paprika	2 mL
½ tsp	salt, optional	2 mL
¼ tsp	freshly ground black pepper	1 mL
4	skinless, boneless chicken breasts	4
1	egg	1
2 tbsp	margarine or butter	25 mL
1	clove garlic, minced	1

1. In a food processor, combine cracker crumbs, Parmesan cheese, basil, marjoram, paprika, optional salt and pepper. Process to make fine crumbs. Place in a shallow bowl.

2. Cut chicken breasts into four strips each. In a bowl, beat egg; add chicken strips. Using a fork, dip chicken strips in crumb mixture until evenly coated. Arrange on greased rack set on baking sheet. In small bowl, microwave butter and garlic at High for 45 seconds or until melted. Brush chicken strips with melted butter.

3. Bake in preheated oven for 15 minutes or until no longer pink in center. (If frozen, bake for up to 25 minutes.)

Choices Per Serving

| ½ | Carbohydrate |
| 3 | Meat & Alternatives |

Nutritional Analysis Per Serving

Calories	236	Fat, total	12 g
Carbohydrate	10 g	Fat, saturated	6 g
Fiber	1 g	Sodium	400 mg
Protein	22 g	Cholesterol	114 mg

Tips

Kids will love eating
these "fingers" with
their fingers.

This honey dip adds
about 20 g carbohydrate
or 1½ Carbohydrates
choices to the meal.
Choosing another type
of dip, such as salsa,
barbecue sauce or low-fat
dressing can eliminate
these from the recipe.

Make Ahead

The chicken fingers and
honey dip can be made
up to 4 hours ahead,
covered and refrigerated.

Sesame Chicken Fingers with Honey Dip

HONEY DIP

⅓ cup	light mayonnaise	75 mL
3 tbsp	liquid honey	45 mL
1 tbsp	fresh lemon juice	15 mL
¼ cup	light mayonnaise	50 mL
2 tbsp	Dijon mustard	25 mL
2 tbsp	fresh lemon juice	25 mL
⅓ cup	dry bread crumbs	75 mL
3 tbsp	sesame seeds	45 mL
1 tsp	dried Italian herb seasoning	5 mL
1 lb	skinless boneless chicken breasts, cut into strips 2 inches (5 cm) long by ½ inch (1 cm) wide	500 g

1. *Honey Dip:* In a bowl, stir together mayonnaise, honey and lemon juice until well combined. Refrigerate if making ahead.

2. In a bowl combine mayonnaise, Dijon mustard and lemon juice.

3. On waxed paper or in a bowl, combine bread crumbs, sesame seeds and Italian seasoning.

4. Coat chicken with mayonnaise mixture, then with bread crumb mixture. Place on prepared cookie sheet. Bake in preheated oven, turning once, for 15 to 20 minutes or until golden brown and chicken is no longer pink inside. Serve hot with the honey dip.

Choices Per Serving

2 Carbohydrates

4 Meat & Alternatives

Nutritional Analysis Per Serving			
Calories	367	Fat, total	15 g
Carbohydrate	31 g	Fat, saturated	2 g
Fiber	2 g	Sodium	422 mg
Protein	28 g	Cholesterol	66 mg

If your kids don't like rice, serve this dish over 1 lb (500 g) spaghetti. Also, feel free to omit the onions.

Serve with vegetables such as green beans and add a Milk & Alternatives choice to make this a complete meal.

Make Ahead

Make up to 2 days ahead; reheat before serving. Can be frozen for up to 6 weeks. Great for leftovers.

Sweet-and-Sour Chicken Meatballs over Rice

12 oz	ground chicken	375 g
¼ cup	finely chopped onions	50 mL
2 tbsp	ketchup	25 mL
2 tbsp	bread crumbs	25 mL
1	egg	1
2 tsp	olive oil	10 mL
2 tsp	minced garlic	10 mL
⅓ cup	chopped onions	75 mL
2 cups	tomato juice	500 mL
2 cups	pineapple juice	500 mL
½ cup	chili sauce	125 mL
2 cups	white rice	500 mL

1. In a bowl combine chicken, onions, ketchup, bread crumbs and egg; mix well. Form each 1 tbsp (15 mL) mixture into a meatball; set aside.

2. In a large saucepan, heat oil over medium heat. Add garlic and onions; cook for 3 minutes or until softened. Add tomato juice, pineapple juice, chili sauce and meatballs. Simmer, covered, for 30 to 40 minutes or until meatballs are tender.

3. Meanwhile, bring 4 cups (1 L) water to boil; add rice. Reduce heat; simmer, covered, for 20 minutes or until liquid is absorbed. Remove from heat; let stand for 5 minutes, covered. Serve meatballs and sauce over rice.

Choices Per Serving

3½ Carbohydrates

1 Meat & Alternative

½ Fat

Nutritional Analysis Per Serving			
Calories	346	Fat, total	8 g
Carbohydrate	54 g	Fat, saturated	1 g
Fiber	2 g	Sodium	422 mg
Protein	13 g	Cholesterol	27 mg

Preheat oven to
400°F (200°C)

Baking sheet sprayed
with vegetable spray

· · · · · · · · · · · · · ·

Tip

Use bran flakes instead
of natural bran; they
have a sweetness that
children love.

· · · · · · · · · · · · · ·

Make Ahead

Coat the drumsticks
up to 1 day ahead. They
can be baked a few
hours in advance and
then gently reheated.
Great for leftovers.

Crunchy Cheese and Herb Drumsticks

1½ cups	bran or corn flakes cereal	375 mL
1½ tbsp	fresh chopped parsley	20 mL
2½ tbsp	grated Parmesan cheese	35 mL
1 tsp	minced garlic	5 mL
¾ tsp	dried basil (or ½ tsp/2 mL dried)	4 mL
½ tsp	chili powder	2 mL
⅛ tsp	ground black pepper	0.5 mL
1	egg	1
2 tbsp	milk or water	25 mL
8	skinless chicken drumsticks	8

1. In a food processor combine bran flakes, parsley, Parmesan, garlic, basil, chili powder and pepper; process into fine crumbs. Set aside.

2. In a bowl whisk together egg and milk. Dip each drumstick into egg wash, then roll in crumbs; place on prepared baking sheet. Bake, turning halfway, for 35 minutes or until browned and chicken is cooked through.

Choices Per Serving

½   Carbohydrate

4   Meat & Alternatives

Nutritional Analysis Per Serving

Calories	238	Fat, total	9 g
Carbohydrate	11 g	Fat, saturated	3 g
Fiber	2 g	Sodium	186 mg
Protein	28 g	Cholesterol	151 mg

Tips

Children love this version of packaged Beefaroni. It is not only more delicious, it is healthier for them.

Double this recipe and serve it to a group.

Substitute ground chicken or veal for the beef.

This casserole is an excellent source of iron and zinc.

Make Ahead

Cook and refrigerate up to a day before, then reheat to serve.

Beef, Macaroni and Cheese Casserole

1½ tsp	vegetable oil	7 mL
2 tsp	crushed garlic	10 mL
½ cup	chopped onion	125 mL
12 oz	lean ground beef	375 g
1	can (19 oz/540 mL) tomatoes, crushed	1
1 tsp	dried basil	5 mL
1 tsp	dried oregano	5 mL
1 cup	macaroni	250 mL
2 tbsp	grated Parmesan cheese	25 mL

1. In a large nonstick skillet, heat oil; sauté garlic and onion for 3 minutes. Add beef and sauté until no longer pink, stirring constantly to break up beef.

2. Add tomatoes, basil and oregano; cover and cook for 15 minutes, stirring occasionally.

3. Meanwhile, cook macaroni according to package directions or until firm to the bite. Drain and place in serving bowl. Toss with sauce and sprinkle with cheese.

Choices
Per Serving

2	Carbohydrates
2½	Meat & Alternatives
½	Fat

Nutritional Analysis Per Serving			
Calories	359	Fat, total	16 g
Carbohydrate	32 g	Fat, saturated	6 g
Fiber	3 g	Sodium	436 mg
Protein	22 g	Cholesterol	50 mg

Updated Sloppy Joes

1 lb	lean ground beef	500 g
1	small onion, chopped	1
1	clove garlic, minced	1
1	sweet green pepper, diced	1
1	sweet yellow pepper, diced	1
1	can (14 oz/398 mL) tomato sauce	1
1 tbsp	red wine vinegar	15 mL
1 tbsp	fresh lemon juice	15 mL
1 tbsp	Worcestershire sauce	15 mL
1 tbsp	packed brown sugar	15 mL
1 tsp	Dijon mustard	5 mL
1 tsp	paprika	5 mL
1 tsp	Tabasco sauce	5 mL
	Salt and pepper	
4	Kaiser buns, split and toasted	4

1. In medium saucepan or large skillet, cook beef, onion, garlic and sweet peppers over medium-high heat, breaking up meat with spoon, until meat is no longer pink, about 10 minutes. Drain off any fat. Stir in tomato sauce, vinegar, lemon juice, Worcestershire sauce, brown sugar, mustard, paprika, Tabasco sauce, and salt and pepper to taste; bring to boil. Reduce heat and simmer, uncovered and stirring occasionally, until thickened, about 20 minutes. Spoon over buns.

Choices Per Serving

3	Carbohydrates
3½	Meat & Alternatives
½	Fat

Nutritional Analysis Per Serving

Calories	489	Fat, total	20 g
Carbohydrate	48 g	Fat, saturated	7 g
Fiber	2 g	Sodium	1006 mg
Protein	30 g	Cholesterol	64 mg

....

Preheat oven to
400°F (200°C)

Shallow baking dish

....

Tip

How to bake potatoes:
Scrub baking potatoes
(10 oz/300 g each) well
and pierce skins with a
fork in several places to
allow steam to escape.
Place in 400°F (200°C)
oven for 1 hour or until
potatoes give slightly
when squeezed.

Beef-Stuffed Spuds

4	large potatoes (about 10 oz/300 g each)	4
8 oz	lean ground beef or ground veal	250 g
⅓ cup	finely chopped onions	75 mL
1	clove garlic, minced	1
1 tsp	Worcestershire sauce	5 mL
	Salt and pepper	
½ cup	sour cream or plain yogurt or buttermilk (approx.)	125 mL
2 tbsp	chopped parsley	25 mL
1 cup	shredded reduced-fat Cheddar cheese	250 mL

1. Bake potatoes as directed (see tip).

2. In a large nonstick skillet over medium-high heat, cook beef, breaking up with back of spoon, for 4 minutes or until no longer pink.

3. Reduce heat to medium. Add onions, garlic and Worcestershire sauce; season with salt and pepper. Cook, stirring often, for 4 minutes or until onions are softened.

4. Cut warm potatoes into half lengthwise. Carefully scoop out each potato, leaving a ¼-inch (5 mm) shell; set aside.

5. In a bowl mash potatoes with a potato masher or fork; beat in enough sour cream to make smooth. Stir in beef mixture, parsley and half the cheese; season to taste with salt and pepper. Spoon into potato shells; top with remaining cheese.

6. Arrange in baking dish; bake in preheated oven for 15 minutes or until cheese is melted. Alternatively, place on microwave-safe rack or large serving plate; microwave at Medium-High for 5 to 7 minutes or until heated through and cheese melts.

**Choices
Per Serving**

2 Carbohydrates

1 Meat & Alternative

Nutritional Analysis Per Serving

Calories	227	Fat, total	6 g
Carbohydrate	31 g	Fat, saturated	3 g
Fiber	3 g	Sodium	101 mg
Protein	12 g	Cholesterol	22 mg

Potato Wedge Fries

Tip

If children like spicier
fries, use chili powder
instead of paprika.

Make Ahead

Cut potatoes early in
the day and leave in
cold water so they
don't discolor.

3	potatoes (about 10 oz/300 g each)	3
2 tbsp	melted margarine or butter	25 mL
1 tsp	minced garlic	5 mL
2 tbsp	grated Parmesan cheese	25 mL
¼ tsp	paprika	1 mL

1. Scrub potatoes and cut lengthwise into 8 wedges. Put on prepared baking sheet. Combine margarine and garlic in a small bowl. Combine Parmesan and paprika in another small bowl.

2. Brush potato wedges with half of the margarine and cheese mixture. Bake for 20 minutes, turn the wedges, brush with remaining margarine mixture (reheat if necessary). Sprinkle on remaining Parmesan mixture, and bake for another 20 minutes or just until potatoes are tender and crisp.

**Choices
Per Serving**

1   Carbohydrate

1   Fat

Nutritional Analysis Per Serving			
Calories	118	Fat, total	5 g
Carbohydrate	17 g	Fat, saturated	1 g
Fiber	1 g	Sodium	92 mg
Protein	3 g	Cholesterol	2 mg

● ● ● ● ● ● ● ● ● ● ● ● ● ● ●

Preheat oven to
375°F (190°C)

12 muffin cups sprayed
with vegetable spray

● ● ● ● ● ● ● ● ● ● ● ● ● ● ●

Tips

These muffins are
a heavenly treat for
children. What a
combination — peanut
butter, bananas
and chocolate!

Using 1/3 cup (75 mL)
granulated sugar and
1/3 cup (75 mL) sugar
substitute will change the
texture of the muffins
somewhat, but will
reduce the carbohydrate
content by 5 g/serving.

● ● ● ● ● ● ● ● ● ● ● ● ● ● ●

Make Ahead

Prepare up to a day
ahead. These freeze
well up to 4 weeks.

Banana Peanut Butter Chip Muffins

2/3 cup	granulated sugar	150 mL
3 tbsp	vegetable oil	45 mL
3 tbsp	peanut butter	45 mL
1	large banana, mashed	1
1	egg	1
1 tsp	vanilla	5 mL
3/4 cup	all-purpose flour	175 mL
3/4 tsp	baking powder	4 mL
3/4 tsp	baking soda	4 mL
1/4 cup	2% yogurt	50 mL
3 tbsp	semi-sweet chocolate chips	45 mL

1. In large bowl or food processor, combine sugar, oil, peanut butter, banana, egg and vanilla; mix until well blended. In another bowl combine flour, baking powder and baking soda; add to batter and mix just until blended. Stir in yogurt and chocolate chips.

2. Fill muffin cups half-full. Bake for 15 to 18 minutes, or until tops are firm to the touch and cake tester inserted in the center comes out dry.

Choices
Per Serving

1½ Carbohydrates

1½ Fats

Nutritional Analysis Per Serving			
Calories	169	Fat, total	8 g
Carbohydrate	24 g	Fat, saturated	2 g
Fiber	1 g	Sodium	90 mg
Protein	3 g	Cholesterol	18 mg

Peanut Butter-Coconut-Raisin Granola Bars

Tips

Chopped dates can
replace raisins.

Use a no-sugar-added
smooth or chunky
peanut butter.

Do not overcook the
peanut butter mixture.

Make Ahead

Prepare these up to
2 days ahead and keep
tightly closed in a cookie
tin. These freeze for
up to 2 weeks.

1⅓ cups	rolled oats	325 mL
⅔ cup	raisins	150 mL
½ cup	bran flakes	125 mL
⅓ cup	unsweetened coconut	75 mL
3 tbsp	chocolate chips	45 mL
2 tbsp	chopped pecans	25 mL
1 tsp	baking soda	5 mL
¼ cup	peanut butter	50 mL
¼ cup	brown sugar	50 mL
3 tbsp	margarine or butter	45 mL
3 tbsp	honey	45 mL
1 tsp	vanilla	5 mL

1. Put oats, raisins, bran flakes, coconut, chocolate chips, pecans and baking soda in bowl. Combine until well mixed.

2. In small saucepan, whisk together peanut butter, brown sugar, margarine, honey and vanilla over medium heat for approximately 30 seconds or just until sugar dissolves and mixture is smooth. Pour over dry ingredients and stir to combine. Press into prepared pan and bake for 15 to 20 minutes or until browned. Let cool completely before cutting into bars.

Choices Per Serving

1 Carbohydrate

1 Fat

Nutritional Analysis Per Serving			
Calories	97	Fat, total	5 g
Carbohydrate	13 g	Fat, saturated	2 g
Fiber	1 g	Sodium	77 mg
Protein	2 g	Cholesterol	0 mg

Breads, Biscuits, Muffins and More

Lower-fat muffins and breads are fabulous alternatives to traditional baked goods. These delicious goodies are great for breakfast, as part of a quick lunch, or as an accompaniment to a main course. Once your family tastes these treats, they'll be asking for more!

Preheat oven to
350°F (180°C)

9- by 5-inch (2 L) loaf
pan, lightly greased

Tips

Fat-free and easy to
prepare, this loaf has a
delicate yeast flavor that
works well with soups,
salads and egg dishes.

Any type of beer
works well in this recipe
— whether cold or
at room temperature,
flat or foamy.

Variation

Increase the quantity
of one dried herb to
bring out the flavor
you like best.

Low-Fat Herbed Beer Bread

2¾ cups	all-purpose flour	675 mL
2 tbsp	granulated sugar	25 mL
2 tbsp	baking powder	25 mL
1 tsp	salt	5 mL
½ tsp	dried marjoram	2 mL
½ tsp	dried oregano	2 mL
½ tsp	dried thyme	2 mL
Pinch	dried dill	Pinch
1	can (13 oz/355 mL) beer	1

1. In a large bowl, stir together flour, sugar, baking powder, salt, marjoram, oregano, thyme and dill. Add beer and stir just until combined. Spoon into prepared pan.

2. Bake in preheated oven for 70 to 80 minutes or until a cake tester inserted in the center comes out clean. Let cool in pan on rack for 10 minutes. Remove from pan and serve warm.

Choices Per Serving

1   Carbohydrate

Nutritional Analysis Per Serving

Calories	96	Fat, total	0 g
Carbohydrate	19 g	Fat, saturated	0 g
Fiber	1 g	Sodium	231 mg
Protein	2 g	Cholesterol	0 mg

Preheat oven to
400°F (200°C)

Baking sheet,
lightly greased

Tip

Score the top of the
round at least $\frac{1}{2}$ inch
(1 cm) deep. This will
ensure it breaks easily
into wedges.

Irish Whole Wheat Soda Bread

2 cups	whole wheat flour	500 mL
1 cup	all-purpose flour	250 mL
1 tbsp	granulated sugar	15 mL
1 tsp	baking powder	5 mL
1 tsp	baking soda	5 mL
1 tsp	salt	5 mL
1½ cups	buttermilk	375 mL

1. In a large bowl, stir together whole wheat flour, flour, sugar, baking powder, baking soda and salt. Add buttermilk all at once, stirring with a fork to make a soft, but slightly sticky dough.

2. With lightly floured hands, form dough into a ball. On a lightly floured surface, knead the dough gently for 8 to 10 times. Pat the dough into a 6-inch (15 cm) thick round, with a slightly flattened top.

3. Place dough on prepared baking sheet. With a shape knife or pizza cutter, score the top in the shape of a cross or large X. Bake in preheated oven for 35 to 45 minutes. Remove from baking sheet onto a cooling rack immediately. Dust top with rice flour. Serve warm from the oven.

Choices Per Serving

1½ Carbohydrates

Nutritional Analysis Per Serving			
Calories	123	Fat, total	1 g
Carbohydrate	25 g	Fat, saturated	0 g
Fiber	3 g	Sodium	335 mg
Protein	5 g	Cholesterol	1 mg

Preheat oven to
350°F (180°C)

9- by 5-inch (2 L)
loaf pan, lightly greased

Tip

Leave blueberries in the
freezer until just before
using. This will help to
prevent them from
"bleeding" into the bread.

Variation

Try substituting half or
all of the blueberries with
frozen sour cherries
or cranberries.

Blueberry Buckwheat Bread

1⅔ cups	all-purpose flour	400 mL
⅓ cup	buckwheat flour	75 mL
1 tbsp	baking powder	15 mL
½ tsp	salt	2 mL
1 tsp	grated lemon zest	5 mL
3 tbsp	vegetable oil	45 mL
2	egg whites	2
1¼ cups	plain yogurt	300 mL
⅓ cup	honey	75 mL
½ cup	frozen blueberries	125 mL

1. In a large bowl, stir together flour, buckwheat flour, baking powder, salt and zest.

2. In a separate bowl, using an electric mixer, beat oil, eggs, yogurt and honey until combined. Pour mixture over dry ingredients and stir just until combined. Gently fold in frozen blueberries. Spoon into prepared pan.

3. Bake in preheated oven for 70 to 80 minutes or until a cake tester inserted in the center comes out clean. Let cool in pan on rack for 10 minutes. Remove from pan and let cool completely on rack.

Choices
Per Serving

2   Carbohydrates

½   Fat

Nutritional Analysis Per Serving

Calories	158	Fat, total	4 g
Carbohydrate	28 g	Fat, saturated	0 g
Fiber	1 g	Sodium	181 mg
Protein	4 g	Cholesterol	0 mg

Preheat oven to
350°F (180°C)

9- by 5-inch (2 L)
loaf pan, lightly greased

Tips

Barm brack, meaning
"yeast bread" in Gaelic,
is an Irish bread with
raisins or currants and
candied fruit peel —
although it is not always
made with yeast. Try
this fruited version
made with tea, apricots
and cranberries.

Snip dried apricots into
¼-inch (5 mm) pieces
with sharp scissors.

Variation

Try replacing one or
more of the fruits with
an equal quantity of
dried cherries, dried
apples or fresh dates.

Fruited Barm Brack

2 cups	all-purpose flour	500 mL
½ cup	packed brown sugar	125 mL
2 tsp	baking powder	10 mL
½ tsp	baking soda	2 mL
½ tsp	salt	2 mL
1 tsp	ground cinnamon	5 mL
1 tsp	ground nutmeg	5 mL
½ cup	snipped dried apricots	125 mL
½ cup	currants	125 mL
½ cup	dried cranberries	125 mL
2 tbsp	vegetable oil	25 mL
1	egg	1
1 cup	tea (at room temperature)	250 mL

1. In a large bowl, stir together flour, brown sugar, baking powder, baking soda, salt, cinnamon and nutmeg. Stir in dried apricots, currants and dried cranberries.

2. In a separate bowl, using an electric mixer, beat oil, egg and tea until combined. Pour mixture over dry ingredients and stir just until combined. Spoon into prepared pan.

3. Bake in preheated oven for 70 to 80 minutes or until a cake tester inserted in the center comes out clean. Let cool in pan on rack for 10 minutes. Remove from pan and let cool completely on rack.

Choices
Per Serving

2½ Carbohydrates

½ Fat

Nutritional Analysis Per Serving			
Calories	186	Fat, total	3 g
Carbohydrate	37 g	Fat, saturated	0 g
Fiber	2 g	Sodium	192 mg
Protein	3 g	Cholesterol	18 mg

Preheat oven to
350°F (180°C)

9- by 5-inch (2 L)
loaf pan, lightly greased

Tip

Instead of using
egg whites, try using
1 whole egg. This will
increase the fat content
slightly, but it yields
a softer-textured loaf.

Variation

Substitute dates
for raisins and ground
ginger or nutmeg for
the cinnamon.

Low-Fat Applesauce Raisin Bread

2 cups	all-purpose flour	500 mL
½ cup	granulated sugar	125 mL
1 tsp	baking powder	5 mL
½ tsp	baking soda	2 mL
¼ tsp	salt	1 mL
½ tsp	ground cinnamon	2 mL
1 cup	raisins	250 mL
2	egg whites	2
1¼ cups	unsweetened applesauce	300 mL

1. In a large bowl, stir together flour, sugar, baking powder, baking soda, salt and cinnamon. Stir in raisins.

2. In a separate bowl, using an electric mixer, beat egg whites and applesauce until combined. Pour mixture over dry ingredients and stir just until combined. Spoon into prepared pan.

3. Bake in preheated oven for 70 to 80 minutes or until a cake tester inserted in the center comes out clean. Let cool in pan on rack for 10 minutes. Remove from pan and let cool completely on rack.

Choices
Per Serving

2 Carbohydrates

Nutritional Analysis Per Serving

Calories	123	Fat, total	0 g
Carbohydrate	29 g	Fat, saturated	0 g
Fiber	1 g	Sodium	95 mg
Protein	2 g	Cholesterol	0 mg

• • • • • • • • • • • • • •

Preheat oven to
350°F (180°C)

9- by 5-inch (2 L)
loaf pan, lightly greased

• • • • • • • • • • • • • •

Variation

Substitute sesame
or flaxseeds for the
poppy seeds.

Poppy Seed Oat Bread

1 cup	whole wheat flour	250 mL
1 cup	all-purpose flour	250 mL
1 cup	quick-cooking oats	250 mL
1 tsp	baking powder	5 mL
1 tsp	baking soda	5 mL
½ tsp	salt	2 mL
¼ cup	poppy seeds	50 mL
1	egg	1
1¾ cups	buttermilk	425 mL
⅓ cup	honey	75 mL

1. In a large bowl, stir together whole wheat flour, flour, oats, baking powder, baking soda, salt and poppy seeds.

2. In a separate bowl, using an electric mixer, beat egg and buttermilk until combined. Add honey while mixing. Pour mixture over dry ingredients and stir just until combined. Spoon into prepared pan.

3. Bake in preheated oven for 70 to 80 minutes or until a cake tester inserted in the center comes out clean. Let cool in pan on rack for 10 minutes. Remove from pan and let cool completely on rack.

**Choices
Per Serving**

2   Carbohydrates

½   Fat

Nutritional Analysis Per Serving

Calories	174	Fat, total	3 g
Carbohydrate	32 g	Fat, saturated	1 g
Fiber	2 g	Sodium	254 mg
Protein	6 g	Cholesterol	19 mg

Preheat oven to
350°F (180°C)

9- by 5-inch (2 L)
loaf pan, lightly greased

Tips

Leave blueberries in
the freezer until just
before using. This will
help to prevent them
from "bleeding" into
the bread.

Use ripe bananas for the
best flavor.

Variation

Try natural wheat bran
instead of the oat bran.

Blueberry Banana Oat Bread

1¾ cups	all-purpose flour	425 mL
¼ cup	quick-cooking oats	50 mL
2 tbsp	oat bran	25 mL
½ cup	granulated sugar	125 mL
2 tsp	baking powder	10 mL
½ tsp	salt	2 mL
2 tbsp	vegetable oil	25 mL
1	egg	1
1½ cups	mashed bananas	375 mL
¾ cup	frozen blueberries (see Tip)	175 mL

1. In a large bowl, stir together flour, oats, oat bran, sugar, baking powder and salt.

2. In a separate bowl, using an electric mixer, beat oil, egg and banana until combined. Pour mixture over dry ingredients and stir just until combined. Gently fold in frozen blueberries. Spoon into prepared pan.

3. Bake in preheated oven for 70 to 80 minutes or until a cake tester inserted in the center comes out clean. Let cool in pan on rack for 10 minutes. Remove from pan and serve warm.

Choices Per Serving

2	Carbohydrates
½	Fat

Nutritional Analysis Per Serving

Calories	169	Fat, total	3 g
Carbohydrate	32 g	Fat, saturated	0 g
Fiber	2 g	Sodium	138 mg
Protein	3 g	Cholesterol	18 mg

Preheat oven to
350°F (180°C)

9- by 5-inch (2 L)
loaf pan, lightly greased

Tip

The rhubarb must
be finely chopped;
otherwise, the finished
loaf tends to crumble
when sliced.

Variation

Substitute pecans
or pistachios for the
walnuts and lemon
zest for the orange.

Rhubarb Orange Bread

1¾ cups	finely chopped rhubarb	425 mL
⅓ cup	granulated sugar	75 mL
2 cups	all-purpose flour	500 mL
2 tsp	baking powder	10 mL
¾ tsp	baking soda	4 mL
½ tsp	salt	2 mL
2 tbsp	grated orange zest	25 mL
½ cup	chopped walnuts	125 mL
3 tbsp	vegetable oil	45 mL
1	egg	1
⅔ cup	orange juice	150 mL
1 tsp	vanilla extract	5 mL

1. In a bowl combine rhubarb and sugar; set aside for
10 to 15 minutes.

2. In a large bowl, stir together flour, baking powder,
baking soda, salt and zest. Stir in walnuts.

3. In a separate bowl, using an electric mixer, beat oil, egg,
juice and vanilla extract until combined. Stir in reserved
rhubarb mixture. Pour over dry ingredients and stir
just until combined. Spoon into prepared pan.

4. Bake in preheated oven for 70 to 80 minutes or until
a cake tester inserted in the center comes out clean.
Let cool in pan on rack for 10 minutes. Remove from
pan and let cool completely on rack.

Choices
Per Serving

1½ Carbohydrates

1½ Fats

Nutritional Analysis Per Serving			
Calories	178	Fat, total	7 g
Carbohydrate	25 g	Fat, saturated	1 g
Fiber	1 g	Sodium	214 mg
Protein	4 g	Cholesterol	18 mg

• • • • • • • • • • • • • •

Preheat oven to
350°F (180°C)

9- by 5-inch (2 L)
loaf pan, lightly greased

• • • • • • • • • • • • • •

Tip

Blueberries are
becoming very popular as
a source of antioxidants
with disease-fighting
properties.

• • • • • • • • • • • • • •

Variation

For a milder spice flavor,
use mace or nutmeg
instead of the cardamom.

Peach Blueberry Quick Bread

1¾ cups	all-purpose flour	425 mL
2½ tsp	baking powder	12 mL
¾ tsp	salt	4 mL
½ tsp	ground cardamom	2 mL
⅓ cup	margarine	75 mL
⅔ cup	granulated sugar	150 mL
2	eggs	2
⅓ cup	milk	75 mL
1 cup	chopped fresh peaches	250 mL
½ cup	fresh or frozen blueberries	125 mL

1. In a large bowl, stir together flour, baking powder, salt and cardamom.

2. In a separate large bowl, using an electric mixer, cream margarine, sugar and eggs until light and fluffy. Stir in dry ingredients alternately with milk, making 3 additions of dry ingredients and 2 of milk; stir just until combined. Gently fold in peaches and blueberries. Spoon into prepared pan.

3. Bake in preheated oven for 70 to 80 minutes or until a cake tester inserted in the center comes out clean. Let cool in pan on rack for 10 minutes. Remove from pan and let cool completely on rack.

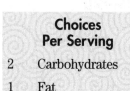

Choices Per Serving	
2	Carbohydrates
1	Fat

Nutritional Analysis Per Serving			
Calories	180	Fat, total	6 g
Carbohydrate	28 g	Fat, saturated	1 g
Fiber	1 g	Sodium	266 mg
Protein	3 g	Cholesterol	36 mg

Preheat oven to
375°F (190°C)

9- by 5-inch (2 L) loaf
pan sprayed with
nonstick vegetable spray

Tip

If you like muffins, fill
12 muffin cups and
bake approximately
20 minutes or until tops
are firm to the touch.

Make Ahead

Make up to 2 days in
advance or freeze for
up to 2 months.

Banana Nut Raisin Loaf

2	large ripe bananas	2
⅓ cup	soft margarine	75 mL
½ cup	granulated sugar	125 mL
1	egg	1
1	egg white	1
¼ cup	hot water	50 mL
1⅓ cups	whole wheat flour	325 mL
¾ tsp	baking soda	4 mL
¼ cup	raisins	50 mL
⅓ cup	chopped pecans or walnuts	75 mL

1. In bowl or food processor, beat bananas and margarine; beat in sugar, egg, egg white and water until smooth.

2. Combine flour and baking soda; stir into batter along with raisins and all but a few of the pecans, mixing just until blended. Do not overmix. Pour into pan; arrange reserved nuts down middle of mixture. Bake for 35 to 45 minutes or until tester inserted into center comes out dry.

**Choices
Per Serving**

1   Carbohydrate

1   Fat

Nutritional Analysis Per Serving

Calories	107	Fat, total	5 g
Carbohydrate	16 g	Fat, saturated	1 g
Fiber	1 g	Sodium	84 mg
Protein	2 g	Cholesterol	11 mg

Carrot Pineapple Zucchini Loaf

Preheat oven to
350°F (180°C)

9- by 5-inch (2 L) loaf
pan sprayed with
nonstick vegetable spray

Tips

If you like muffins, fill
12 muffin cups and
bake approximately
20 minutes or until tops
are firm to the touch.

The carrots in this loaf
make this recipe a good
source of vitamin A.

Lower-fat loaves such
as this one will dry out
more quickly, so should
be frozen after slicing if
they will not be used
within a couple of days.

Make Ahead

Make up to 2 days in
advance or freeze for
up to 2 months.

¼ cup	margarine	50 mL
1 cup	granulated sugar	250 mL
1	egg	1
1	egg white	1
2 tsp	cinnamon	10 mL
1½ tsp	vanilla	7 mL
¼ tsp	nutmeg	1 mL
¾ cup	grated carrot	175 mL
¾ cup	grated zucchini	175 mL
½ cup	drained crushed pineapple	125 mL
⅓ cup	raisins	75 mL
1¼ cups	all-purpose flour	300 mL
½ cup	whole wheat flour	125 mL
1 tsp	baking powder	5 mL
1 tsp	baking soda	5 mL

1. In large bowl or food processor, cream margarine
with sugar. Add egg, egg white, cinnamon, vanilla and
nutmeg; beat well. Stir in carrot, zucchini, pineapple
and raisins, blending until well combined.

2. Combine all-purpose and whole wheat flours, baking
powder and soda; add to bowl and mix just until
combined. Pour into loaf pan and bake for 35 to
45 minutes or until tester inserted into center comes
out dry.

Choices Per Serving

1½ Carbohydrate

½ Fat

Nutritional Analysis Per Serving

Calories	119	Fat, total	3 g
Carbohydrate	22 g	Fat, saturated	0 g
Fiber	3 g	Sodium	116 mg
Protein	2 g	Cholesterol	11 mg

Moors and Christians *page 268*
Overleaf: Polenta with Chèvre and
Roasted Vegetables *page 282*

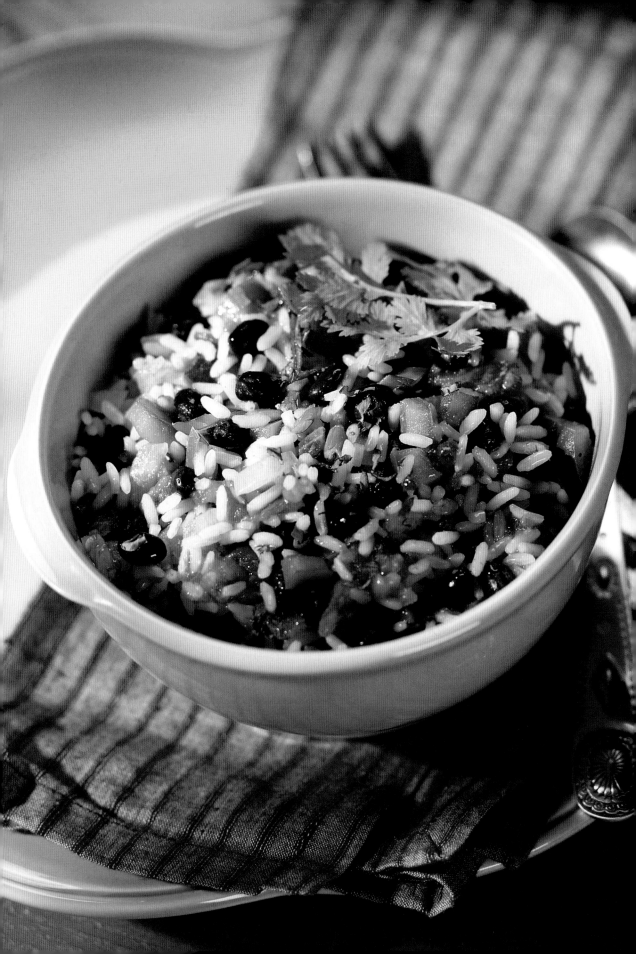

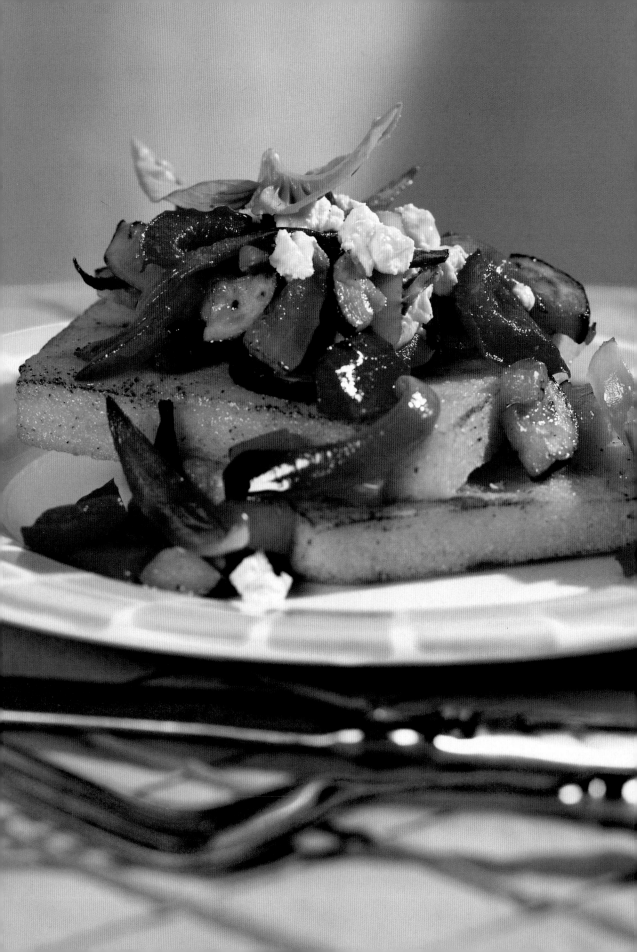

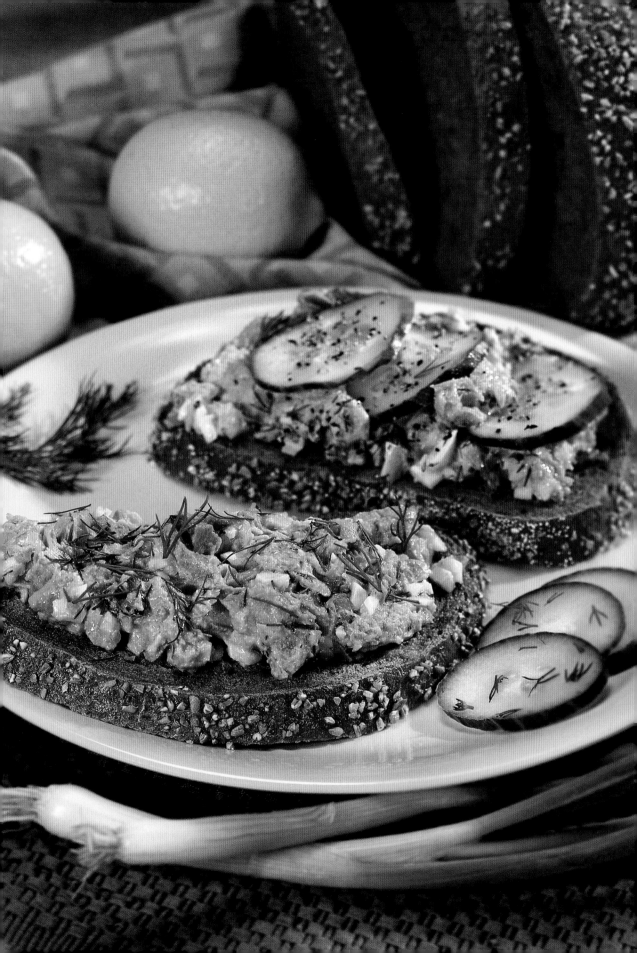

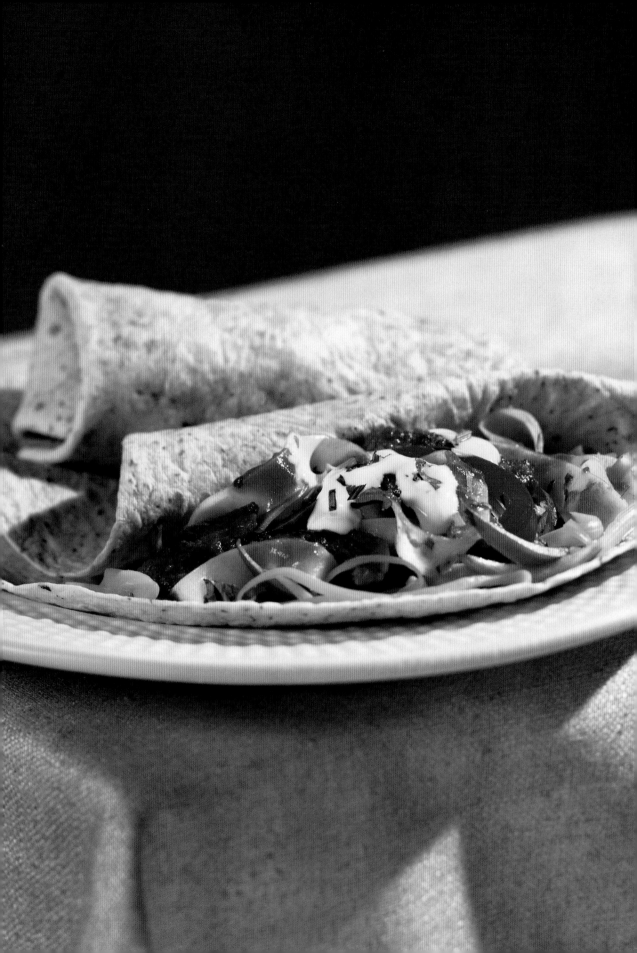

● ● ● ● ● ● ● ● ● ● ● ● ● ● ● ●

Preheat oven to
350°F (180°C)

9- by 5-inch (2 L) loaf
pan sprayed with
vegetable spray

● ● ● ● ● ● ● ● ● ● ● ● ● ● ● ●

Tips

Grate carrots or chop and
process them in food
processor just until finely
diced. Chopped, pitted
dates can replace raisins.

Orange fruits and
vegetables such carrots,
squash and mangoes
are good sources of beta
carotene or vitamin A.

● ● ● ● ● ● ● ● ● ● ● ● ● ● ● ●

Make Ahead

Prepare up to a day
ahead, or freeze up to
4 weeks.

Carrot, Apple and Coconut Loaf

⅔ cup	granulated sugar	150 mL
¼ cup	margarine or butter	50 mL
2	eggs	2
1½ tsp	cinnamon	7 mL
¼ tsp	nutmeg	1 mL
1 tsp	vanilla	5 mL
1¼ cup	grated carrots	300 mL
⅔ cup	peeled, finely chopped apples	150 mL
⅓ cup	unsweetened shredded coconut	75 mL
⅓ cup	raisins	75 mL
⅔ cup	all-purpose flour	150 mL
½ cup	whole wheat flour	125 mL
1 tsp	baking powder	5 mL
1 tsp	baking soda	5 mL
⅓ cup	2% yogurt	75 mL

1. In large bowl or food processor, cream together sugar
   and margarine. Add eggs, cinnamon, nutmeg and
   vanilla; beat well. Stir in carrots, apples, coconut
   and raisins.

2. In bowl, combine flour, whole wheat flour, baking
   powder and baking soda; add to batter alternately
   with yogurt, mixing until just combined. Pour batter
   into loaf pan; bake for 40 to 45 minutes or until tester
   inserted in center comes out clean.

Choices Per Serving

1   Carbohydrate

1   Fat

Nutritional Analysis Per Serving			
Calories	111	Fat, total	4 g
Carbohydrate	17 g	Fat, saturated	2 g
Fiber	1 g	Sodium	121 mg
Protein	2 g	Cholesterol	22 mg

Pork Fajitas with Salsa, Onions and Rice Noodles page 289
Overleaf: Dilled Salmon and Egg Salad
on Pumpernickel page 284

Lemon Poppy Seed Loaf

Preheat oven to
350°F (180°C)

9- by 5-inch (2 L) loaf
pan sprayed with
nonstick vegetable spray

Tips

You can also make
muffins by pouring batter
into 12 cups and baking
in 375°F (190°C) oven
for 15 to 20 minutes.

If you like a strong lemon
taste, use 1 tsp (5 mL)
more lemon rind.

In this recipe, granulated
sugar is used in the loaf
and icing sugar is used in
the glaze.

Make Ahead

Bake a day before or
freeze for up to 6 weeks.

¾ cup	granulated sugar	175 mL
⅓ cup	soft margarine	75 mL
1	egg	1
2 tsp	grated lemon rind	10 mL
3 tbsp	lemon juice	45 mL
⅓ cup	2% milk	75 mL
1¼ cups	all-purpose flour	300 mL
1 tbsp	poppy seeds	15 mL
1 tsp	baking powder	5 mL
½ tsp	baking soda	2 mL
⅓ cup	2% yogurt or light sour cream	75 mL

GLAZE

¼ cup	icing sugar	50 mL
2 tbsp	lemon juice	25 mL

1. In large bowl or food processor, beat together sugar,
margarine, egg, lemon rind and juice, mixing well.
Add milk, mixing well.

2. Combine flour, poppy seeds, baking powder and baking
soda; add to bowl alternately with yogurt, mixing just
until incorporated. Do not overmix. Pour into pan and
bake for 35 to 40 minutes or until tester inserted into
center comes out dry.

3. *Glaze:* Prick holes in top of loaf with fork. Combine
icing sugar with lemon juice; pour over loaf.

Choices Per Serving	
1	Carbohydrate
½	Fat

Nutritional Analysis Per Serving			
Calories	102	Fat, total	4 g
Carbohydrate	16 g	Fat, saturated	1 g
Fiber	1 g	Sodium	88 mg
Protein	2 g	Cholesterol	11 mg

Crêpe pan or frypan,
lightly greased

Tip

Blini can be prepared in
a frypan, crêpe pan or on
a grill. The choice is up to
you. For fluffier pancakes,
warm egg whites to room
temperature before using.

Variation

For a stronger buckwheat
flavor, increase the
buckwheat flour to 3 tbsp
(45 mL) and decrease the
flour to ¼ cup (50 mL).

Russian Blini

⅓ cup	milk	75 mL
½ tsp	granulated sugar	2 mL
½ tsp	instant yeast	2 mL
1	egg yolk	1
1 tsp	vegetable oil	5 mL
⅓ cup	all-purpose flour	75 mL
2 tbsp	buckwheat flour	25 mL
¼ tsp	salt	1 mL
2	egg whites	2
Pinch	cream of tartar	Pinch

1. In a small microwaveable bowl, heat milk to lukewarm. Stir in sugar and yeast.

2. In another bowl, whisk together egg yolk and oil. Add yeast mixture, flour, buckwheat flour and salt stirring until smooth. Cover and set in a pan of warm water for 1¼ hours.

3. In a separate bowl, using an electric mixer, beat egg whites and cream of tartar until stiff (but not dry) peaks form; using a spatula, fold whites gently into batter.

4. Heat pan until medium hot. Using 2 tbsp (25 mL) batter, spoon into hot pan. Spread batter, with the back of a spoon, for thinner blini. When the underside is brown, turn and cook about 30 to 60 seconds longer or until the second side is golden brown. Repeat with remaining batter.

Nutritional Analysis Per Serving			
Calories	42	Fat, total	1 g
Carbohydrate	6 g	Fat, saturated	0 g
Fiber	0 g	Sodium	78 mg
Protein	2 g	Cholesterol	24 mg

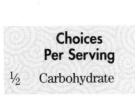

**Choices
Per Serving**

½ Carbohydrate

Scottish Oatmeal Scones

1 cup	whole wheat flour	250 mL
1¼ cups	all-purpose flour	300 mL
½ cup	quick-cooking oats	125 mL
2 tsp	baking powder	10 mL
¾ tsp	salt	4 mL
⅓ cup	margarine	75 mL
1	egg	1
¾ cup	buttermilk	175 mL

Preheat oven to
425°F (220°C)

Baking sheet,
lightly greased

Tip

To enjoy the next day,
split scones in half and
reheat in a toaster oven.

Variation

For a heavier, more
traditional oatmeal
biscuit, omit the
margarine. This will
eliminate the Fat choice.

1. In a large bowl, stir together whole wheat flour, flour, oats, baking powder and salt. Using a pastry blender, cut in margarine until mixture resembles coarse crumbs.

2. In a small bowl, whisk together egg and buttermilk. Pour over dry ingredients all at once, stirring with a fork to make a soft, but slightly sticky dough.

3. With lightly floured hands, form dough into a ball. On a lightly floured surface, knead the dough gently for 8 to 10 times. Pat or roll out the dough into a 1-inch (2.5 cm) thick round.

4. Using a 2-inch (5 cm) floured biscuit cutter, cut out as many rounds as possible. Place on baking sheet. Gently form scraps into a ball, flatten and cut out rounds.

5. Bake in preheated oven for 12 to 15 minutes. Remove from baking sheet onto a cooling rack immediately. Serve warm.

**Choices
Per Serving**

1 Carbohydrate

1 Fat

Nutritional Analysis Per Serving

Calories	133	Fat, total	5 g
Carbohydrate	18 g	Fat, saturated	1 g
Fiber	2 g	Sodium	225 mg
Protein	4 g	Cholesterol	16 mg

● ● ● ● ● ● ● ● ● ● ● ● ● ● ● ● ●

Preheat oven to
425°F (220°C)

Baking sheet,
lightly greased

● ● ● ● ● ● ● ● ● ● ● ● ● ● ● ● ●

Tip

Adjust the quantity of
poppy seeds to your
taste. For browner,
crisper tops, bake
biscuits in the upper
third of the oven.

● ● ● ● ● ● ● ● ● ● ● ● ● ● ● ● ●

Variation

Poppy seeds can
be replaced with any
other small seed — such
as sesame, caraway,
fennel, anise or mini
sunflower seeds. For
stronger-flavored seeds,
you may wish to reduce
the quantity used.

Whole Wheat Poppy Biscuits

1½ cups	whole wheat flour	375 mL
1 cup	all-purpose flour	250 mL
¼ cup	granulated sugar	50 mL
¼ cup	poppy seeds	50 mL
1 tbsp	baking powder	15 mL
½ tsp	baking soda	2 mL
½ tsp	salt	2 mL
⅓ cup	margarine	75 mL
1 cup	buttermilk	250 mL

1. In a large bowl, stir together whole wheat flour, flour, sugar, poppy seeds, baking powder, baking soda and salt. Using a pastry blender, cut in margarine until mixture resembles coarse crumbs. Add buttermilk all at once, stirring with a fork to make a soft, but slightly sticky dough.

2. With lightly floured hands, form dough into a ball. On a lightly floured surface, knead the dough gently for 8 to 10 times. Pat or roll out the dough into a ½-inch (1 cm) thick round.

3. Using a 2-inch (5 cm) floured biscuit cutter, cut out as many rounds as possible. Place on baking sheet. Gently form scraps into a ball, flatten and cut out rounds.

4. Bake in preheated oven for 12 to 15 minutes. Remove from baking sheet onto a cooling rack immediately. Serve warm.

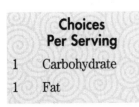

Choices Per Serving	
1	Carbohydrate
1	Fat

Nutritional Analysis Per Serving			
Calories	117	Fat, total	5 g
Carbohydrate	17 g	Fat, saturated	1 g
Fiber	2 g	Sodium	193 mg
Protein	3 g	Cholesterol	0 mg

● ● ● ● ● ● ● ● ● ● ● ● ● ● ● ●

Preheat oven to
425°F (220°C)

Baking sheet, ungreased

Lemon Yogurt Biscuits

2 cups	all-purpose flour	500 mL
2 tbsp	granulated sugar	25 mL
1 tbsp	baking powder	15 mL
½ tsp	baking soda	2 mL
½ tsp	salt	2 mL
2 tsp	grated lemon zest	10 mL
⅓ cup	cold margarine or butter	75 mL
1 cup	plain yogurt	250 mL

1. In a large bowl, stir together flour, sugar, baking powder, baking soda, salt and zest. Using a pastry blender, cut in margarine until mixture resembles coarse crumbs. Add yogurt all at once, stirring with a fork to make a soft, but slightly sticky dough.

2. With lightly floured hands, form dough into a ball. On a lightly floured surface, knead the dough gently for 8 to 10 times. Pat or roll out the dough into a 1-inch (2.5 cm) thick round. Using a 2-inch (5 cm) floured cutter, cut out as many rounds as possible. Place on baking sheet. Gently form scraps into a ball, flatten and cut out rounds.

3. Bake in preheated oven for 12 to 15 minutes. Remove from baking sheet onto a cooling rack immediately.

Choices Per Serving

1½ Carbohydrates

1 Fat

Nutritional Analysis Per Serving

Calories	141	Fat, total	5 g
Carbohydrate	20 g	Fat, saturated	1 g
Fiber	1 g	Sodium	281 mg
Protein	3 g	Cholesterol	0 mg

Wheat Muffins

Preheat oven to
400°F (200°C)

12-cup muffin tin,
sprayed with low-fat
cooking spray or
paper-lined

Tip

To keep muffins at their
best, freeze any which
won't be used in the first
2 days after baking. Thaw
at room temperature or
reheat in the microwave.

1 cup	all-purpose flour	250 mL
1 cup	unsifted whole-wheat flour	250 mL
2 tsp	baking powder	10 mL
1 tsp	salt	5 mL
1	egg, slightly beaten	1
¼ cup	molasses	50 mL
1 cup	milk	250 mL
¼ cup	margarine or butter, melted	50 mL

1. In a large bowl, combine all-purpose flour, whole-wheat flour, baking powder and salt. Make a well in the center.

2. In another bowl, combine egg, molasses, milk and margarine. Add to flour mixture, stirring just until blended. Do not overmix.

3. Spoon batter into prepared muffin tin, filling cups three-quarters full. Bake in preheated oven for 25 minutes or until golden brown.

Choices Per Serving

1½ Carbohydrates

1 Fat

Nutritional Analysis Per Serving

Calories	138	Fat, total	5 g
Carbohydrate	21 g	Fat, saturated	1 g
Fiber	2 g	Sodium	290 mg
Protein	4 g	Cholesterol	18 mg

● ● ● ● ● ● ● ● ● ● ● ● ● ●

Preheat oven to
400°F (200°C)

12-cup muffin tin,
sprayed with low-fat
cooking spray or
paper-lined

Honey Whole Wheat Muffins

1 cup	whole wheat flour	250 mL
1 cup	all-purpose flour	250 mL
3 tsp	baking powder	15 mL
1 tsp	salt	5 mL
1	egg	1
1 cup	milk	250 mL
¼ cup	vegetable oil	50 mL
¼ cup	honey	50 mL

1. In a large bowl, combine whole-wheat flour, all-purpose flour, baking powder and salt. Make a well in the center.

2. In another bowl, whisk together egg, milk and oil. Add the honey. Stir into flour mixture until moist and lumpy.

3. Spoon batter into prepared muffin tin, dividing evenly. Bake in preheated oven for 20 to 25 minutes or until lightly browned.

**Choices
Per Serving**

1½ Carbohydrates

1 Fat

Nutritional Analysis Per Serving			
Calories	152	Fat, total	5 g
Carbohydrate	23 g	Fat, saturated	1 g
Fiber	2 g	Sodium	260 mg
Protein	4 g	Cholesterol	18 mg

• • • • • • • • • • • • • • • • •

Preheat oven to
400°F (200°C)

12-cup muffin tin,
sprayed with low-fat
cooking spray or
paper-lined

Blueberry Wheat Germ Muffins

1¾ cups	all-purpose flour	425 mL
⅓ cup	wheat germ	75 mL
⅓ cup	granulated sugar	75 mL
1 tbsp	baking powder	15 mL
1½ tsp	grated lemon zest	7 mL
½ tsp	salt	2 mL
1	egg	1
1 cup	milk	250 mL
¼ cup	vegetable oil	50 mL
1 cup	fresh blueberries or frozen blueberries, drained	250 mL

1. In a large bowl, combine flour, wheat germ, sugar, baking powder, zest and salt. Make a well in the center.

2. In another bowl, whisk together egg, milk and oil. Add to dry ingredients, stirring just until moist and blended. Fold in berries.

3. Spoon batter into prepared muffin tin, filling cups three-quarters full. Bake in preheated oven for 20 to 25 minutes.

Choices Per Serving

1½ Carbohydrates

1 Fat

Nutritional Analysis Per Serving			
Calories	161	Fat, total	6 g
Carbohydrate	24 g	Fat, saturated	1 g
Fiber	1 g	Sodium	170 mg
Protein	4 g	Cholesterol	18 mg

Preheat oven to
400°F (200°C)

12-cup muffin tin,
sprayed with low-fat
cooking spray or
paper-lined

Peanut Butter
Surprise Muffins

1 cup	all-purpose flour	250 mL
½ tsp	salt	2 mL
3 tsp	baking powder	15 mL
1 tbsp	granulated sugar	15 mL
½ cup	cornmeal	125 mL
1 cup	milk	250 mL
1	egg, beaten	1
¼ cup	peanut butter	50 mL
1 tbsp	margarine or butter, melted	15 mL

1. In a large bowl, combine flour, salt, baking powder and sugar. Stir in cornmeal, mixing to blend well.

2. In a small bowl, combine milk, egg, peanut butter and melted margarine. Add to dry ingredients, stirring until moistened and blended.

3. Spoon batter into prepared muffin tin, filling cups three-quarters full. Bake in preheated oven for about 20 minutes.

Choices
Per Serving

1   Carbohydrate

1   Fat

Nutritional Analysis Per Serving

Calories	120	Fat, total	5 g
Carbohydrate	16 g	Fat, saturated	1 g
Fiber	1 g	Sodium	170 mg
Protein	4 g	Cholesterol	18 mg

● ● ● ● ● ● ● ● ● ● ● ● ● ● ● ●

Preheat oven to
400°F (200°C)

12-cup muffin tin,
sprayed with low-fat
cooking spray or
paper-lined

Kiwi Raspberry Muffins

1 cup	all-purpose flour	250 mL
1 cup	whole-wheat flour	250 mL
1 tbsp	baking powder	15 mL
½ tsp	baking soda	2 mL
2	peeled chopped kiwi	2
½ cup	fresh raspberries (or frozen)	125 mL
1	egg, lightly beaten	1
¼ cup	margarine or butter	50 mL
⅓ cup	skim milk	75 mL
1 tsp	vanilla	5 mL

1. In a large bowl, mix together all-purpose flour, whole-wheat flour, baking powder and baking soda. Add kiwi and raspberries, mixing well. Make a well in the center.

2. In another bowl, combine egg, margarine, milk and vanilla. Add to the flour mixture, stirring only until moistened and blended. Do not overmix.

3. Spoon batter into prepared muffin tin, filling cups to the top. Bake in preheated oven for 15 to 20 minutes.

Choices Per Serving

1   Carbohydrate

1   Fat

Nutritional Analysis Per Serving

Calories	126	Fat, total	5 g
Carbohydrate	19 g	Fat, saturated	1 g
Fiber	2 g	Sodium	219 mg
Protein	3 g	Cholesterol	18 mg

Preheat oven to
375°F (190°C)

12 muffin cups sprayed
with nonstick vegetable
spray

Tips

These delicious muffins
are a nice finish to a
low-fat lunch.

For a change, bake in
9- by 5-inch (2 L) loaf
pan. Check loaf at
15 minutes for doneness.

Use unsweetened
applesauce.

Make Ahead

Prepare up to a day
before. Freeze for up
to 6 weeks.

Choices Per Serving

| 1½ | Carbohydrates |
| 1 | Fat |

Streusel Apple Muffins

½ cup	brown sugar	125 mL
½ cup	applesauce	125 mL
¼ cup	vegetable oil	50 mL
1	egg	1
1 tsp	vanilla	5 mL
1 cup	all-purpose flour	250 mL
1 tsp	baking soda	5 mL
1 tsp	baking powder	5 mL
½ tsp	cinnamon	2 mL
¾ cup	diced peeled apple	175 mL

TOPPING

2 tbsp	brown sugar	25 mL
2 tsp	all-purpose flour	10 mL
½ tsp	cinnamon	2 mL
1 tsp	margarine	5 mL

1. In large bowl, combine sugar, applesauce, oil, egg and
   vanilla until well mixed. Combine flour, baking soda,
   baking powder and cinnamon; stir into bowl just until
   incorporated. Stir in apple. Pour into muffin cups, filling
   two-thirds full.

2. *Topping:* In small bowl, combine sugar, flour and
   cinnamon; cut in margarine until crumbly. Sprinkle
   evenly over muffins. Bake for 20 minutes or until tops
   are firm to the touch.

Nutritional Analysis Per Serving			
Calories	156	Fat, total	6 g
Carbohydrate	26 g	Fat, saturated	1 g
Fiber	1 g	Sodium	144 mg
Protein	2 g	Cholesterol	8 mg

. . . .

Preheat oven to
375°F (190°C)

12 muffin cups
sprayed with nonstick
vegetable spray

. . . .

Tips

A 9- by 5-inch (2 L) loaf
pan can also be used;
bake for 30 to 40 minutes
or until tester comes
out dry.

Use the ripest bananas
possible for the best
flavor.

. . . .

Make Ahead

Bake a day before or
freeze for up to 6 weeks.

Blueberry Banana Muffins

¾ cup	puréed bananas (about 1½ bananas)	175 mL
½ cup	granulated sugar	125 mL
⅓ cup	vegetable oil	75 mL
1	egg	1
1 tsp	vanilla	5 mL
1 cup	all-purpose flour	250 mL
1 tsp	baking powder	5 mL
1 tsp	baking soda	5 mL
¼ cup	2% yogurt or light sour cream	50 mL
½ cup	blueberries	125 mL

1. In large bowl, beat together bananas, sugar, oil, egg and vanilla until well mixed.

2. Combine flour, baking powder and baking soda; stir into bowl. Stir in yogurt; fold in blueberries.

3. Pour batter into muffin cups; bake for approximately 20 minutes or until tops are firm to the touch.

Choices Per Serving

1½ Carbohydrates

1½ Fats

Nutritional Analysis Per Serving

Calories	151	Fat, total	7 g
Carbohydrate	21 g	Fat, saturated	1 g
Fiber	1 g	Sodium	138 mg
Protein	2 g	Cholesterol	18 mg

Preheat oven to
350°F (180°C)

9-inch (2.5 L) springform
pan, lightly greased

Tips

Be sure to buy pumpkin
purée, not pumpkin pie
filling, which is too
sweet and contains
too much moisture for
this snacking cake.

Substitute 2 to
3 tsp (10 to 15 mL)
pumpkin pie spice for
the individual spices.

Orange Pumpkin Snacking Cake

1 cup	whole wheat flour	250 mL
2 cups	all-purpose flour	500 mL
¾ cup	packed brown sugar	175 mL
1 tbsp	grated orange zest	15 mL
1 tbsp	baking powder	15 mL
1 tsp	baking soda	5 mL
1 tsp	ground cinnamon	5 mL
½ tsp	ground allspice	2 mL
½ tsp	ground ginger	2 mL
½ tsp	ground nutmeg	2 mL
¼ tsp	ground cloves	1 mL
½ cup	vegetable oil	125 mL
3	eggs	3
1¼ cups	canned pumpkin purée (not pie filling)	300 mL
½ cup	orange juice	125 mL
1 cup	chopped pecans	250 mL

1. In a large bowl, stir together whole wheat flour, flour, brown sugar, zest, baking powder, baking soda, cinnamon, allspice, ginger, nutmeg and cloves; set aside.

2. In a separate bowl, using an electric mixer, beat oil, eggs, pumpkin purée and orange juice until combined. Pour mixture over dry ingredients and stir just until combined. Stir in pecans. Spoon into prepared pan.

3. Bake in preheated oven for 60 to 70 minutes or until a cake tester inserted in the center comes out clean. Immediately invert on a cooling rack. Remove pan and let cool completely.

Choices Per Serving

2   Carbohydrates

2½   Fats

Nutritional Analysis Per Serving

Calories	253	Fat, total	13 g
Carbohydrate	32 g	Fat, saturated	1 g
Fiber	2 g	Sodium	139 mg
Protein	5 g	Cholesterol	40 mg

Desserts

The Canadian Diabetes Association's nutrition guidelines for diabetes suggest that up to 10% of the total calories in the diet can come from "added sugars." The recipes contained in this section use regular sugar instead of sugar substitutes. Using sugar substitutes can maintain the sweetness, but may alter the texture in baked goods.

If you wish to reduce the sugar or carbohydrate content of these recipes, begin by choosing recipes such as Mango Blueberry Strudel (page 355) or the Individual Miniature Cheesecakes (page 357). One quarter cup (50 mL) of sugar contains 50 g of carbohydrate. Keep this in mind when making alterations to the carbohydrate content of the recipes.

continued on next page

Preheat oven to
350°F (180°C)

Baking sheet sprayed
with nonstick
vegetable spray

Tip

This cookie dough can
be chilled, then rolled
out and cut into various
patterns.

Make Ahead

Dough can be frozen
for up to 2 weeks.

Cinnamon Ginger Cookies

¼ cup	brown sugar	50 mL
3 tbsp	margarine, melted	45 mL
2 tbsp	molasses	25 mL
2 tbsp	2% yogurt	25 mL
1 tsp	vanilla	5 mL
1 cup	all-purpose flour	250 mL
½ tsp	baking soda	2 mL
½ tsp	ginger	2 mL
½ tsp	cinnamon	2 mL
Pinch	nutmeg	Pinch
1½ tsp	brown sugar	7 mL

1. In bowl, combine ¼ cup (50 mL) brown sugar,
margarine, molasses, yogurt and vanilla until
well mixed.

2. Combine flour, baking soda, ginger, cinnamon and
nutmeg; stir into bowl just until combined.

3. Using teaspoon, form dough into small balls and place
on baking sheet. Press flat with fork; sprinkle with
1½ tsp (7 mL) brown sugar. Bake for 10 to 12 minutes.

Choices Per Serving

1   Carbohydrate

½   Fat

Nutritional Analysis Per Serving

Calories	76	Fat, total	2 g
Carbohydrate	12 g	Fat, saturated	0 g
Fiber	0 g	Sodium	68 mg
Protein	1 g	Cholesterol	0 mg

• • • • • • • • • • • • • •

Preheat oven to
375°F (190°C)

Greased cookie sheet

• • • • • • • • • • • • • •

Tip

Freeze cranberries before
chopping or grinding
them to ease cleanup.

Cranberry Orange Oatmeal Cookies

2 cups	all-purpose flour	500 mL
1 tsp	baking powder	5 mL
¼ tsp	baking soda	1 mL
½ tsp	salt	2 mL
2 cups	quick-cooking oats	500 mL
1 cup	softened margarine or butter	250 mL
1½ cups	granulated sugar	375 mL
2	eggs	2
1 tsp	vanilla	5 mL
1 cup	raisins	250 mL
1 cup	coarsely chopped cranberries, fresh or frozen	250 mL
1 tbsp	grated orange zest	15 mL

1. In a bowl, mix together flour, baking powder, baking soda, salt and oats.

2. In another bowl, beat margarine and sugar until smooth and creamy. Beat in eggs, one at a time, until well incorporated. Mix in vanilla. Add flour mixture and mix well. Fold in raisins, cranberries and orange zest.

3. Drop by rounded teaspoonfuls (5 mL), about 2 inches (5 cm) apart, onto prepared cookie sheet. Bake in preheated oven for 10 to 12 minutes or until edges are lightly browned. Immediately transfer to wire racks to cool.

**Choices
Per Serving**

1 Carbohydrate

½ Fat

Nutritional Analysis Per Serving			
Calories	86	Fat, total	4 g
Carbohydrate	13 g	Fat, saturated	1 g
Fiber	1 g	Sodium	69 mg
Protein	1 g	Cholesterol	7 mg

● ● ● ● ● ● ● ● ● ● ● ● ● ● ●

Preheat oven to
350°F (180°C)

Cookie sheet lined
with foil, bright side up

Oatmeal Lace Pennies

1 cup	old-fashioned rolled oats	250 mL
1 cup	granulated sugar	250 mL
3 tbsp	all-purpose flour	45 mL
¼ tsp	baking powder	1 mL
½ tsp	salt	2 mL
1	egg, beaten	1
½ cup	margarine or butter, melted	125 mL
½ tsp	vanilla	2 mL

1. In a bowl, mix together oats, sugar, flour, baking powder and salt.

2. In another bowl, beat egg, margarine and vanilla. Add flour mixture and mix well. (If dough seems too soft, chill for 15 to 20 minutes to firm.)

3. Drop by rounded teaspoonfuls (5 mL), about 2 inches (5 cm) apart, onto prepared cookie sheet. Bake in preheated oven for 8 to 10 minutes. Cool for 2 minutes on foil, then transfer to wire racks to cool completely.

Choices
Per Serving

½	Carbohydrate
½	Fat

Nutritional Analysis Per Serving			
Calories	64	Fat, total	3 g
Carbohydrate	8 g	Fat, saturated	2 g
Fiber	0 g	Sodium	64 mg
Protein	1 g	Cholesterol	14 mg

Preheat oven to
350°F (180°C)

Baking sheets sprayed
with nonstick
vegetable spray

Tips

These cookies are soft
and chewy if baked for
a shorter time; crisp if
baked longer.

If wheat germ is
unavailable, substitute
another ¼ cup (50 mL)
rolled oats.

Two of these cookies
provide 1 Carbohydrate
choice and 1 Fat choice.
A tasty option to finish
a meal or for an evening
snack.

Make Ahead

Dough can be frozen for
up to 2 weeks.

Oatmeal Raisin Pecan Cookies

½ cup	brown sugar	125 mL
¼ cup	soft margarine	50 mL
1	egg	1
1 tsp	vanilla	5 mL
½ cup	rolled oats	125 mL
¼ cup	whole wheat flour	50 mL
¼ cup	wheat germ	50 mL
¼ cup	pecan pieces	50 mL
¼ cup	raisins	50 mL
½ tsp	baking powder	2 mL

1. In large bowl or food processor, beat together sugar, margarine, egg and vanilla until well blended.

2. Add rolled oats, flour, wheat germ, pecans, raisins and baking powder; mix just until incorporated.

3. Drop by heaping teaspoonfuls (5 mL) 2 inches (5 cm) apart onto baking sheets. Bake for 12 to 15 minutes or until browned.

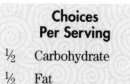

**Choices
Per Serving**

½   Carbohydrate

½   Fat

Nutritional Analysis Per Serving

Calories	57	Fat, total	3 g
Carbohydrate	8 g	Fat, saturated	0 g
Fiber	0 g	Sodium	27 mg
Protein	1 g	Cholesterol	7 mg

Preheat oven to
350°F (180°C)

Baking sheets sprayed
with nonstick
vegetable spray

Tips

The longer they bake, the
crispier the cookies.

Use natural peanut butter
made from peanuts only.

Make Ahead

Dough can be frozen
up to 2 weeks. Bake
just before eating for
best flavor.

Peanut Butter Chocolate Chip Cookies

½ cup	brown sugar	125 mL
⅓ cup	granulated sugar	75 mL
⅓ cup	peanut butter	75 mL
⅓ cup	2% milk	75 mL
¼ cup	soft margarine	50 mL
1	egg	1
1 tsp	vanilla	5 mL
½ cup	all-purpose flour	125 mL
⅓ cup	whole wheat flour	75 mL
1 tsp	baking soda	5 mL
⅓ cup	chocolate chips	75 mL
¼ cup	raisins	50 mL

1. In large bowl or food processor, beat together brown and granulated sugars, peanut butter, milk, margarine, egg and vanilla until well blended.

2. Combine all-purpose and whole wheat flours and baking soda; add to bowl and mix just until incorporated. Do not overmix. Stir in chocolate chips and raisins.

3. Drop by heaping teaspoonfuls (5 mL) 2 inches (5 cm) apart onto baking sheets. Bake for 12 to 15 minutes or until browned.

Choices Per Serving

½ Carbohydrate

½ Fat

Nutritional Analysis Per Serving			
Calories	70	Fat, total	3 g
Carbohydrate	10 g	Fat, saturated	1 g
Fiber	1 g	Sodium	51 mg
Protein	1 g	Cholesterol	6 mg

Diced Rhubarb Cookies

Preheat oven to
350°F (180°C)

Greased cookie sheet

Tip

If you are lactose
intolerant, use
lactose-reduced milk
in baking. It can be
substituted for regular
milk and will not
affect the results.

2 cups	all-purpose flour or whole wheat flour or a combination of both	500 mL
2 tsp	baking powder	10 mL
Pinch	salt	Pinch
1 tsp	cinnamon	5 mL
½ tsp	nutmeg	2 mL
½ tsp	cloves	2 mL
½ cup	softened margarine or butter	125 mL
1 cup	lightly packed brown sugar	250 mL
1	egg	1
¼ cup	milk	50 mL
1 cup	diced rhubarb	250 mL
1 cup	chopped walnuts	250 mL

1. In a bowl, combine flour, baking powder, salt, cinnamon, nutmeg and cloves.

2. In another bowl, beat margarine and sugar until smooth and creamy. Beat in egg until well incorporated. Mix in milk. Add flour mixture and beat until smooth. Fold in rhubarb and walnuts until well combined.

3. Drop by rounded teaspoonfuls (5 mL), 2 inches (5 cm) apart, onto prepared cookie sheet. Bake in preheated oven for 18 to 20 minutes or until crisp and lightly browned. Immediately transfer to wire racks to cool.

**Choices
Per Serving**

½ Carbohydrate

1 Fat

Nutritional Analysis Per Serving			
Calories	83	Fat, total	4 g
Carbohydrate	11 g	Fat, saturated	2 g
Fiber	0 g	Sodium	48 mg
Protein	1 g	Cholesterol	11 mg

● ● ● ● ● ● ● ● ● ● ● ● ● ● ● ●

Preheat oven to
350°F (180°C)

Lightly greased
cookie sheet

Sesame Seed Cookies

1½ cups	whole wheat flour	375 mL
1 tsp	baking powder	5 mL
¼ tsp	salt	1 mL
¼ cup	softened margarine or butter	50 mL
¼ cup	liquid honey	50 mL
¼ cup	sesame paste (tahini)	50 mL
½ tsp	almond extract	2 mL
½ cup	sesame seeds, toasted	125 mL

1. In a bowl, mix together flour, baking powder and salt.

2. In another bowl, beat margarine, honey, sesame paste and almond extract until smooth. Add flour mixture and mix well. Stir in sesame seeds.

3. Shape dough into 1-inch (2.5 cm) balls and place about 2 inches (5 cm) apart on prepared cookie sheet. Using the tines of a fork dipped in flour, flatten, or using your hands, mold into crescent shapes. (Wet your hands first, if using to mold the dough.) Bake in preheated oven for 10 to 12 minutes or until lightly browned. Immediately transfer to wire racks to cool.

Choices Per Serving

½	Carbohydrate
1	Fat

Nutritional Analysis Per Serving			
Calories	87	Fat, total	5 g
Carbohydrate	10 g	Fat, saturated	1 g
Fiber	2 g	Sodium	51 mg
Protein	2 g	Cholesterol	0 mg

• • • • • • • • • • • • • • • • •

Preheat oven to
350°F (180°C)

Lightly greased
cookie sheet

Whole Wheat Spice Cookies

¼ cup	vegetable oil	50 mL
¼ cup	molasses	50 mL
½ cup	granulated sugar	125 mL
¼ cup	packed brown sugar	50 mL
2	eggs	2
½ cup	whole wheat flour	125 mL
1½ cups	all-purpose flour	375 mL
2 tsp	baking soda	10 mL
¼ tsp	salt	1 mL
1 tsp	ginger	5 mL
1 tsp	cinnamon	5 mL
1 tsp	cloves	5 mL

1. In a bowl, whisk oil, molasses, sugars and eggs until blended.

2. In a large bowl, mix together flours, baking soda, salt, ginger, cinnamon and cloves. Make a well in the center and add the molasses mixture, mixing until thoroughly blended.

3. Drop by teaspoonfuls (5 mL), about 2 inches (5 cm) apart, onto prepared cookie sheets. Bake in preheated oven for 8 to 10 minutes or until cookies are firm to the touch. Cool on sheets for 5 minutes, then transfer to wire racks to cool completely.

Choices Per Serving

½ Carbohydrate

½ Fat

Nutritional Analysis Per Serving			
Calories	65	Fat, total	2 g
Carbohydrate	11 g	Fat, saturated	0 g
Fiber	0 g	Sodium	87 mg
Protein	1 g	Cholesterol	12 mg

Preheat oven to
350°F (180°C)

Cookie sheet, lined
with parchment paper
or lightly greased
aluminum foil

Variation

Try with half black
sesame seeds or
flaxseeds and half
white sesame seeds.

Sesame Snap Wafers

⅔ cup	all-purpose flour	150 mL
¼ tsp	baking powder	1 mL
½ cup	margarine or butter, softened	125 mL
1 cup	packed brown sugar	250 mL
1	egg	1
1 tsp	vanilla	5 mL
1¼ cups	sesame seeds, toasted	300 mL

1. Combine flour and baking powder.

2. Cream margarine, sugar, egg and vanilla. Add flour mixture. Mix until combined. Stir in seeds.

3. Drop by teaspoonfuls (5 mL) about 2 inches (5 cm) apart onto prepared cookie sheet. Bake for 6 to 9 minutes or until lightly browned. Cool for 5 minutes on sheet, then transfer to rack and cool completely.

**Choices
Per Serving**

½	Carbohydrate
1	Fat

Nutritional Analysis Per Serving			
Calories	43	Fat, total	3 g
Carbohydrate	5 g	Fat, saturated	0 g
Fiber	1 g	Sodium	20 mg
Protein	1 g	Cholesterol	3 mg

• • • • • • • • • • • • • •

Preheat oven to
300°F (150°C)

Cookie sheet, ungreased

Cookie cutters

• • • • • • • • • • • • • •

Tip

Shortbreads are one of
the few cookies that
are altered significantly
when made with
margarine. Although
butter and margarine
contribute the same
amount of total fat to the
recipe, butter contains
more saturated fat than
most soft margarine.

Oatmeal Shortbread

¾ cup	all-purpose flour	175 mL
⅔ cup	oats	150 mL
½ cup	cornstarch	125 mL
½ cup	confectioner's (icing) sugar, sifted	125 mL
¾ cup	butter, softened	175 mL

1. Combine flour, oats, cornstarch and confectioner's sugar in large bowl. With large spoon, blend in butter. Work with hands until soft, smooth dough forms. Shape into ball. If necessary, refrigerate for 30 minutes or until easy to handle.

2. Roll out dough to ¼-inch (5 mm) thickness. Cut into shapes with cookie cutters. Place on cookie sheet. Decorate if desired. Bake for 15 to 25 minutes or until edges are lightly browned. (Time will depend on cookie size.) Cool for 5 minutes on sheet, then transfer to rack and cool completely. Store in tightly covered container.

**Choices
Per Serving**

½   Carbohydrate

1   Fat

Nutritional Analysis Per Serving			
Calories	76	Fat, total	5 g
Carbohydrate	8 g	Fat, saturated	3 g
Fiber	0 g	Sodium	45 mg
Protein	1 g	Cholesterol	12 mg

○ ○ ○ ○ ○ ○ ○ ○ ○ ○ ○ ○ ○ ○

Preheat oven to
325°F (160°C)

Greased cookie sheet

Lemon Almond Biscotti

1¾ cups	all-purpose flour	425 mL
¾ cup	granulated sugar	175 mL
1 tbsp	baking powder	15 mL
2 tbsp	finely grated lemon zest	25 mL
¾ cup	coarsely chopped almonds	175 mL
2	eggs	2
⅓ cup	olive oil	75 mL
1 tsp	vanilla	5 mL
½ tsp	almond extract	2 mL

1. In a bowl, mix together flour, sugar, baking powder, lemon zest and almonds. Make a well in the center.

2. In another bowl, whisk eggs, oil, vanilla and almond extract. Pour into well and mix until a soft, sticky dough forms.

3. Divide dough in half. Shape into two rolls about 10 inches (25 cm) long. Place about 2 inches (5 cm) apart on prepared cookie sheet. Bake in preheated oven for 20 minutes.

4. Cool on sheet for 5 minutes, then cut into slices ½ inch (1 cm) thick. Return to sheet and bake for 10 minutes. Turn slices over and bake for 10 minutes more. Immediately transfer to wire racks.

**Choices
Per Serving**

½ Carbohydrate

½ Fat

Nutritional Analysis Per Serving			
Calories	78	Fat, total	4 g
Carbohydrate	10 g	Fat, saturated	1 g
Fiber	1 g	Sodium	24 mg
Protein	2 g	Cholesterol	12 mg

Two-Tone Chocolate Orange Biscotti

Preheat oven to
350°F (180°C)

Baking sheet sprayed
with vegetable spray

Tips

If dough is sticky when
forming into logs, try
wetting your fingers.

Two colors of dough
make these cookies
very attractive.

Make Ahead

Freeze in containers for
up to 6 weeks.

1¼ cups	granulated sugar	300 mL
⅓ cup	margarine or butter	75 mL
2	eggs	2
2 tbsp	orange juice concentrate	25 mL
1 tbsp	grated orange zest	15 mL
2⅔ cups	all-purpose flour	650 mL
2½ tsp	baking powder	12 mL
3 tbsp	cocoa	45 mL

1. In a food processor or in a bowl with an electric mixer, beat together sugar, margarine, eggs, orange juice concentrate and orange zest until smooth. Add flour and baking powder; mix just until combined.

2. Divide dough in half; to one half, add cocoa and mix well. Divide chocolate and plain doughs in half to produce 4 doughs. Roll each piece into a long thin rope approximately 12 inches (30 cm) long and 1 inch (2.5 cm) wide. Use extra flour if too sticky. Place 1 cocoa dough on top of (or beside) each plain dough. (Ensure the plain and cocoa doughs touch one another.)

3. Bake 20 minutes. Cool 10 minutes. Cut logs on an angle into ½-inch (1 cm) slices. Bake another 20 minutes.

Choices Per Serving

½ Carbohydrate

½ Fat

Nutritional Analysis Per Serving			
Calories	61	Fat, total	2 g
Carbohydrate	11 g	Fat, saturated	0 g
Fiber	0 g	Sodium	32 mg
Protein	1 g	Cholesterol	9 mg

Preheat oven to
400°F (200°C)

9-inch (2.5 L) round
or square baking dish

Tips

If using frozen fruit,
there's no need to defrost
before using.

If you prefer to
bake the cobbler earlier
in the day, reheat in
350°F (180°C) oven for
about 15 minutes.

This dessert is high in
carbohydrate. To reduce
this, replace the ¾ cup
(175 mL) sugar in the
fruit portion with a sugar
substitute. This will
reduce the carbohydrate
content by almost
20 g/serving.

Strawberry-Rhubarb Cobbler

4 cups	chopped fresh rhubarb	1 L
2 cups	sliced strawberries	500 mL
¾ cup	granulated sugar	175 mL
2 tbsp	cornstarch	25 mL
1 tsp	grated orange zest	5 mL

BISCUIT TOPPING

1 cup	all-purpose flour	250 mL
¼ cup	granulated sugar	50 mL
1½ tsp	baking powder	7 mL
¼ tsp	salt	1 mL
¼ cup	cold margarine or butter, cut into pieces	50 mL
½ cup	milk	125 mL
1 tsp	vanilla	5 mL
	Additional granulated sugar	

1. Place rhubarb and strawberries in baking dish. In a small bowl, combine sugar, cornstarch and orange zest; sprinkle over fruit and gently toss.

2. Bake in preheated oven for 20 to 25 minutes (increase to 30 minutes if using frozen fruit) until hot and bubbles appear around edges.

3. *Biscuit Topping:* In a bowl, combine flour, sugar, baking powder and salt. Cut in margarine using a pastry blender or fork to make coarse crumbs. In a glass measure, combine milk and vanilla; stir into dry ingredients to make a soft sticky dough.

4. Using a large spoon, drop eight separate spoonfuls of dough onto hot fruit; sprinkle with 2 tsp (10 mL) sugar.

5. Bake in preheated oven for 25 to 30 minutes or until top is golden and fruit is bubbly.

Choices Per Serving

3   Carbohydrates

1   Fat

Nutritional Analysis Per Serving			
Calories	246	Fat, total	6 g
Carbohydrate	46 g	Fat, saturated	1 g
Fiber	2 g	Sodium	198 mg
Protein	3 g	Cholesterol	0 mg

Preheat oven to
425°F (220°C)

9-inch (23 cm) flan pan
with removable bottom

Tips

Try this recipe using
wild or low-bush
blueberries when they
are in season. They have
a delicious and more
intense flavor than the
cultivated variety.

Blueberries are gaining
in popularity because
of their antioxidant
properties. This delicious
flan contains a minimal
amount of fat.

*This recipe courtesy
of dietitians Pamela
Good and Carrie Roach.*

Blueberry Flan

1½ cups	all-purpose flour	375 mL
¼ cup	granulated sugar	50 mL
1½ tsp	baking powder	7 mL
¼ cup	soft margarine	50 mL
2	egg whites	2
¼ tsp	almond extract	1 mL

FILLING

3 cups	fresh blueberries	750 mL
⅓ cup	granulated sugar	75 mL
1 tbsp	all-purpose flour	15 mL
1 tbsp	lemon juice	15 mL
2 tsp	ground cinnamon	10 mL

1. In a bowl, combine flour, sugar and baking powder; stir in margarine, egg whites and almond extract to form dough. Press into 9-inch (23 cm) flan pan with removable bottom. Freeze for 15 minutes.

2. *Filling:* In a bowl, mix together blueberries, sugar, flour, lemon juice and cinnamon; pour over crust. Bake in preheated oven for 15 minutes. Reduce temperature to 350°F (180°C); bake for 20 to 25 minutes longer. Cool on rack. Refrigerate for at least 1 hour before serving.

Choices Per Serving

2½	Carbohydrates
1	Fat

Nutritional Analysis Per Serving

Calories	234	Fat, total	6 g
Carbohydrate	42 g	Fat, saturated	1 g
Fiber	2 g	Sodium	135 mg
Protein	4 g	Cholesterol	0 mg

Lemon Poppy Seed Loaf *page 322*

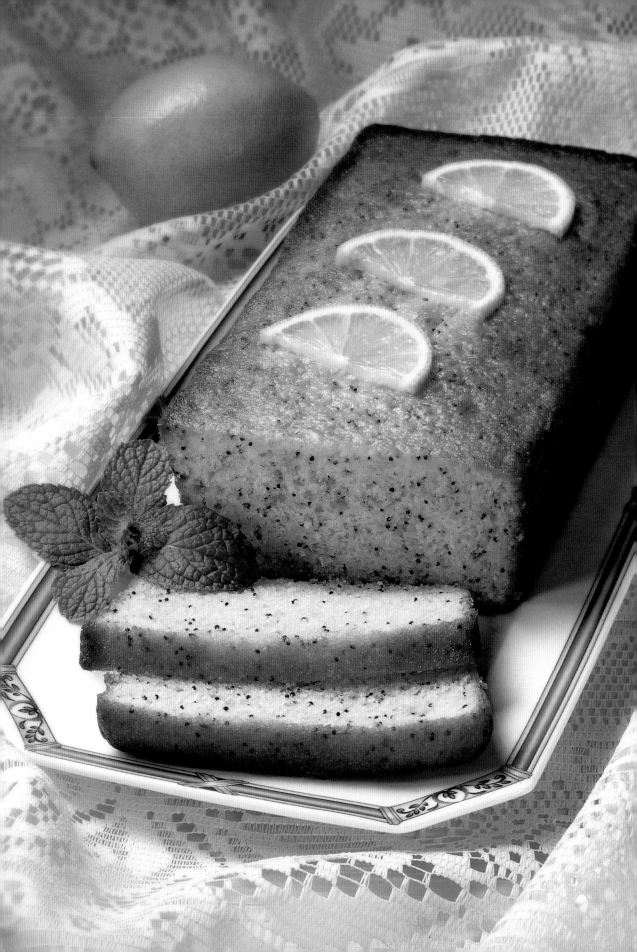

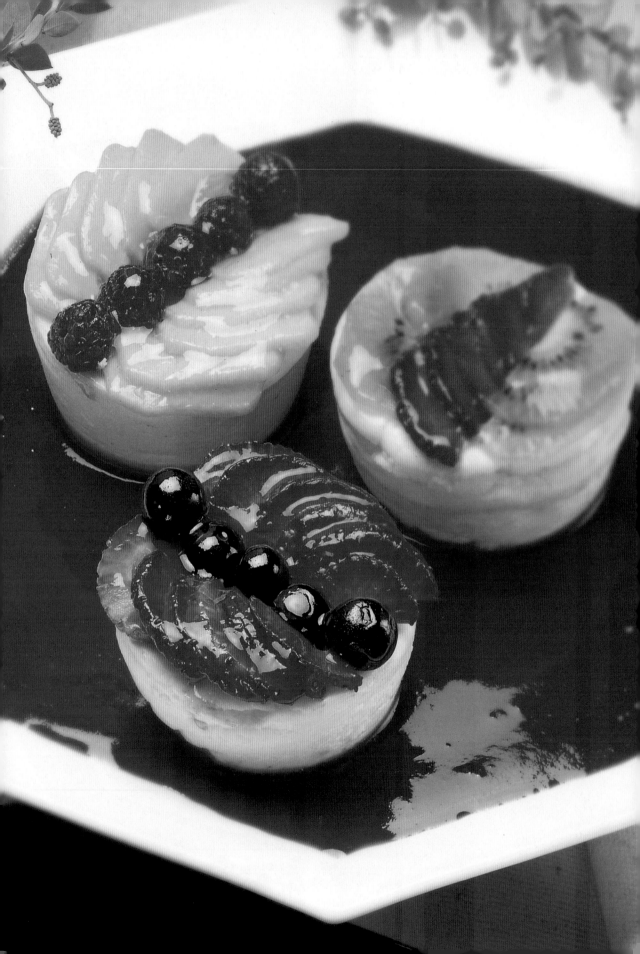

Preheat oven to
325°F (160°C)

4 large or 6 small
custard cups

Tips

Most baked custards
have 2 or more eggs.
This custard uses
2% evaporated milk
and 1 egg to create a
slightly softer version.

This is a superb way
to use up all the
pumpkin you scooped
out when making the
jack-o'-lantern for
Halloween. The custard
is rich in vitamin A
and calcium and makes
a good finish for a
lighter meal.

*This recipe courtesy
of Cynthia Chace,
Dietitian.*

Pumpkin Custard

1 cup	2% evaporated milk	250 mL
1 cup	pumpkin purée (not pie filling, if using canned)	250 mL
2 tbsp	granulated sugar	25 mL
1	egg	1
¼ tsp	ground nutmeg	1 mL
¼ tsp	ground ginger	1 mL

1. In a blender or food processor, combine milk, pumpkin, sugar, egg and spices. Process until well blended; pour into 4 large or 6 small custard cups. Bake in preheated oven for about 30 minutes or until knife inserted in center comes out clean. Serve warm or cold.

Choices Per Serving

1   Carbohydrate

½   Fat

Nutritional Analysis Per Serving

Calories	82	Fat, total	2 g
Carbohydrate	12 g	Fat, saturated	1 g
Fiber	1 g	Sodium	56 mg
Protein	5 g	Cholesterol	39 mg

Individual Miniature Cheesecakes page 357

- - - - - - - - - - - - - - -

Preheat oven to
350°F (180°C)

Baking sheet sprayed
with nonstick
vegetable spray

- - - - - - - - - - - - - - -

Tips

This decadent strudel
is a wonderful finish to
a dinner with guests.

Ripen pears at room
temperature in a bowl
or paper bag.

- - - - - - - - - - - - - - -

Make Ahead

Filling can be prepared
a couple of hours before
baking. Keep covered.
Do not assemble strudel
until ready to bake.

Pear, Apple and Raisin Strudel

2²⁄₃ cups	chopped peeled apples	650 mL
2²⁄₃ cups	chopped peeled pears	650 mL
⅓ cup	raisins	75 mL
2 tbsp	chopped pecans or walnuts	25 mL
2 tbsp	brown sugar	25 mL
1 tbsp	lemon juice	15 mL
1 tbsp	honey	15 mL
1 tsp	cinnamon	5 mL
6	phyllo sheets	6
4 tsp	margarine, melted	20 mL

1. In bowl, combine apples, pears, raisins, pecans, sugar, lemon juice, honey and cinnamon; mix well.

2. Lay out 2 sheets of phyllo; brush with some margarine. Place 2 more sheets over top; brush with margarine again. Top with remaining 2 sheets phyllo.

3. Spread filling over phyllo, leaving 1-inch (2.5 cm) border uncovered. Roll up like jelly roll and place seam down on baking sheet. Brush with remaining margarine. Bake for 40 to 50 minutes or until golden and fruit is tender.

Choices Per Serving	
2	Carbohydrates
½	Fat

Nutritional Analysis Per Serving			
Calories	142	Fat, total	3 g
Carbohydrate	29 g	Fat, saturated	0 g
Fiber	3 g	Sodium	75 mg
Protein	1 g	Cholesterol	0 mg

Mango Blueberry Strudel

2 cups	fresh blueberries (or frozen, thawed and drained)	500 mL
1 tbsp	all-purpose flour	15 mL
2½ cups	peeled chopped ripe mango	625 mL
¼ cup	granulated sugar	50 mL
1 tbsp	lemon juice	15 mL
½ tsp	cinnamon	2 mL
6	sheets phyllo pastry	6
2 tsp	melted margarine or butter	10 mL

1. Toss blueberries with flour. In large bowl, combine mango, blueberries, sugar, lemon juice and cinnamon.

2. Lay 2 phyllo sheets one on top of the other; brush with melted margarine. Layer another 2 phyllo sheets on top and brush with melted margarine. Layer last 2 sheets on top. Put fruit filling along long end of phyllo; gently roll over until all of filling is enclosed, fold sides in, and continue to roll. Put on prepared baking sheet, brush with remaining margarine and bake for 20 to 25 minutes or until golden. Sprinkle with icing sugar.

Tips

Mango can be replaced with ripe peaches or even pears.

Phyllo pastry is located in the freezer section of store. Handle quickly so the sheets do not dry out. Cover those not being used with a slightly damp cloth.

Make Ahead

Prepare filling early in the day. For best results, do not fill until just ready to bake. If in a hurry, fill phyllo, cover and refrigerate. Bake just ahead serving.

Choices Per Serving

2 Carbohydrates

½ Fat

Nutritional Analysis Per Serving

Calories	147	Fat, total	2 g
Carbohydrate	31 g	Fat, saturated	0 g
Fiber	2 g	Sodium	101 mg
Protein	2 g	Cholesterol	0 mg

Chocolate Coffee Tiramisu

1½ cups	5% ricotta cheese	375 mL
½ cup	light cream cheese	125 mL
½ cup	granulated sugar	125 mL
3 tbsp	cocoa	45 mL
1	egg yolk	1
1 tsp	vanilla	5 mL
3	egg whites	3
⅓ cup	granulated sugar	75 mL
¾ cup	strong, prepared coffee	175 mL
3 tbsp	chocolate or coffee-flavored liqueur	45 mL
16	lady finger cookies	16

9-inch (2.5 L) square baking dish sprayed with vegetable spray

Tips

Sift some cocoa on top of each portion just before serving. This tiramisu tastes so decadent, you'll never believe it hasn't the same calories and fat as the one made with mascarpone.

Spongy or harder lady fingers can be used.

The longer this chills, the better it is. The liqueur-coffee mixture penetrates the cookies.

Make Ahead

Prepare up to 2 days ahead. It tastes best after 8 hours of refrigeration.

1. In food processor, combine ricotta cheese, cream cheese, sugar, cocoa, egg yolk and vanilla until smooth; transfer to a bowl.
2. In bowl, beat egg whites until soft peaks form. Gradually add sugar and continue to beat until stiff peaks form. Gently fold the whites into the ricotta mixture.
3. Combine coffee and liqueur in a small bowl.
4. Put half of lady fingers in bottom of dish. Sprinkle with half of coffee-liqueur mixture. Spread half of ricotta mixture on top. Repeat layers. Cover and chill for at least 3 hours, or overnight.

Choices Per Serving

1½ Carbohydrate
½ Meat & Alternative
½ Fat

Nutritional Analysis Per Serving			
Calories	150	Fat, total	5 g
Carbohydrate	21 g	Fat, saturated	2 g
Fiber	0 g	Sodium	102 mg
Protein	6 g	Cholesterol	66 mg

Preheat oven to
350°F (180°C)

Line 10 muffin cups with
muffin paper cups

Tips

Substitute one 8-oz
(250 g) package of light
cream cheese for the
ricotta cheese.

Decorate cheesecakes
with berries and sliced
fresh fruit; glaze with
2 tbsp (25 mL) no-sugar-
added apricot spread.

Count fruit topping as
a Carbohydrate choice.

Individual Miniature Cheesecakes

1 cup	5% ricotta cheese	250 mL
1 cup	low-fat cottage cheese	250 mL
1/3 cup	granulated sugar	75 mL
1	medium egg	1
1/4 cup	light sour cream	50 mL
1/2 tsp	cornstarch	2 mL
1/8 tsp	vanilla extract	0.5 mL
	Fruit purée (optional)	

1. In a food processor, combine ricotta cheese, cottage cheese and sugar; purée until smooth. Beat in egg. Blend in sour cream, cornstarch and vanilla until well mixed. Divide batter among muffin cups. Set muffin tin in larger pan; pour in enough hot water to come half way up sides. Bake 30 to 35 minutes or until tester inserted in center comes out clean. Remove from water bath; cool on wire rack. Chill.

2. Serve with fruit purée, if desired.

Choices Per Serving

1/2	Carbohydrate
1	Meat & Alternative
1/2	Fat

Nutritional Analysis Per Serving

Calories	127	Fat, total	8 g
Carbohydrate	9 g	Fat, saturated	4 g
Fiber	0 g	Sodium	268 mg
Protein	6 g	Cholesterol	42 mg

Tip

Here's a great recipe
for when you need a
decadent dessert but
don't have time to fuss.
Small amounts of
unsalted butter and
bittersweet chocolate
add 6 g of saturated fat,
so save this for special
occasions.

Fried Pineapple

1	ripe pineapple	1
2 tbsp	sugar	25 mL
2 tbsp	unsalted butter	25 mL
2 tbsp	sultana raisins	25 mL
1 oz	bittersweet chocolate, shaved	25 g
4	sprigs fresh mint	4

1. With a sharp knife cut off top half of pineapple, reserving it for another use. Remove rind from the bottom (sweeter) half and slice pineapple into 4 rounds, each ½ inch (1 cm) thick. Spread sugar on a plate and dredge the pineapple slices in the sugar.

2. In a large frying pan melt butter over high heat until foaming. Add the dredged pineapple slices and fry for 2 minutes. Flip the slices and spread raisins around them; fry for another 2 to 3 minutes until pineapple has browned and raisins are swollen. Remove from heat and transfer one pineapple slice to each of 4 dessert plates, flipping them so the more attractively browned side faces upward. Spoon some raisins onto each plate and top with a bit of the sauce from the pan. Garnish with chocolate shavings and mint. Serve immediately.

Choices Per Serving

2 Carbohydrates

2 Fats

Nutritional Analysis Per Serving

Calories	212	Fat, total	10 g
Carbohydrate	34 g	Fat, saturated	6 g
Fiber	3 g	Sodium	4 mg
Protein	2 g	Cholesterol	16 mg

Tips

Use fresh ripe strawberries or unsweetened frozen berries; if using frozen, thaw and drain before using.

For attractive orange segments, peel a whole orange with a sharp knife, removing zest, pith and membrane; cut on both sides of dividing membranes to release segments.

This mousse is an excellent source of vitamin C, providing half of the daily recommended amount.

Banana-Strawberry Mousse

3	small ripe bananas	3
1 cup	orange juice	250 mL
1 cup	strawberries	250 mL
6 tbsp	lemon juice	90 mL
½ cup	cold water	125 mL
1	pkg (1 tbsp/7 g) gelatin	1
	Orange segments or sliced strawberries	

1. In a blender, combine bananas, orange juice, strawberries and lemon juice; purée until smooth. Put water in a small saucepan; sprinkle with gelatin. Let stand 1 minute. Heat gently, stirring until gelatin dissolves. With motor running, pour hot gelatin through blender feed tube; purée until smooth. Divide among 6 individual dessert dishes or champagne coupes.

2. Chill 2 hours. Serve garnished with orange segments or sliced strawberries.

Choices Per Serving

1½ Carbohydrates

Nutritional Analysis Per Serving			
Calories	88	Fat, total	0.4 g
Carbohydrate	21 g	Fat, saturated	0 g
Fiber	2 g	Sodium	4 mg
Protein	2 g	Cholesterol	0 mg

8 small custard cups

Tips

This is similar to a frozen soufflé but is lighter and lower in calories.

Because of the risk of salmonella poisoning, raw eggs should be used with caution. Cracked eggs should be avoided. Recipes calling for raw eggs should be prepared as close to serving time as possible and kept well refrigerated.

Make this light, lower-calorie, low-fat dessert a staple in your recipe repertoire. Not only does it complement any meal, it is rich in vitamins C and A as well as in calcium from the skim-milk powder.

This recipe courtesy of Joan Gallant, Dietitian.

Lemon Sherbet

½ cup	granulated sugar	125 mL
⅓ cup	lemon juice	75 mL
2 tsp	grated lemon zest	10 mL
2	eggs, separated	2
⅔ cup	skim-milk powder	150 mL
⅔ cup	cold water	150 mL

1. Whisk together sugar, lemon juice, zest and egg yolks; set aside.

2. With an electric mixer, beat egg whites, skim-milk powder and water on high speed for 3 to 5 minutes or until stiff peaks form. Fold in lemon mixture. Pour into 8 small custard cups; cover and freeze for about 3 hours or until firm. Transfer from freezer to refrigerator about 15 minutes before serving.

Choices Per Serving

| 1 | Carbohydrate |
| ½ | Meat & Alternative |

Nutritional Analysis Per Serving

Calories	90	Fat, total	1 g
Carbohydrate	17 g	Fat, saturated	0 g
Fiber	0 g	Sodium	47 mg
Protein	4 g	Cholesterol	55 mg

8-inch (2 L) square pan

Tips

The perfect low-fat ending to any meal, this sorbet can be made with virtually any fruit. Try raspberries, peaches, blueberries, kiwi fruit, cantaloupe or any other seasonal fruit.

Beating the sorbet during the freezing process helps to keep it from becoming too solid and helps to reduce the formation of ice crystals.

Sorbet is a cool and elegant way to serve fruit and end any meal, particularly during the summer. The strawberries in this recipe are a good source of vitamin C.

This recipe courtesy of Vicki McKay, Dietitian.

Strawberry Sorbet

1½ cups	fresh or frozen unsweetened strawberries	375 mL
2 cups	unsweetened apple juice	500 mL
¼ cup	granulated sugar	50 mL
¼ tsp	ground cinnamon	1 mL
2 tbsp	cold water	25 mL
4 tsp	cornstarch	20 mL

1. Wash and hull fresh strawberries or thaw frozen strawberries. In a blender or food processor, blend strawberries and apple juice until almost smooth.

2. In a medium saucepan over medium heat, cook strawberry mixture, sugar and cinnamon, stirring frequently, for about 5 minutes or until sugar is dissolved. Combine water and cornstarch; stir into hot mixture. Cook for about 3 minutes or until thickened and clear. Chill for 1 hour. Pour into 8-inch (2 L) square pan; cover and freeze for about 3 hours or until firm.

3. Break frozen mixture into chunks; beat with electric mixer at medium speed until fluffy. Transfer to an airtight container and freeze until firm. Transfer from freezer to refrigerator about 15 minutes before serving.

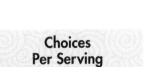

**Choices
Per Serving**

1½   Carbohydrates

Nutritional Analysis Per Serving			
Calories	91	Fat, total	0 g
Carbohydrate	23 g	Fat, saturated	0 g
Fiber	1 g	Sodium	3 mg
Protein	0 g	Cholesterol	0 mg

....

Tips

This is a delicious tropical low-fat finish to a meal.

If you don't have an ice cream maker, pour into a baking dish and freeze until solid. Break into small pieces; in a food processor, pulse on and off until smooth. Store in freezer until ready to serve.

Purée canned crushed pineapple for the smoothest texture.

Pineapple Lime Sorbet

1¼ cups	pineapple purée	300 mL
2 tsp	grated lime or lemon zest	10 mL
¾ cup	freshly squeezed lime or lemon juice	175 mL
¼ cup	water	50 mL
	Thin slices lime or lemon	

1. In a bowl, stir together pineapple purée, lime zest and juice, water and, if desired, sugar.

2. In an ice cream maker, freeze according to manufacturer's directions.

3. Divide among 4 individual dessert dishes. Serve garnished with thin slices of lime.

Choices Per Serving

½ Carbohydrate

Nutritional Analysis Per Serving

Calories	38	Fat, total	0 g
Carbohydrate	11 g	Fat, saturated	0 g
Fiber	1 g	Sodium	1 mg
Protein	1 g	Cholesterol	0 mg

Frozen Vanilla Yogurt

1	egg	1
1/3 cup	brown sugar	75 mL
1/2 cup	2% milk	125 mL
1 1/2 cups	2% yogurt	375 mL
1 1/2 tsp	vanilla	7 mL

1. In bowl, beat egg with sugar until combined; set aside. In saucepan, heat milk just until bubbles appear around side of pan. Stir a little into egg mixture, then pour back into saucepan. Cook over low heat, stirring, just until thickened, 2 to 4 minutes. (Do not let boil or egg will curdle.) Remove from heat and let cool completely.

2. Beat yogurt and vanilla into cooled mixture. Freeze in ice-cream machine according to manufacturer's directions. (Or pour into cake pan and freeze until nearly solid. Chop into chunks and beat with electric mixer or process in food processor until smooth. Freeze again until solid.)

Tip

Add 1 tsp (5 mL) each lemon extract and grated lemon rind to make lemon yogurt.

Make Ahead

This dessert can be prepared up to 2 days in advance, but it is best if served right after freezing.

Choices Per Serving

1   Carbohydrate

1/2   Meat & Alternative

Nutritional Analysis Per Serving			
Calories	114	Fat, total	3 g
Carbohydrate	17 g	Fat, saturated	2 g
Fiber	0 g	Sodium	60 mg
Protein	5 g	Cholesterol	43 mg

Contributing Authors

The New Vegetarian Gourmet
Byron Ayanoglu
Recipes from this book can be found on pages 42, 45, 70, 86, 246, 248, 253

Simply Mediterranean Cooking
Byron Ayanoglu
A recipe from this book can be found on page 220

Another 250 Best Muffin Recipes
Esther Brody
Recipes from this book can be found on pages 327–31

The 250 Best Cookie Recipes
Esther Brody
Recipes from this book can be found on pages 340, 341, 344–46, 349

The Comfort Food Cookbook
Johanna Burkhard
Recipes from this book can be found on pages 50, 80, 96, 99, 169, 172, 204, 207, 218, 227, 249, 252

Fast and Easy Cooking
Johanna Burkhard
Recipes from this book can be found on pages 160, 223

300 Best Comfort Food Recipes
Johanna Burkhard
Recipes from this book can be found on pages 65, 66, 82, 119, 139, 241, 244, 251, 272, 274, 284, 288, 299, 351

Dietitians of Canada
Cook Great Food
Dietitians of Canada
Recipes from this book can be found on pages 352, 353, 360, 361

Delicious and Dependable
Slow Cooker Recipes
Judith Finlayson
A recipe from this book can be found on page 256

The 150 Best Slow Cooker Recipes
Judith Finlayson
Recipes from this book can be found on pages 75, 210, 224, 247, 257, 262, 268

125 Best Casseroles
and One-Pot Meals
Rose Murray
Recipes from this book can be found on pages 83, 130, 173, 201, 208, 216, 266, 278, 304

125 Best Quick Bread Recipes
Donna Washburn and Heather Butt
Recipes from this book can be found on pages 310–18, 223–26, 334

The Robert Rose
Book of Classic Pasta
Recipes from this book can be found on pages 137, 140, 154

Robert Rose's Favorite
Cooking for Kids
Recipes from this book can be found on pages 300–302, 305

Library and Archives Canada Cataloguing in Publication

Complete Canadian diabetes cookbook / edited by Katherine E. Younker.

Published in cooperation with the Canadian Diabetes Association.
Includes index.
ISBN 0-7788-0108-X

1. Diabetes — Diet therapy — Recipes.
I. Younker, Katherine E. II. Canadian Diabetic Association

RC662.C64 2005   641.5'6314   C2004-906540-8

Index

Also Available
from Robert Rose

Canada's Best Cookbook
for
Kids with Diabetes

Features the
NEW
CDA Beyond
the Basics
Meal Planning
Guide

Colleen Bartley
Introduction by
Doreen Yasui, RD, CDE

Published in cooperation with

CANADIAN
DIABETES
ASSOCIATION
ASSOCIATION
CANADIENNE
DU DIABÈTE

Robert
ROSE